Cardiac Muscle:
The Regulation of
Excitation and Contraction

Research Topics in Physiology

Charles D. Barnes, *Editor*
Department of Veterinary and Comparative Anatomy,
Pharmacology and Physiology
College of Veterinary Medicine
Washington State University
Pullman, Washington

1. Donald G. Davies and Charles D. Barnes (Editors). Regulation of Ventilation and Gas Exchange, 1978

2. Maysie J. Hughes and Charles D. Barnes (Editors). Neural Control of Circulation, 1980

3. John Orem and Charles D. Barnes (Editors). Physiology in Sleep, 1981

4. M. F. Crass, III, and C. D. Barnes (Editors). Vascular Smooth Muscle: Metabolic, Ionic, and Contractile Mechanisms, 1982

5. James J. McGrath and Charles D. Barnes (Editors). Air Pollution—Physiological Effects, 1982

6. Charles D. Barnes (Editor). Brainstem Control of Spinal Cord Function, 1984

7. Herbert F. Janssen and Charles D. Barnes (Editors). Circulatory Shock: Basic and Clinical Implications, 1985

8. Richard D. Nathan (Editor). Cardiac Muscle: The Regulation of Excitation and Contraction, 1986

Cardiac Muscle:
The Regulation of
Excitation and Contraction

Edited by

RICHARD D. NATHAN

Department of Physiology
Texas Tech University Health Sciences Center
School of Medicine
Lubbock, Texas

1986

ACADEMIC PRESS, INC.
Harcourt Brace Jovanovich, Publishers

Orlando   San Diego   New York
Austin   Boston   London   Sydney
Tokyo   Toronto

ACADEMIC PRESS, INC.
Orlando, Florida 32887

United Kingdom Edition published by
ACADEMIC PRESS INC. (LONDON) LTD.
24–28 Oval Road, London NW1 7DX

Library of Congress Cataloging in Publication Data
Main entry under title:

Cardiac muscle.

    Includes index.
    1. Heart—Muscle.   2. Heart—Contraction.   I. Nathan,
Richard D.   [DNLM: 1. Calcium—metabolism.   2. Heart—
physiology.   3. Ion Channels—physiology.   4. Myocardial
Contraction—drug effects.   W1 RE235E v.8 / WG 280 C2665]
QP113.2.C38   1986   612'.171   85-20004
ISBN 0–12–514370–2 (alk. paper)

PRINTED IN THE UNITED STATES OF AMERICA

86 87 88 89   9 8 7 6 5 4 3 2 1

Contents

7. Some Experimental Studies of Na–Ca Exchange in Heart Muscle

Harry A. Fozzard

8. The Regulation of Tension in Heart Muscle by Intracellular Sodium

W. J. Lederer, R. D. Vaughan-Jones, D. A. Eisner, S-S. Sheu, and M. B. Cannell

9. Cardiac Glycosides: Regulation of Force and Rhythm

Mario Vassalle

Contributors

Numbers in parentheses indicate the pages on which the authors' contributions begin.

Brinda L. Bailey (297), Department of Physiological Chemistry, The Ohio State University Medical Center, Columbus, Ohio 43210

M. B. Cannell (217), Department of Physiology, University of Maryland School of Medicine, Baltimore, Maryland 21201

Robert L. DeHaan (129), Department of Anatomy, Woodruff Health Sciences Center, Emory University, Atlanta, Georgia 30322

D. A. Eisner (217), Department of Physiology, University College London, London WC1E 6BT, England

Alexandre Fabiato (283), Department of Physiology and Biophysics, Medical College of Virginia, Richmond, Virginia 23298

Harry A. Fozzard (201), Departments of Medicine and Pharmacological and Physiological Sciences, The University of Chicago, Chicago, Illinois 60637

Wayne Giles (1), Department of Medical Physiology, University of Calgary School of Medicine, Calgary, Alberta, Canada T2N 4N1

Theodore J. Grieshop (297), Department of Physiological Chemistry, The Ohio State University Medical Center, Columbus, Ohio 43210

J. David Johnson (297), Department of Physiological Chemistry, The Ohio State University Medical Center, Columbus, Ohio 43210

Robert S. Kass (29), Department of Physiology, University of Rochester School of Medicine and Dentistry, Rochester, New York 14642

Elias J. Khabbaza (297), Department of Physiological Chemistry, The Ohio State University Medical Center, Columbus, Ohio 43210

Douglas S. Krafte (29), Department of Physiology, University of Rochester School of Medicine and Dentistry, Rochester, New York 14642

G. A. Langer (269), Departments of Medicine and Physiology and the Cardiovascular Research Laboratories, Center for the Health Sciences, University of California, Los Angeles, School of Medicine, Los Angeles, California 90024

W. J. Lederer (217), Department of Physiology, University of Maryland School of Medicine, Baltimore, Maryland 21201

Richard D. Nathan (55), Department of Physiology, Texas Tech University Health Sciences Center, School of Medicine, Lubbock, Texas 79430

Denis Noble (171), University Laboratory of Physiology, University of Oxford, Oxford OX1 3PT, England

W. Osterrieder (87), Hoffman-La Roche Co. & AG., Basel, Switzerland

Michael C. Sanguinetti (29), Department of Physiology, University of Rochester School of Medicine and Dentistry, Rochester, New York 14642

S-S. Sheu (217), Department of Pharmacology, University of Rochester School of Medicine and Dentistry, Rochester, New York 14642

E. F. Shibata (1), Department of Medical Physiology, University of Calgary School of Medicine, Calgary, Alberta, Canada T2N 4N1

W. Trautwein (87), II. Physiologisches Institut der Universität des Saarlandes, D-6650 Homburg/Saar, Federal Republic of Germany

Mario Vassalle (237), Department of Physiology, State University of New York, Downstate Medical Center, Brooklyn, New York 11203

R. D. Vaughan-Jones (217), University Laboratory of Physiology, University of Oxford, Oxford OX1 3PT, England

A. van Ginneken[1] (1), Department of Medical Physiology, University of Calgary School of Medicine, Calgary, Alberta, Canada T2N 4N1

[1]Present address: Department of Physiology, University of Amsterdam, Meibergdreef 15, 1105AZ Amsterdam, The Netherlands.

Preface

The eighth volume of the *Research Topics in Physiology* series is a collection of both recent and past findings characterizing the ionic and molecular mechanisms that subserve or regulate excitation and contraction of cardiac muscle. The authors review eight interrelated topics of current interest: (1) the ionic currents underlying diastolic depolarization and pacing of the heart; (2) the mechanisms of action of calcium-channel antagonists and how calcium influx is regulated by indigenous factors such as voltage- or calcium-mediated inactivation; (3) the identification of fixed negative charges on the surface of the sarcolemma and how such charges regulate the gating and permeability of ion channels; (4) the molecular and ionic mechanisms that underlie the electrophysiologic actions of adrenergic and cholinergic neurotransmitters and peptide hormones; (5) theoretical and experimental studies of the sodium–calcium exchange process, its stoichiometry, and how the exchanger might contribute to current flow during or after the action potential; (6) the mechanism whereby cardiac glycosides and intracellular sodium regulate twitch and tonic tension and whereby toxic concentrations induce cardiac arrhythmias; (7) identification of sarcolemmal binding sites for calcium, the likelihood that such binding or the release of calcium from the sarcoplasmic reticulum plays a role in the regulation of contraction, and how calcium might be released from the sarcoplasmic reticulum; and (8) structural similarities among calcium-binding proteins of the contractile apparatus (calmodulin and troponin C) and the calcium channel and how these and other calcium-binding proteins (such as the sodium–calcium exchanger) regulate contraction.

Because of the comprehensive nature of the chapters and the authors' suggestions of questions for future research, this volume should be useful not only to researchers and clinicians who study the physiology and pathophysiology of the heart but also to students who have an interest in its function.

I wish to thank Judith Keeling for her invaluable help in editing the manuscripts and Christina Bridges for typing the chapters.

Richard D. Nathan

Cardiac Muscle:
The Regulation of
Excitation and Contraction

1

Ionic Currents Underlying Cardiac Pacemaker Activity: A Summary of Voltage-Clamp Data from Single Cells

Wayne Giles, A. van Ginneken, and E. F. Shibata

I. FOREWORD

The ionic basis of cardiac pacemaker activity has intrigued electrophysiologists for more than 100 years. Although the pioneering microelectrode recordings that first described the intracellular events underlying cardiac pacemaker activity were done more than 30 years ago (Draper and Weidmann, 1951; Trautwein and Zink, 1952), the ionic mechanism of pacing was not explored with voltage-clamp techniques until the mid 1960s. Much of this early work was done on *secondary* or *subsidiary* pacemaker tissue, cardiac Purkinje fibers, because this preparation was easily isolated from the heart and could be induced to beat spontaneously either by lowering extracellular potassium, $(K^+)_o$, or, for example, by adding norepinephrine to the superfusing Tyrode solution. Only quite recently have investigators succeeded in voltage-clamping small strips of cardiac pacemaker tissue from the bullfrog sinus venosus (Brown *et al.*, 1977) or from the rabbit sinoatrial (SA) node (for review see Irisawa, 1978; Brown, 1982). These studies have yielded useful qualitative data concerning the types of ionic currents that underlie the pacemaker potential or the action potential (for review, see Irisawa, 1978, 1984; Giles *et al.*, 1982; Brown, 1982). Unfortunately, however, as a result of (1) the technical difficulty in obtaining these data (i.e., of maintaining two separate microelectrode impalements in contracting muscle) and

1

(2) the uncertainties in interpretation caused, for example, by voltage-clamp nonuniformity and extracellular depletion or accumulation of K^+ (cf. Attwell *et al.*, 1979), it has not been possible to assign functional significance unequivocally to many of these ionic currents (cf. Brown *et al.*, 1982, 1984b).

Within the last five years, techniques have been developed for voltage-clamping single cells from either amphibian or mammalian cardiac pacemaker tissue. These preparations have provided the possibility of studying quantitatively each of the transmembrane ionic currents that generate the pacemaker potential and/or the action potential. The aim of this chapter is to summarize the data that have been obtained from these cardiac pacemaker single-cell preparations. Comprehensive reviews describing the results of previous experiments on multicellular, cardiac pacemaker tissue may be found in the recent articles by Irisawa (1978), Giles *et al.* (1982), and Brown (1982).

II. INTRODUCTION

In principle, the ability to voltage-clamp single spontaneously active cardiac pacemaker cells provides a very powerful method for determining the mechanism of pacemaker activity in the heart. At a minimum (Hume and Giles, 1981, 1983), this new type of preparation provides a substantial improvement over multicellular strips or trabeculae in terms of (1) assessing and ensuring voltage-clamp uniformity and (2) significantly reducing $(K^+)_o$ accumulation or depletion during the voltage-clamp experiments.

A general concern regarding this technology is that the enzymatic dispersion procedure used for isolation of these spontaneously active single cells may damage them. In addition, the pacemaker activity within the anatomical SA node of the rabbit heart has been shown to be very heterogeneous (cf. Janse *et al.*, 1978; Bleeker *et al.*, 1980). Thus, in these single-cell experiments, the precise source of the ''donor'' tissue must be determined with care.

Recently, in single-cell studies, very substantial progress has been made in analyzing the ion transfer properties and the kinetics of many of the ionic currents that have been identified previously in multicellular cardiac pacemaker tissue. In some cases, these data provide conclusive information concerning the functional role of these currents. More often, however, the results are only suggestive, and important quantitative aspects are still missing.

III. METHODS

A. Recording Techniques

A suction pipette method for recording whole-cell currents from isolated cells was developed by Neher and Sakmann (1976) and later refined to increase the seal resistance to the several gigaohm range (cf. Hamill *et al.,* 1981). The adaptations of this general technique that are in use in our laboratory have been outlined in Hume and Giles (1983), Giles and Shibata (1985), and Giles and van Ginneken (1985, 1986). An additional very significant technical improvement has been made by Noma and his colleagues (Soejima and Noma, 1984). They have developed a method for whole-cell or patch-clamp recording in which it is possible to add controlled amounts of ions or drugs to the intracellular medium via a side port on the microelectrode holder. This is very advantageous. Tests of putative intracellular second messengers or measurements of the concentration dependence of ions or drugs on the activation of voltage-dependent channels or ion pumps are now quite feasible.

It is important to appreciate the difficulty of accurately recording trans-membrane potentials from small cells such as those from the primary pacemaker site in the rabbit SA node. The very high input resistance of these cells (2–10 $G\Omega$) means that without exceedingly high resistance seals between the electrode and the sarcolemma, accurate transmembrane voltages *cannot* be recorded (see Hagiwara and Jaffe, 1979; Pelzer *et al.,* 1984). Second, because very small (2–5 pA) current changes can dramatically alter membrane potential values, very carefully balanced preamplifiers must be used for whole-cell recordings. In addition, a number of the solutions used for filling the suction microelectrodes may give rise to significant (>10 mV) tip potentials (Nakayama *et al.,* 1984); these must be measured and corrected for. Finally, the access resistance to the cell interior can increase substantially during an experiment. When relatively large (>500 pA) currents are being recorded, this series resistance can produce significant potential recording errors as well as prolong the time needed for the cell to be space-clamped, that is, for the command potential to settle (see Hume and Giles, 1983).

B. Cell Morphology

The two most commonly used cardiac pacemaker cell preparations are derived from the rabbit sinoatrial node and from the bullfrog sinus venosus. Representative photomicrographs of each of these cell types are shown in Fig. 1, panels A and B, respectively. In electrophysiological investigations of single cells, the cell morphology should be considered very carefully. Very long thin cells can in principle give rise to voltage nonuniformity. Cells having fenestrated surfaces caused by the presence of caveolae (Masson-Pévet *et al.,* 1980) may exhibit phenomena such as accumulation or depletion of ions (cf. Scheid and Fay, 1980), which normally would *not* be expected in isolated single-cell experiments. As noted previously, Bleeker *et al.* (1980) have pointed out that the rabbit SA node is a very heterogeneous structure both anatomically and electrophysiologically, that is, there is a considerable variety of pacemaker cell types. The cell type that is thought to exhibit primary or leading pacemaker

A

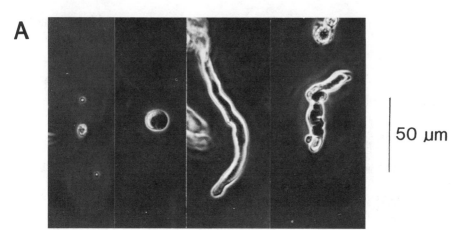

50 μm

B

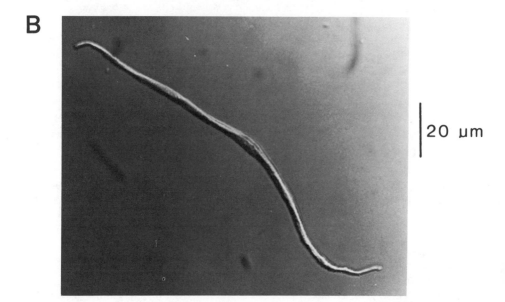

20 um

Fig. 1. Phase contrast micrographs of isolated single cells from the pacemaker region of the rabbit SA node (panel A) and the bullfrog sinus venosus (panel B). The cells from the bullfrog sinus venosus are long, striated, and spindle shaped (approximately 7 μm in maximum diameter and 200–250 μm in length). The cells used in our experiments are spontaneously active. In contrast, the cells from the anatomical rabbit SA node (panel A) assume a variety of shapes in normal Ca^{2+}-containing Tyrode solutions. Characteristic sinus node-like pacemaker depolarizations and action potentials can be recorded from each of these cell types. The partially rounded-up rabbit cells (panel B) have been used in our preliminary experiments (Giles and van Ginneken, 1986) in which I_{Ca}, I_f, and the delayed rectifier potassium current have been studied.

activity (cf. Masson-Pévet *et al.*, 1982) is very small and spherical (6–7 μm in diameter) and has very few cross striations. Other more abundant cells are more rod shaped, about 8 μm in diameter and 100 μm in length. These rod-shaped cells are thought to be secondary or subsidiary pacemaker myocytes. Morphologically, they are somewhat similar to those from the right atrium and/or the crista terminalis (Giles and van Ginneken, 1985, 1986). Thus, careful attention must be paid to the exact source of the single-cell preparations. Second, investigators must ensure that their enzymatically isolated preparations are in fact single cells. Failure to do so will result in significant errors in calculations of ionic current densities; it is precisely these quantitative data that are still lacking in cardiac electrophysiology.

In experiments using single cells from rabbit SA node (but not from bullfrog sinus venosus), an additional somewhat perplexing problem is encountered consistently. After the isolation procedure, when normal Ca^{2+}-containing Tyrode is reintroduced, these cells round-up, becoming spherical or nearly so (Irisawa and Nakayama, 1984; Nakayama *et al*, 1984). This phenomenon may be similar to the Ca^{2+} paradox state seen sometimes in ventricular cells (cf. Dow *et al.*, 1981; Farmer *et al.*, 1983). Interestingly, however, Taniguchi *et al.* (1981) and Nakayama *et al.* (1984) find that these cells exhibit quite normal spontaneous electrical activity. Recent work by Giles and van Ginneken (1986) and by Nathan and Roberts (1985) has confirmed this observation, although in the latter two studies the isolated cells rounded-up only partially, instead of assuming spherical shapes.

It is possible, however, that rounding-up of these cells does *not* indicate that contracture was caused by abnormally high $[Ca^{2+}]_i$. Primary pacemaker cells contain only very little contractile protein and few cytoskeletal elements. Hence, removal of the supporting matrix of extracellular connective tissue during the enzymatic dispersion procedure may allow these cells to collapse. Although this explanation may be suitable, it does not address the effects that such a removal could have on the ionic currents in these cells. Fukuda *et al.* (1981) have shown previously that Na^+ and Ca^{2+} spikes in cultured mammalian neurones *can* be altered significantly after treatment with agents that alter or remove the cytoskeletal elements selectively. Furthermore, alterations in or removal of the glycocalyx may also modify ionic currents, for example, by changing the surface charge on the cells (see Barry *et al.*, 1978; Frank *et al.*, 1982; but compare Isenberg and Klöckner, 1980). The following is an example of the uncertainties this may introduce: Nakayama *et al.* (1984) observed the slow inward current I_f (see section IV, B,3) in only approximately half of the rounded pacemaker cells that they isolated and studied; in contrast, Giles and van Ginneken (1986) found that I_f was present in each acceptable cell, provided that the cell was isolated from near the center of the rabbit SA node.

In summary, the mammalian cardiac pacemaker cells now being used in electrophysiological work exhibit normal spontaneous electrical activity; however, they round-up (at least partially) in normal Tyrode. Corresponding single-cell preparations from the bullfrog heart—sinus venosus single cells (Giles and Shibata, 1985)—do *not* show this phenomenon; therefore, they have been studied in detail in our laboratory.

IV. RESULTS

A. Background Currents

Giles *et al.* (1982) have reviewed the evidence for time-independent or background current(s) carried by Na^+, K^+, Cl^-, and possibly Ca^{2+} in cardiac pacemaker tissue. Evidence for a time-independent *inward* background current is still indirect: although the delayed rectifier current is very selective for K^+, the maximum diastolic potential is 20–25 mV positive to the reversal potential for K^+ (approximately -90 mV). Thus, there must be a steady inward current in these spontaneously active cells. Conventional electrophysiological and radionuclide tracer experiments in intact pacemaker tissue have strongly suggested that there is a steady influx of Na^+ (cf. Irisawa, 1978); however, Walker and Ladle (1973) and Seyama (1978) have pointed out that both amphibian and mammalian cardiac pacemaker tissue also exhibit a significant permeability to Cl^-. Ion-sensitive microelectrode data (Ladle and Walker, 1975) show that the equilibrium potential for chloride ions is approximately -40 mV; therefore, Cl^- moves out of the cell negative to this potential, causing an inward current to be recorded.

Recent data obtained from single cardiac pacemaker cells have provided one very important new result with respect to background currents. Data from multicellular strips showed that the "resting potential" of quiescent rabbit SA node preparations was relatively insensitive to changes in $(K^+)_o$; therefore, it was suggested that membrane permeability to sodium (P_{Na}) may be relatively large (cf. Giles *et al.*, 1982). However, Shibata and Giles (1984, 1985) and Irisawa and his colleagues (cf. Irisawa, 1984; Noma *et al.*, 1984) have shown independently that in cells derived from the bullfrog sinus venosus and rabbit sinoatrial node, there is no measurable inwardly rectifying background K^+ current (I_{K_1}). Furthermore, Shibata and Giles (1985) have drawn attention to a striking contrast between the anatomical pacemaker region, the sinus venosus, and immediately adjacent atrial tissue. Cells from atrial tissue have an inwardly rectifying background K^+ current; in contrast, primary or subsidiary pacemaker cells appear to have either no or very, very little I_{K_1} (see Fig. 2).

One important consequence of the absence of I_{K_1} is that single cardiac pacemaker cells have very high input resistances—approximately 1.0–5.0 GΩ. For voltage-clamp experiments, this is very advantageous; the dc space constant in

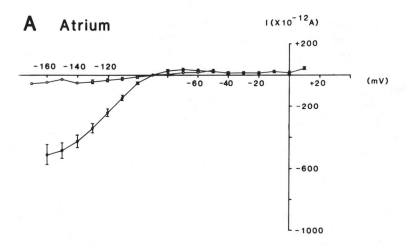

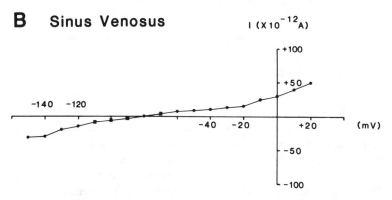

Fig. 2. Comparison of the background K$^+$ currents in single cells from bullfrog atrium (panel A) and the pacemaker region of the bullfrog heart, the sinus venosus (panel B). In these experiments, the transient inward currents, I_{Na} and I_{Ca}, were blocked with tetrodotoxin (TTX, $10^{-6}\,M$) and $CdCl_2$ (1 mM), and the instantaneous currents elicited by 100-msec depolarizations or hyperpolarizations from a holding potential of -80 (atrial cells) or -40 mV (sinus venosus cells) were measured. The two different atrial cell background current–voltage relationships in panel A represent the control I_{K1} records (•) and the current obtained (∘) after the complete blockade of I_{K1} ($5.0 \times 10^{-4}\,M$ BaCl$_2$). In panel B, the control data for the sinus venosus is shown. Note that the background currents in sinus venosus are very similar to those in atrium *after* I_{K1} has been blocked. These data also illustrate that the sinus venosus has an exceedingly high input resistance (approximately 5 GΩ). [From Shibata and Giles (1985).]

cells from rabbit crista terminalis is 30–40 times the length of a single cell (Giles and van Ginneken, 1985). A second very important consequence of the lack of I_{K1} in cardiac pacemaker tissue is that only very tiny net currents are needed to produce the voltage changes that correspond to the pacemaker potential. The total capacitance of a mammalian cardiac pacemaker cell is approximately 60 pF, and the maximum rate of change of voltage (dV/dt) during the pacemaker potential is between 0.02 and 0.05 V/sec; thus, only 1–3 pA of net inward current will generate the pacemaker potential in a uniformly polarized cell (see Giles and van Ginneken, 1986).

In summary, recent voltage-clamp data from single-cell preparations from cardiac pacemaker tissue have shown that (1) the input resistance of these cells is exceedingly high, (2) these cells lack an inwardly rectifying background K^+ current, and (3) tiny current changes will produce the pacemaker potential. Thus, although the P_{Na}/P_K ratio may be much larger than it is in atrium, the Na^+ flux itself is expected to be very small. In the future, it will be very important to define further the ionic nature and the size of the background current(s) in cardiac pacemaker cells. Careful attention must be paid also to sources of transmembrane current other than conventional channels. Either electrogenic Na^+/K^+ pumps or Na^+/Ca^{2+} or Na^+/H^+ ion exchanger mechanisms can, in principle, modulate significantly cardiac pacemaker activity.

B. Time- and Voltage-Dependent Inward Currents

1. Transient Inward Na$^+$ Current, I$_{Na}$

Evidence concerning the presence or absence of a conventional TTX-sensitive transient inward current in mammalian cardiac pacemaker tissue has been reviewed previously (Giles *et al.*, 1982). Recent voltage-clamp studies using single cardiac pacemaker cells from bullfrog heart have failed to identify any TTX-sensitive, transient inward current. For example, Shibata (1983) has studied the transient inward current(s) in bullfrog sinus venosus cells extensively and found that in this preparation no TTX-sensitive inward Na^+ current is present (see Figs. 3 and 4).

The data from mammalian cardiac pacemaker cells are less extensive but appear (Nakayama *et al.*, 1984) to agree with the results from bullfrog in showing that there is no TTX-sensitive, inward Na^+ current. In these experiments, however, relatively positive (e.g., -40 mV) holding potentials were used. (The maximum diastolic potential in rabbit SA node is approximately -65 mV.) At a holding potential of -40 mV, a conventional Na^+ current should be inhibited almost completely as a result of voltage-dependent inactivation of I_{Na}. Recently, we (W. Giles and A. van Ginneken, unpublished) have found that in the peripheral part of the rabbit SA node and in the crista terminalis there is a very substantial TTX-sensitive, fast inward Na^+ current. (This current is so large and fast that it cannot be voltage-clamped adequately by the one microelectrode suction pipette method.) However, in our preliminary studies of cells isolated from the center of the rabbit SA node, no I_{Na} was observed, even when long (500 msec) hyperpolarizing prepulses to -90 mV were applied. These results may explain why in man-made SA node strips (part of which come from the periphery of the node) the dV/dt of the action potential is sensitive to $(Na^+)_o$, and TTX-sensitive Na^+ currents are observed in some experiments.

In summary, the data from single cells isolated from (1) the bullfrog sinus venosus or (2) near the center of the rabbit SA node suggest strongly that there is no conventional TTX-sensitive Na^+ current in these cells. This is consistent with the very small dV/dt_{max} of the action potential upstroke. In the mammalian single-cell preparations, however, more complete investigations with careful determination of the exact anatomical source of the tissue are needed. In these experiments, more hyperpolarized holding potentials should be used consistently so that the possibility of the inhibition of a TTX-sensitive Na^+ current from slow inactivation, for example, can be assessed.

2.   Transient Inward Calcium Current, I_{Ca}

A TTX-insensitive, transient, inward calcium current is consistently present in single, cardiac pacemaker cells. Shibata (1983) has analyzed this current, I_{Ca}, in frog sinus venosus cells. These results agree in general with previous data on the ion selectivity, kinetics, and pharmacological modulation of the TTX-resistant, transient inward current in small strips of cells from the rabbit SA node (cf. Brown, 1982; Giles *et al.*, 1982). Thus, I_{Ca} in bullfrog sinus venosus appears to be carried almost entirely by Ca^{2+}; it is increased by isoproterenol, and it is inhibited by standard ionic (Cd^{2+}, Mn^{2+}, La^{3+}) and organic (D-600, nitren-dipine) blockers. Recently, a somewhat similar I_{Ca} has been recorded from single cells from the rabbit SA node (Nakayama *et al.* (1984) and AV node (Kokubun *et al.*, 1982).

Figure 3 (panel A) shows a family of current records within the activation range of I_{Ca}, as well as a current–voltage (I–V) relationship for this current in sinus venosus cells (panel B). The voltage dependence of the current agrees well with that determined previously from multicellular cardiac preparations, including trabeculae from frog sinus venosus (Brown *et al.*, 1977). In addition, the averaged I–V data from six cells show a number of very interesting features. First, the reversal potential for the current lies far below that of a pure Ca^{2+} electrode, although the slope of the change in reversal potential versus the change in $[Ca^{2+}]_o$ *is* approximately 28 mV per 10-fold change in $[Ca^{2+}]$ (see Figs. 4 and 5). Second, the threshold for activation of the current is at a relatively negative potential; that is, there is a significant (5 or more pA) activation of inward current at all potentials positive to -60 mV. Recently, Shibata and Giles (1985) have pointed out that since I_{Ca} is activated within the pacemaker range of potentials, it must help to depolarize the cells during the last portion of the pacemaker potential, as well as during the upstroke of the action potential.

A

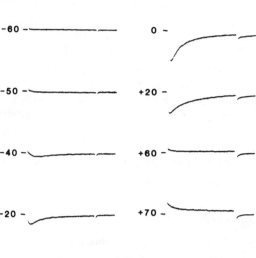

B

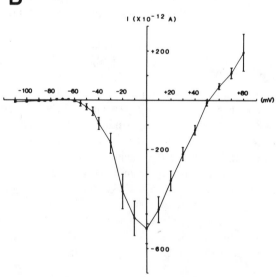

The available I_{Ca} data from the mammalian, pacemaker single-cell preparations agree in general with those from the bullfrog sinus venosus; however, a number of possible differences should be noted: (1) According to Nakayama *et al.* (1984), the inactivation of I_{Ca} in rabbit SA node cells is a two-exponential process. (2) Although the delayed rectifier potassium current (see below) is not very large in the mammalian preparations, it is much faster than that in the bullfrog; hence, it may overlap the calcium current to some extent. (3) In preparations of subsidiary pacemaker tissue (e.g., crista terminalis; Giles and van Ginneken, 1985) in which a substantial transient outward current (I_A) exists, quantitative analysis of I_{Ca} will require either complete inactivation or pharmacological inhibition of this current. (4) Recent data from SA node-strip preparations suggest that I_{Ca} in this preparation may be generated by contributions from two kinetically and pharmacologically distinct types of channels (Brown *et al.,* 1984a). (5) The inactivation mechanism of I_{Ca} in the mammalian preparations, and in most other excitable tissues (cf. Hagiwara and Byerly, 1981; Tsien, 1983), appears to involve both current-dependent and voltage-dependent components.

Further, more quantitative data on these points will be difficult to obtain in cardiac pacemaker tissue. The small size of the cells in these preparations limits severely the type of recording pipette that can be used. In particular, it seems very difficult to use the rather large pipettes that are optimal for internal dialysis or perfusion. Control of the intracellular medium is often desirable and sometimes essential for full quantitative study of I_{Ca} in excitable tissues.

3.   Inward Current Activated by Hyperpolarization, I_f

The work of DiFrancesco and Ojéda (1980) in cardiac Purkinje fibers and rabbit SA node was the first to draw attention to a very slow but relatively large *inward* current, I_f, which is activated within (or very near) the pacemaker range of potentials. DiFrancesco (1981a) pointed out that in the Purkinje fiber this is the same current that Noble and Tsien (1968) described originally as an *outward* potassium current. Recently, I_f currents have been recorded in single pacemaker cells from the rabbit SA node by Nakayama *et al.* (1984) and also by Giles and

---

Fig. 3.   Measurement of the TTX-insensitive, transient inward calcium current, I_{Ca}, in a bullfrog sinus venosus pacemaker cell. Panel A shows raw data obtained by voltage-clamping the cell at -70 mV and then applying 150-msec depolarizing steps to the potential shown beside each record. Note that in this experiment a measurable inward current was seen first at -50 mV and that this current reversed at approximately $+50$ mV. Panel B shows an averaged current–voltage relationship obtained by plotting the peak inward or minimum outward current from six experiments such as the one illustrated in panel A. Note that the threshold for activation of I_{Ca} is near -60 mV and that the apparent reversal potential is approximately $+50$ mV in normal Ca^{2+}-containing (2.5 mM) Ringers. [From Shibata and Giles (1985).]

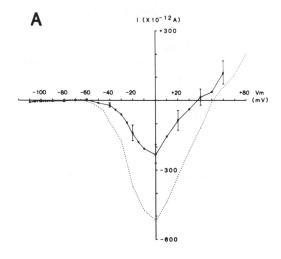

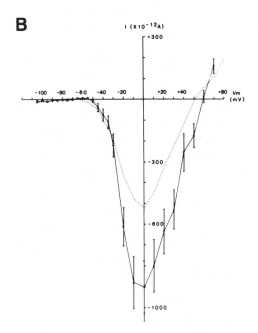

Fig. 4. Test of the selectivity of the TTX-insensitive, transient inward current, I_{Ca}, in bullfrog sinus venosus pacemaker cells. Panel A illustrates the effect on the I_{Ca} I–V relation of reducing $[Ca^{2+}]_o$ from 2.5 to 1.25 mM while keeping the external divalent cation concentration constant by replacing $CaCl_2$ with $MgCl_2$. Note that the peak current (plotted from Fig. 3) is reduced by approximately 50% and that the reversal potential shifts in the hyperpolarizing direction. Panel B illustrates the converse experiment in which $[Ca^{2+}]_o$ has been increased from 2.5 to 7.5 mM (5 cells). Note that the current doubles approximately in size and that the reversal potential shifts in the depolarizing direction. In these experiments as well as those shown in Figs. 3 and 5 the possibility of a contaminating influence by a conventional sodium current was removed by application of a relatively high dose of tetrodotoxin (10^{-6} M).

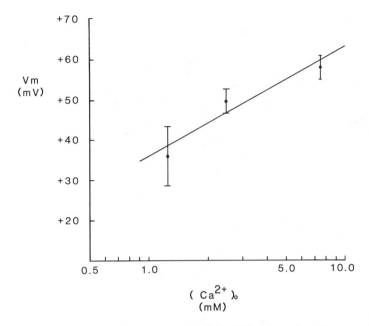

Fig. 5. Dependence of the reversal potential of the TTX-resistant inward current, I_{Ca}, on $[Ca^{2+}]_o$ in bullfrog sinus venosus pacemaker cells. The data points represent the mean ± S.E. from 8 cells in 2.5 mM $[Ca^{2+}]_o$, 5 cells in 1.2 mM $[Ca^{2+}]_o$, and 5 cells in 7.5 mM $[Ca^{2+}]_o$. The best-fitting straight line has a slope of approximately 27 mV per 10-fold change in $(Ca^{2+})_o$. These data suggest that Ca^{2+} is the major charge carrier during the flow of this inward current; however, the absolute value of the reversal potential is not near that calculated from the Nernstian equation.

van Ginneken (1986). As noted previously, however, Nakayama *et al.* (1984) reported that I_f was present in only approximately 50% of their single-cell preparations.

A typical pattern of I_f current changes in a rabbit pacemaker cell is shown in panel B of Fig. 6. Panel C of Fig. 6 shows that I_f can be blocked almost completely by addition of CsCl (1 mM) to the superfusing solution.

The capability to record I_f consistently in single-cell preparations is of considerable interest and importance; in these preparations it is very unlikely that I_f arises from current changes caused mainly (or entirely) by accumulation or depletion of K^+, in small extracellular spaces. Recently, Giles and van Ginneken (1985) have confirmed the original observation of DiFrancesco (1981a) that activation of this current is accompanied by a substantial increase in conductance. These findings and the ability to identify a reproducible reversal potential between -30 and -20 mV provide further evidence against the hypothesis that I_f arises entirely from accumulation or depletion of extracellular K^+ (see Maylie *et al.*, 1981) or intracellular Na^+. However, in sheep cardiac Purkinje fibers Glitsch *et al.* (1985) have shown that activation of I_f is accompanied by a significant increase in

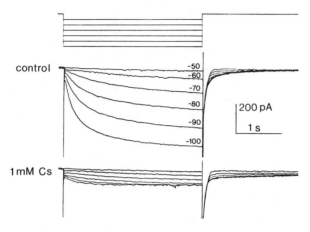

Fig. 6.   Illustration of the slow inward current activated by hyperpolarizing pulses in a single cell from the SA node of the rabbit. The top panel illustrates the voltage-clamp protocol. The holding potential was -40 mV, and relatively long (4-sec), 10-mV steps from -50 to -100 mV were applied. In the control data (shown in panel B), these hyperpolarizations elicited a substantial time- and voltage-dependent inward current. The data in panel C illustrate that 1 m*M* CsCl inhibits this current substantially. As noted in the text, primary cardiac pacemaker cells exhibit I_f consistently in this range of potentials.

intracellular Na^+ activity. The value of the reversal potential indicates that the ion transfer mechanism of I_f may be approximately equally selective for Na^+ and K^+ (DiFrancesco, 1981b); however, at present, $(Cl^-)_o$ replacement experiments have not been done systematically in single-cell preparations.

Perhaps the most important question with respect to I_f in cardiac pacemaker activity is whether this current is activated within the pacemaker range of potentials (cf. Brown *et al.*, 1984b). Much of the existing data indicate that the voltage dependence of I_f, that is, its activation range, lies negative or hyperpolarized to the normal pacemaker potential range. This conclusion depends critically, however, on an accurate assessment of the maximum diastolic potential in the tissue of interest and on having reproducible data regarding the steady-state voltage dependence and kinetics of I_f. In the recent study of Nakayama *et al.* (1984), there is very large cell-to-cell variability in the voltage dependence of I_f. We (Giles and van Ginneken, 1986) have reinvestigated this recently and have found much less variability. Our data suggest strongly that a small but significant amount of I_f *is activated* within the pacemaker range of potentials in cells from the SA node. Although this change in I_f is very small (5–10 pA), it *can*, for reasons given previously, be very important in modulating cardiac pacemaker activity. Our recent results are, therefore, in disagreement with some of those from multicellular strips of rabbit SA node, which suggested that the activation of I_f was *not significant* in the genesis of normal primary pacemaker activity

(Noma *et al.*, 1983). Noma *et al.* (1983) found that the activation range of I_f was negative to the maximum diastolic potential, and that I_f could *not* be observed in approximately 50% of the strips studied.

Although recent work has shown convincingly that I_f can be identified in mammalian cardiac pacemaker cells, the functional role of I_f will not be completely clear until more data on the selectivity of this channel and more detailed kinetic results have been obtained (cf. Maylie and Morad, 1984). It is worth recalling also that although I_f-like currents were demonstrated originally in trabeculae from bullfrog sinus venosus (Brown *et al.*, 1977), no I_f-like current can be identified in spontaneously active single cells from the bullfrog sinus venosus (Giles and Shibata, 1985). At present there is no satisfactory explanation for why this current change is *not* observed in single cells. As noted previously, it is not clear either why I_f is absent from approximately 50% of the single cells studied by Irisawa, Noma, and colleagues. Perhaps only pacemaker cells from near the center of the sinoatrial node or sinus venosus exhibit I_f.

C.   Outward Currents

1.   Time- and Voltage-Dependent Outward Current, I_K

A substantial time- and voltage-dependent outward current (the delayed rectifier) is consistently present in single cells isolated from both amphibian and mammalian cardiac pacemaker tissue (Shibata and Giles, 1984; Nakayama *et al.*, 1984; Giles and Shibata, 1985). In both of these preparations, this delayed rectifier current appears to be carried mainly by potassium ions (see Fig. 7) (although the data from the mammalian preparation (cf. Nakayama *et al.*, 1984) are only suggestive because of a 10- to 15-mV uncertainty in the exact value of the junction potential and, hence, transmembrane potential in those experiments). Nevertheless, in both preparations the size and the kinetics of this current make it very likely that (1) its activation is important in repolarization of the action potential and (2) its decay is one of the significant factors in regulating the development of the pacemaker potential and, hence, heart rate. For these reasons, the kinetics of this current have been studied in some detail; interestingly, the data from the amphibian preparation appear to differ from those obtained from the rabbit SA node. In single cells from the bullfrog sinus venosus, the activation and decay of I_K are best described as single-exponential processes (see Fig. 8). A sigmoid time course of activation is observed, but this can be readily accounted for by raising the exponential kinetic function to the second power (Giles and Shibata, 1985). In contrast, data from the mammalian single-cell preparations exhibit two exponentials consistently in the I_K decay tails. Nakayama *et al.* (1984) have argued that although one of these time constants is

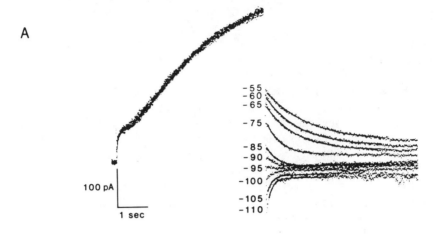

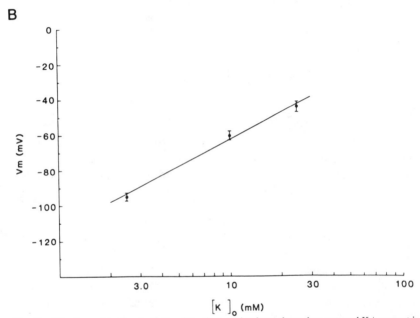

Fig. 7. Kinetics and ionic selectivity of the time- and voltage-dependent outward K^+ current in an isolated cardiac pacemaker cell from the bullfrog sinus venosus. The 10 superimposed records in part A show a measurement of the reversal potential of this current in normal Ringers (2.5 mM K_o^+). A double pulse protocol was used: P_I depolarized the cell from the holding potential, -75 mV, to $+30$ mV for 5 sec; P_{II} lasted 5 sec and was varied from -55 to -110 mV in 5-mV steps. Note that the reversal potential is between -95 and -100 mV, very near E_K. The kinetics of decay of each current tail were determined by fitting it with a function consisting of a sum of exponentials. Using the criteria developed by Provencher (1976), a single exponential function (denoted as the solid black curve) was shown consistently (in 80–85% of all trials) to give the best fit. Part B illustrates the change in E_{rev} as a function of $[K^+]_o$. The data points denote the mean $\pm$ S.E. ($n=4$). The best-fitting straight line has a slope of 51 mV per 10-fold change in $[K^+]_o$, suggesting strongly that this time- and voltage-dependent outward current is carried mainly by K^+. [From Shibata and Giles (1985).]

16

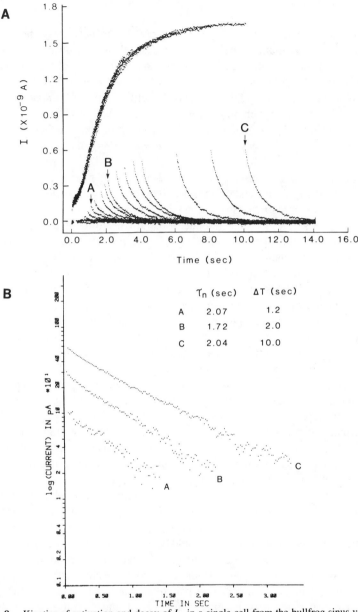

Fig. 8. Kinetics of activation and decay of I_K in a single cell from the bullfrog sinus venosus. Depolarizing pulses from the holding potential (-60 to $+30$ mV) were applied, and the pulse duration was varied from 200 msec to 10 sec. In part A, the onsets, or activation phases, of I_K are superimposed; the resulting current tails are plotted as relaxations back to the baseline. The current tails denoted by the letters are shown on semilogarithmic coordinates in part B. The linear decay and nearly constant slope of these data (which differ by approximately threefold in initial amplitude) suggests that only a single Hodgkin–Huxley conductance-component mechanism underlies I_K. [From Giles and Shibata (1985).]

rather slow (700 msec to 1 sec at -40 mV), it is not likely the result of extracellular accumulation of K^+. Nonetheless, their data do not rule this out completely; as noted earlier, the caveolae in the sarcolemma of these cells could certainly give rise to such accumulation (Scheid and Fay, 1980). On the other hand, recent quantitative studies of delayed rectification in frog node of Ranvier have yielded results much more complex than those described originally as simple exponential kinetics of a uniform population of channels having only one conductance level. (Dubois, 1983; Conti *et al.*, 1984) of a single, time- and voltage-dependent K^+ channel.

Recently, somewhat similar, rather complex, results have also been obtained from squid axon (White and Bezanilla, 1985), patches of skeletal muscle sarcolemma (Standen *et al.*, 1985), and bovine chromaffin cells (Marty and Neher, 1985). Further studies have been made of the kinetics of delayed rectification in cardiac Purkinje fibers (Bennett *et al.*, 1985) and in single cells from dog cardiac Purkinje fibers (Cohen *et al.*, 1984). In both cases the decay of the delayed rectifier current was found to be biexponential and the results were interpreted using a model involving one type of channel which can exist in three (two closed, one open) conformational states connected by voltage dependent rate constants.

One plausible explanation for the rather slow time course of this K^+ current in cardiac pacemaker tissue and for the sigmoidicity in its onset is that an increase in $(Ca^{2+})_i$, possibly brought about the Ca^{2+} influx during I_{Ca}, triggers or activates I_K. In the sinus venosus cells from the frog heart, Giles and Shibata (1985) have shown, however, that complete inhibition of I_{Ca} produces no significant change in I_K. At present, corresponding experiments in the mammalian single-cell preparation have not been reported.

One puzzling feature of this I_K in cardiac single-cell preparations is the following: although a substantial I_K can be recorded from every successfully impaled cell, it is very difficult (if not impossible) in patch-clamp experiments to identify the single-channel events underlying this current. The reason(s) for this is not known; however, plots of the fully activated current–voltage relation and knowledge of the single-channel conductance of this type of channel in a variety of other preparations (e.g., embryonic heart, approximately 60 pS; Clapham and DeFelice, 1984) suggest that there should be approximately 500 channels per cell or 1 channel/5 μm^2. It is possible, therefore, that our failure to identify single-channel events underlying I_K is a statistical problem resulting, for example, from clustering of these channels in one part of the cell. Alternatively, the single-channel conductance may be exceedingly small and therefore not within the resolution of our recordings ($\sim$0.5 pA at 500 Hz). Our preliminary noise experiments in bullfrog atrial cells (R. B. Clark, W. Giles, and E. F. Shibata, unpublished data) suggest that the latter explanation is more likely: a small number of channels with relatively large conductances in a single cell, whether they are clustered or not, would be expected to give rise to significant current noise, and we have failed to observe this.

2. Transient Outward Current, I_A

Very recently, a transient outward current, I_A, has been identified in two types of subsidiary cardiac pacemaker tissue: the rabbit AV node (Nakayama and Irisawa, 1985) and rabbit crista terminalis (Giles and van Ginneken, 1985). In both of these preparations, this current appears to be carried mainly by K^+ and can be blocked selectively by external application of 4-aminopyridine (3 mM). Furthermore, as it does in various neurones, I_A exhibits voltage-dependent inactivation (see Fig. 9). The kinetics and voltage dependence of (1) the activation of I_A, (2) the development of inactivation, and (3) the subsequent removal of inactivation produce a significant frequency-dependent modulation of the size of I_A and hence the duration of the action potential. Because this current is relatively large and its activation time course is comparable to that of I_{Ca}, I_A can overlap substantially and neutralize I_{Ca}. In the crista terminalis of the rabbit heart, this can produce very substantial changes in action potential duration and, therefore, in the rate and pattern of firing of this tissue.

We (Giles and van Ginneken, 1985, 1986) have tested whether any I_A-like current is present in cells taken from near the center of the rabbit SA node, where leading or primary pacemaker activity is thought to originate. It appears, however, that there is no I_A current unless the cells are derived from the peripheral

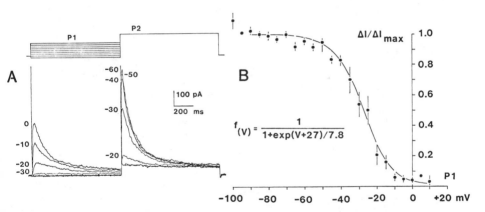

Fig. 9.   Steady-state inactivation of I_A in a single cell from the rabbit crista terminalis. Panel A illustrates the protocol and raw data. The protocol consisted of a variable prepulse (P_1) lasting 1 sec, followed by a fixed test pulse (P_{II}) to +20 mV for 1 sec. Holding potential was −60 mV. P_1 ranged from −100 to +10 mV. Note the saturation of I_A when the P_1 was made more negative than approximately −70 mV. Panel B: Inactivation curve obtained by plotting the fraction of the maximum P_{II} current obtained when P_{II} was preceded by various P_1 voltages. The data are plotted as mean ± S.E.M. ($n=7$) and were fitted by a Boltzman distribution (continuous curve) given by

$$\Delta I / \Delta I_{max} = \frac{1}{1 + \exp[(V + 27)/7.8]}$$

[From Giles and van Ginneken (1985).]

portions of the SA node or from the crista terminalis. Because careful identification and mapping of the anatomical site (source) of the cells now being used as cardiac pacemaker preparations is *not* routinely done, I_A is likely to be present in some of these cells. For example, in pacemaker cells isolated from the mammalian heart and voltage-clamped at a holding potential of -40 mV (as is common in the experiments of Irisawa and his colleagues), I_A would be observed, especially when low cycle times are used.

In summary, a substantial, transient outward current, I_A, is present in the peripheral portions of the rabbit SA node and in the AV node. Its presence must be recognized before data on action potential changes or I_{Ca} kinetics can be interpreted correctly.

D.   Electrogenic Pump and Exchanger Currents

As mentioned previously, the very high input resistance of cardiac pacemaker cells makes it possible for very small current sources to produce significant (5 mV) changes in membrane potential. For this reason, and also because the rates of change of membrane potential in cardiac pacemaker tissue are relatively low, attention must be paid to the possible influence of transmembrane current(s) (generated, for example, by the electrogenic Na^+/K^+ pump) on (1) the development of the pacemaker potential and/or (2) the size and/or duration of the action potential. Recently, a transmembrane current change arising from activation of the Na^+/K^+ pump has been identified, both in single cells from the bullfrog atrium (Shibata *et al.*, 1984) and in myocytes from the guinea pig ventricle (Gadsby *et al.*, 1985). In most respects, these data confirm previous findings from multicellular SA node-strip preparations (for review, see Giles *et al.*, 1982).

The data obtained from both single-cell preparations agree in showing that the maximally activated Na^+/K^+ pump current is approximately 100 pA. In addition, Gadsby *et al.* (1985) have shown that this pump current is weakly voltage dependent and that its activity is modulated by changes in intracellular Na^+, with a half-activation concentration of approximately 40 mM. This is very similar to previous data from red blood cells and from a variety of excitable tissues. In addition, we (Shibata *et al.*, 1984) have evidence that the current can be activated also by extracellular potassium with a half-activation concentration near 2 mM.

Because cardiac pacemaker cells have a relatively large surface area to volume ratio, one might expect that substantial, activity-dependent changes in $(Na^+)_i$ or $(K^+)_o$ can occur as a function of changes in heart rate or cell metabolism. In this regard, it is very important to study further whether there is a conventional I_{Na} in cardiac pacemaker tissue. Obviously, in the absence of I_{Na}, large changes in $(Na^+)_i$ are not likely to occur as a function of physiological changes in heart rate. Although changes in $(K^+)_o$ may take place physiologically, these in general will *not* modulate pump activity significantly. The K_a for $(K^+)_o$ activation of the Na^+/K^+ pump is 1.5 to 2 mM. Hence, in mammalian preparations, the expected changes in $(K^+)_o$—from approximately 4.5 to 5.0 or 5.0 to 5.5 mM— would *not* be expected to enhance Na^+/K^+ pump activity significantly. It seems therefore that Na^+/K^+ pump activity in cardiac pacemaker cells would be relatively constant. If so, it should have little direct effect on the pacemaker potential or the action potential.

The recent findings of Kameyama *et al.* (1984) are relevant to the study of Na^+/K^+ pump currents in isolated cardiac cells. These experiments have identified in ventricular myocytes a K^+ channel that is activated by $(Na^+)_i$ greater than 20 mM. If this mechanism is present in cardiac pacemaker tissue, whole-cell measurements of Na^+/K^+ pump current involving changes in $(Na^+)_i$ must be carried out and interpreted with caution.

In addition, it is important to note that in the rabbit AV node (Kakei and Noma, 1984) and in mammalian ventricular myocytes (Noma, 1983; Trube and Hescheler, 1984) intracellular ATP depletion to levels less than approximately 1 mM unmasks a K^+ current with a relatively large ($\sim$80 pS) single-channel conductance. Under experimental conditions of intense, prolonged Na^+/K^+ pump activation, ATP is hydrolyzed rapidly and an unphysiological depletion may result. This could generate a substantial outward current apart from that generated directly by the Na^+/K^+ pump.

As noted earlier, there is a significant influx of Ca^{2+} during each cardiac cycle. This Ca^{2+} must be extruded subsequently, either by an ATP-requiring Ca^{2+} pump or by an Na^+/Ca^{2+} exchanger mechanism. These processes could be electrogenic; moreover, the Na/Ca^{2+} exchanger could bring about a substantial change in $(Na^+)_i$ and hence modulate indirectly the Na^+/K^+ pump. Evaluation of the functional importance of this working hypothesis must await the unambiguous identification of a current change caused *entirely* by the Na^+/Ca^{2+} exchanger (see Eisner and Lederer, 1985). Finally, it should be remembered that most cells, including cardiac cells, exhibit Na^+/H^+ exchange (cf. Piwnica-Worms *et al.*, 1985). This exchanger, too, could bring about substantial changes in $(Na^+)_i$ and therefore modulate the Na^+/K^+ pump, even though the Na^+/H^+ exchanger itself is thought to be electroneutral.

V. SUMMARY

The work summarized in this chapter shows that viable pacemaker cells can be obtained from both the amphibian and the mammalian heart, and that whole-cell voltage-clamp experiments with these cells are yielding important new insights into the mechanism of pacing. Nonetheless, the interesting quantitative aspects of this work have just begun: a detailed comparison of the cells from the center versus the periphery of the mammalian SA node is needed to understand further the differences between primary and secondary or subsidiary pacemakers. Each of the pacemaker cell types selected for study must be characterized more completely. For example, it is essential to determine the details of the appropriate equivalent circuit for each cell type and to make quantitative measurements of each of the ionic current densities. At present, there are few patch-clamp data from cardiac pacemaker cells (for review, see Clapham, 1985). It will be important to study further, at the single-channel level, each of the macroscopic currents that have been identified. It may still be premature to put forward mechanistic explanations of the pacemaker potential or the action potential; however, recent work from single cells does answer some of the questions that remained when data from only multicellular tissues were available (cf. Brown, 1982; Giles *et al.*, 1982).

A. Ionic Currents Underlying Pacing

The major time- and voltage-dependent currents that underlie pacemaker activity in both the amphibian and the mammalian heart are I_{Ca} and I_K, the delayed rectifier potassium current. An I_f current has not been identified in bullfrog pacemaker cells, nor is it present in the peripheral portions of the rabbit SA node. Because both of these preparations exhibit pacemaker activity, it is not appropriate to describe I_f as "the pacemaker current." Nevertheless, our data illustrate that I_f is present within the pacemaker range of potentials in mammalian cardiac pacemaker tissue. Provided that this is not unique for the rabbit SA node, these data suggest that I_f may be a significant modulator of mammalian primary pacemaker activity. An important new result from single-cell studies is that cardiac pacemaker tissues do not have a conventional, inwardly rectifying, background K^+ current, I_{K_1}. This provides an explanation for the relatively depolarized level of the maximum diastolic potential; furthermore, the absence of I_{K_1} means that only very tiny net inward currents are necessary to depolarize the cell during the development of the pacemaker potential.

B. Ionic Currents Underlying the Action Potential

In primary pacemaker tissue, only two time- and voltage-dependent ionic currents underlie the action potential. I_{Ca} is activated during the last third of the pacemaker potential and appears to have the appropriate kinetics and magnitude to generate the dV/dt of the action potential. Its reversal potential is approximately 10 mV positive to the maximum overshoot of the action potential. The explanation for the relatively long plateau phase of the action potential (100–150 msec at an average potential of $+10$ mV) is not known, but it may arise from a persistent inward current (Hume and Giles, 1983) and/or from the failure of I_{Ca} to inactivate completely at these potentials. Repolarization of the action potential is brought about by the time- and voltage-dependent activation of I_K, the delayed rectifier K^+ current. In contrast to that in atrial tissue (Shibata and Giles, 1984; Giles et al., 1984), in which the inwardly rectifying, background potassium current is a significant factor in the final phase of repolarization, in pacemaker tissue repolarization is brought about entirely by the activation of I_K. In the peripheral portion of the SA node or in subsidiary, cardiac pacemaker tissue, there is also a large and fast, transient outward K^+ current, I_A. I_A can significantly modulate action potential duration. In addition tissue from the periphery of the mammalian SA node exhibits a TTX-sensitive transient inward sodium current, I_{Na}. I_{Na} enhances the excitability and conductance velocity in these regions, and it may also modulate the duration of the plateau of the action potential.

It is also very important to remember that there are electrogenic pump and exchanger mechanisms throughout the heart, including the pacemaker regions. These are capable of generating currents that can change net current balances significantly during both the pacemaker potential and the action potential. However, during normal electrical or cardiac pacemaker activity, these would be expected to be very small; therefore, much of our understanding of their possible effects continues to come from computer simulations of cardiac pacemaker activity. In this regard, the recent work of Noble and Noble (1984) and DiFrancesco and Noble (1985) is of interest. The inclusion in these models of the effects of ion concentration changes (in either the extracellular or intracellular space) and expressions for Na^+/K^+ pump and Na^+/Ca^{2+} exchanger currents represents a significant improvement over previous models in which only classical Hodgkin–Huxley conductance changes or minor modifications thereof were included (Yanagihara et al., 1980; Bristow and Clark, 1982).

Finally, although cardiac pacemaker activity is a myogenic phenomenon, the strong effects of autonomic or purinergic transmitters must often be considered. The actions of these agents on man-made strip preparations have been reviewed previously (Giles and Shibata, 1981; Giles et al., 1982), and relevant findings from single-channel experiments have been summarized recently by Clapham (1985) and Trautwein and Osterrieder (Chapter 4).

ACKNOWLEDGMENTS

This experimental work was supported by grants from the N.I.H. (DHHS-HL-27454, DHHS-HL-33662), the Canadian M.R.C., the Canadian Heart Foundation, the Alberta Heritage Foundation for Medical Research (AHFMR), and the Netherlands Organization for the Advancement of Pure

Research (ZWO). Dr. Giles held an Established Investigator's Award from the American Heart Association and is presently an AHFMR Scholar. Doctors van Ginneken and Shibata were supported by an AHFMR Postdoctoral Fellowship and a NIH Postdoctoral Fellowship, respectively.

REFERENCES

Attwell, D., Eisner, D., and Cohen, I. (1979). Voltage clamp and tracer flux data: Effects of a restricted extracellular space. *Q. Rev. Biophys.* **12**, 213–263.

Barry, W. H., Goldminz, D., Kimball, T., and Fitzgerald, J. W. (1978). Influence of cell dissociation and culture of chick embryo ventricle on inotropic response to calcium and lanthanum. *J. Mol. Cell. Cardiol.* **10**, 967–979.

Bennett, P. B., McKinney, L. C., Kass, R. S., and Begenisich, T. (1985). Delayed rectification in the calf cardiac Purkinje fibre: Evidence for multiple state kinetics. *Biophys. J.,* **48**, 553–567.

Bleeker, W. K., MacKaay, A. J. C., Masson-Pévet, M., Bouman, L. N., and Becker, A. E. (1980). The functional and morphological organization of the rabbit sinus node. *Circ. Res.* **46**, 11–22.

Bristow, D. G., and Clark, J. W. (1982). A mathematical model of primary pacemaking cell in SA node of the heart. *Am. J. Physiol.* **243**, H207-H218.

Brown, H. F. (1982). Electrophysiology of the sinoatrial node. *Physiol. Rev.* **62**, 505–530.

Brown, H. F., Giles, W., and Noble, S. J. (1977). Membrane currents underlying activity in frog sinus venosus. *J. Physiol. (London)* **271**, 783–816.

Brown, H. F., Kimura, J., and Noble, S. (1982). The relative contributions of various time-dependent membrane currents to pacemaker activity in the sinoatrial node. *In:* "Cardiac Rate and Rhythm" (L. N. Bouman and H. J. Jongsma, eds.), pp. 53–68. Martinus Nijhoff Publishing, Boston.

Brown, H. F., Kimura, J., Noble, D., Noble, S. J., and Taupignon, A. (1984a). The slow inward current, i_{si}, in the rabbit sino-atrial node investigated by voltage clamp and computer simulation. *Proc. R. Soc. London B* **222**, 305–328.

Brown, H. F., Kimura, J., Noble, D., Noble, S. J., and Taupignon, A. (1984b). The ionic currents underlying pacemaker activity in rabbit sino-atrial node: Experimental results and computer simulations. *Proc. R. Soc. London B* **222**, 329–347.

Clapham, D. E. (1985). A brief review of single channel measurements from isolated heart cells. *In:* "The Heart Cell in Culture" (A. Pinson, ed.), CRC Reviews.

Clapham, D. E., and DeFelice, L. J. (1984). Voltage-activated K channels in embryonic chick heart. *Biophys. J.* **45**, 40–42.

Cohen, I. S., Daytner, N. B., and Gintant, G. A. (1984). A study of potassium currents in acutely dissociated canine cardiac Purkinje myocytes. *J. Physiol. (London)* **349**, 49p.

Conti, F., Hille, B., and Nonner, W. (1984). Non-stationary fluctuations of the potassium conductance at the node of Ranvier of the frog. *J. Physiol. (London)* **353**, 199–230.

DiFrancesco, D. (1981a). A new interpretation of the pacemaker current in calf Purkinje fibres. *J. Physiol. (London)* **314**, 359–376.

DiFrancesco, D. (1981b). A study of the ionic nature of the pacemaker current in calf Purkinje fibres. *J. Physiol. (London)* **314**, 377–393.

DiFrancesco, D., and Noble, D. (1985). A model of cardiac electrical activity incorporating ionic pumps and concentration changes. *Phil. Trans. R. Soc. London B* **307**, 353–398.

DiFrancesco, D., and Ojéda, C. (1980). Properties of the current i_f in the sinoatrial node of the rabbit compared with those of the current i_{K_2} in Purkinje fibres. *J. Physiol. (London)* **308**, 353–367.

Dow, J. W., Harding, N. G., and Powell, T. (1981). Isolated cardiac myocytes: I. Preparation of adult myocytes and their homology with the intact tissue. *Circ. Res.* **15**, 483–514.

Draper, M. H., and Weidmann, S. (1951). Cardiac resting and action potentials recorded with an intracellular electrode. *J. Physiol. (London)* **115**, 74–94.

Dubois, J. M. (1983). Potassium currents in the frog node of Ranvier. *Prog. Biophys. Mol. Biol.* **42**, 1–21.

Eisner, D. A., and Lederer, W. J. (1985). Na–Ca exchange: stoichiometry and electrogenicity. *Am. J. Physiol.* **248**, C189-C203.

Farmer, B. B., Mancina, M., Williams, E. S., and Watanabe, A. M. (1983). Isolation of calcium tolerant myoctyes from adult rat hearts: Review of the literature and description of a method. *Life Sci.* **33**, 1–18.

Frank, J. S., Rich, T. L., Beydler, S., and Kreman, M. (1982). Calcium depletion in rabbit myocardium. Ultrastructure of the sarcolemma and correlation with the calcium paradox. *Circ. Res.* **51**, 117–130.

Fukuda, J., Kameyama, M., and Yamaguchi, K. (1981). Breakdown of cytoskeletal filaments selectively reduces Na and Ca spikes in cultured mammalian neurons. *Nature (London)* **294**, 82–85.

Gadsby, D. C., Kimura, J., and Noma, A. (1985). Voltage dependence of Na/K pump current in isolated heart cells. *Nature (London)* **315**, 63–65.

Giles, W., and Shibata, E. F. (1981). Autonomic transmitter actions on cardiac pacemaker tissue: A brief review. *Fed. Proc.* **40**, 2618–2624.

Giles, W., and Shibata, E. F. (1985). Voltage clamp of isolated cardiac pacemaker cells from bullfrog sinus venosus: A quantitative analysis of potassium currents. *J. Physiol (London)* **368**, 265–292.

Giles, W., and van Ginneken, A. (1985). A transient outward current in isolated cells from the crista terminalis of rabbit heart. *J. Physiol. (London)*. **368**, 243–264.

Giles, W., and van Ginneken, A. (1986). Voltage clamp analysis of the f-current in isolated cells from the rabbit sinoatrial node: Its role in pacemaking. *J. Physiol. (London)*. Submitted.

Giles, W., Eisner, D. A., and Lederer, W. J. (1982). Sinus pacemaker activity in the heart. *In*: "Cellular Pacemakers" (D. O. Carpenter, ed.), pp. 91–125. John Wiley and Sons, New York.

Giles, W., Robinson, K., Shibata, E. F., and Hume, J. R. (1984). Repolarization in cardiac muscle: An experimental and theoretical study using single cells from bullfrog atrium. *Biophys. J.* **45**, 278a.

Glitsch, H. G., Pusch, H., and Verdonck, F. (1985). The pacemaker current increases the intracellular Na activity in isolated sheep cardiac Purkinje fibres. *J. Physiol. (London)* **366**, 86p.

Hagiwara, S., and Byerly, L. (1981). Calcium channel. *Ann. Rev. Neurosci.* **4**, 69–125.

Hagiwara, S., and Jaffe, L. A. (1979). Electrical properties of egg cell membranes. *Ann Rev. Biophys. Bioeng.* **8**, 385–416.

Hamill, O. P., Marty, A., Neher, E., Sakmann, B., and Sigworth, F. J. (1981). Improved patch clamp techniques for high-resolution current recording from cell and cell-free membrane patches. *Pflügers Arch. ges. Physiol.* **391**, 85–100.

Hume, J. R., and Giles, W. (1981). Active and passive electrical properties of single bullfrog atrial cells. *J. Gen. Physiol.* **78**, 19–42.

Hume, J. R., and Giles, W. (1983). Ionic currents in single isolated bullfrog atrial cells. *J. Gen. Physiol.* **81**, 153–194.

Irisawa, H. (1978). Comparative physiology of the cardiac pacemaker mechanism. *Physiol. Rev.* **58**, 461–487.

Irisawa, H. (1984). Electrophysiology of single cardiac cells. *Jap. J. Physiol.* **34**, 375–388.

Irisawa, H., and Nakayama, T. (1984). Isolation of a single pacemaker cell from rabbit S-A node. *Jikeikai Med. J.* **30**, 65–70.

Isenberg, G., and Klöckner, U. (1980). Glycocalyx is not required for slow inward calcium current in isolated rat heart myocytes. *Nature (London)* **284**, 358–360.

Janse, M. J., Tranum-Jensen, J., Kleber, A. G., and van Capelle, F. J. J. (1978). Techniques and problems in correlating cellular electrophysiology and morphology in cardiac nodal tissues. *In*: "The Sinus Node: Structure, Function, and Clinical Relevance" (F. I. M. Bonke, ed.), pp. 182–194. Martinus Nijhoff Publishing, Boston.

Kakei, M., and Noma, A. (1984). Adenosine-5'-triphosphate-sensitive single potassium channel in the atrioventricular node cell of the rabbit heart. *J. Physiol. (London)* **352**, 265–284.

Kameyama, M., Kakei, M., Sato, R., Shibasaki, T., Matsuda, H., and Irisawa, H. (1984). Intracellular Na^+ activates a K^+ channel in mammalian cardiac cells. *Nature (London)* **309**, 354–356.

Kokubun, S., Nishimura, M., Noma, A., and Irisawa, H. (1982). Membrane currents in the rabbit atrioventricular node cell. *Pflügers Arch. ges. Physiol.* **393**, 15–22.

Ladle, R. O., and Walker, J. L. (1975). Intracellular chloride activity in frog heart. *J. Physiol. (London)* **251**, 549–559.

Marty, A. and Neher, E. (1985). Potassium channels in curtured bovine adrenal chromaffin cells. *J. Physiol. (London)* **367**, 117–141.

Masson-Pévet, M., Gros, D., and Besselsen, E. (1980). The caveolae in rabbit sinus node and atrium. *Cell Tissue Res.* **208**, 183–196.

Masson-Pévet, M., Jongsma, H. J., Bleeker, W. K., Tsjernina, L., van Ginneken, A. G. C., Treijtel, B. W., and Bouman, L. N. (1982). Intact isolated sinus node cells from the adult rabbit heart. *J. Mol. Cell. Cardiol.* **14**, 295–299.

Maylie, J., and Morad, M. (1984). Ionic currents responsible for the generation of the pacemaker current in the rabbit sino-atrial node. *J. Physiol. (London)* **355**, 215–235.

Maylie, J., Morad, M., and Weiss, J. (1981). A study of pacemaker potential in rabbit sinoatrial node: Measurement of potassium activity under voltage clamp conditions. *J. Physiol. (London)* **311**, 161–178.

Nakayama, T., and Irisawa, H. (1985). Transient outward current carried by K^+ and Na^+ in quiescent atrio-ventricular node cells of rabbit. *Circ. Res.* **57**, 65–73.

Nakayama, T., Kurachi, Y., Noma, A., and Irisawa, H. (1984). Action potential and membrane currents of single pacemaker cells of the rabbit heart. *Pflugers Arch. ges. Physiol.* **402**, 248–257.

Nathan, R. D., and Roberts, L. A. (1985). Voltage-gated currents in single cultured pacemaker cells from the sinoatrial node. *Biophys. J.* **47**, 496a.

Neher, E., and Sakmann, B. (1976). Single-channel currents recorded from membrane of denervated frog muscle fibres. *Nature (London)* **260**, 799–802.

Noble, D., and Noble, S. J. (1984). A model of sino-atrial node electrical activity based on a modification of the DiFrancesco–Noble (1984) equations. *Proc. R. Soc. Lond. B* **222**, 295–304.

Noble, D., and Tsien, R. W. (1968). The kinetic and rectifier properties of the slow potassium current in cardiac Purkinje fibres. *J. Physiol. (London)* **195**, 185–214.

Noma, A. (1983). ATP-regulated K^+ channels in cardiac muscle. *Nature (London)* **305**, 147–148.

Noma, A., Morad, M., and Irisawa, H. (1983). Does the "pacemaker current" generate the diastolic depolarization in the rabbit SA node cells? *Pflügers Arch. ges. Physiol.* **397**, 190–194.

Noma, A., Nakayama, T., Kurachi, Y., and Irisawa, H. (1984). Resting K conductances in pacemaker and non-pacemaker heart cells of the rabbit. *Jpn. J. Physiol.* **34**, 245–254.

Pelzer, D., Trube, G., and Piper, H. M. (1984). Low resting potentials in single isolated heart cells due to membrane damage by the recording microelectrode. *Pflügers Arch. ges. Physiol.* **400**, 197–199.

Piwnica-Worms, D., Jacob, R., Horres, C. R., and Lieberman, M. (1985). Na/H exchange in cultured chick heart cells pH_i regulation. *J. Gen. Physiol.* **85**, 43–65.

Provencher, S. W. (1976). A Fourier method for analysis of exponential decay curves. *Biophys. J.* **16**, 27–41.

Scheid, C. R., and Fay, F. S. (1980). Control of ion distribution in isolated smooth muscle cells. I. Potassium. *J. Gen. Physiol.* **75,** 163–182.

Seyama, I. (1978). Which ions are important for the maintenance of the resting membrane potential of the cells of the sinoatrial node of the rabbit? *In:* "The Sinus Node: Structure, Function, and Clinical Relevance" (F. I. M. Bonke, ed.), pp. 339–347. Martinus Nijhoff Publishing, Boston.

Shibata, E. F. (1983). Ionic currents in isolated cardiac pacemaker cells. Ph.D. Thesis. University of Texas Medical Branch, Galveston, Texas, U.S.A.

Shibata, E. F., and Giles, W. (1984). Cardiac pacemaker cells from bullfrog sinus venosus lack an inwardly rectifying background K^+ current. *Biophys. J.* **45,** 136a.

Shibata, E. F., and Giles, W. (1985). Ionic currents which generate the spontaneous diastolic depolarization in individual cardiac pacemaker cells. *Proc. Natl. Acad. Sci. U.S.A.* **82,** 7796–7800.

Shibata, E. F., Momose, Y., and Giles, W. (1984). An electrogenic Na^+/K^+ pump current in individual bullfrog atrial myocytes. *Biophys. J.* **45,** 136a.

Soejima, M., and Noma, A. (1984). Mode of regulation of the ACh-sensitive K-channel by the muscarinic receptor in rabbit atrial cells. *Pflügers Arch. ges. Physiol.* **400,** 424–431.

Standen, N. B., Stanfield, P. R., and Ward, T. A. (1985). Properties of single potassium channels in vesicles formed from the sarcolemma of frog skeletal muscle. *J. Physiol. (London)* **364,** 339–358.

Taniguchi, J., Kokubun, S., Noma, A., and Irisawa, H. (1981). Spontaneously active cells isolated from the sino-atrial and atrioventricular node of the rabbit heart. *Jpn. J. Physiol.* **31,** 547–558.

Trautwein, W., and Zink, K. (1952). Über Membran- und Aktionspotentiale einzelner Myokardfasern des Kalt- und Warmblüterherzens. *Plügers Arch. ges. Physiol.* **256,** 68–84.

Trube, G., and Hescheler, J. (1984). Inward-rectifying channels in isolated patches of heart cell membrane: ATP-dependence and comparison with cell-attached patches. *Pflügers Arch. ges. Physiol.* **401,** 178–184.

Tsien, R. W. (1983). Calcium channels in excitable cell membranes. *Ann. Rev. Physiol.* **45,** 341–358.

Walker, J. L., and Ladle, R. O. (1973). Frog heart intracellular potassium activities measured with potassium microelectrodes. *Am. J. Physiol.* **225,** 263–267.

White, M. M., and Bezanilla, F. (1985). Activation of squid axon K^+ channels. *J. Gen. Physiol.* **85,** 539–554.

Yanagihara, K., Noma, A., and Irisawa, H. (1980). Reconstruction of sinoatrial node pacemaker potential based on the voltage clamp experiments. *Jpn. J. Physiol.* **30,** 841–857.

2

Inactivation and Modulation of Cardiac Ca Channels

Robert S. Kass, Michael C. Sanguinetti, and Douglas S. Krafte

I. INTRODUCTION

It is now generally accepted that the flow of ions through Ca channels is important to the physiological activity of a large number of cells (Hagiwara and Byerly, 1981). Gated influx of calcium ions is crucial to synaptic transmission in nervous tissue and excitation/secretion coupling in GH3 cells and is linked to excitation/contraction coupling in skeletal muscle (Tsien, 1983). In the heart, gated Ca-channel current is essential to normal cardiac function because it has multiple roles. Ca-channel current underlies impulse conduction in nodal tissue, helps maintain the long-lasting plateau phase of the cardiac action potential, and is linked very closely to activation of the contractile proteins (Kass and Scheuer, 1982a, for review). In addition to these roles in the maintenance of normal cardiac function, influx of Ca is now thought to contribute to the genesis of a variety of disturbances of cardiac rhythm (Cranefield, 1977; Hoffman and Rosen, 1981). Thus an understanding of the regulation of Ca influx through gated channels by both indigenous and drug-induced mechanisms is fundamental to our knowledge of the normal heart and to management of certain pathological states.

Ca channels open when the cell membrane is depolarized to voltages more positive than -40 mV (Reuter, 1979; Kass and Sanguinetti, 1984). After opening, many Ca channels close, or inactivate, but recent work suggests that some channels might fail to inactivate even after prolonged depolarization (Kass *et al.*,

29

CARDIAC MUSCLE:
THE REGULATION OF EXCITATION AND CONTRACTION

1976; Matteson and Armstrong, 1984). Ca channels are thought to inactivate through mechanisms regulated by cell membrane potential, intracellular Ca, or a combination of the two. Interest in distinguishing the manner by which this important group of ion channels inactivates has recently increased considerably because of the importance and universality of these channels. In addition, it appears now that certain organic compounds that inhibit Ca fluxes through these channels may exert their effects by interacting preferentially with the inactivated state of the channel.

When a channel inactivates, it becomes unavailable for ion flow. Similarly, a channel is also closed to ion flow when it is blocked by a particular drug. Thus, it is not surprising that the mode of action of certain Ca-channel antagonists (also referred to as Ca-channel blockers) might be closely related to the manner in which the Ca channel inactivates under drug-free conditions.

The purpose of this chapter is to review briefly our understanding of the mechanisms that underlie Ca-channel inactivation in cardiac cells and to discuss the interrelationship between the inactivated state of the channel and block of the channel by Ca-channel antagonists. State-dependent agonism is discussed in addition to state-dependent antagonism of Ca-channel currents.

II. INACTIVATION OF CARDIAC CALCIUM CHANNELS: VOLTAGE- AND CALCIUM-MEDIATED MECHANISMS

Until recently, inactivation of calcium channels in heart as well as other tissues was thought to be governed by a voltage-dependent mechanism similar to that described by Hodgkin and Huxley (1952) for sodium channels in the squid axon. Convincing results reported by Eckert and Tillotson (1981) indicate, however, that Ca-channel inactivation in molluscan neurons can be accounted for completely by a calcium-dependent mechanism that is related only secondarily to membrane potential. In view of this new information, several groups have re-evaluated the inactivation process in cardiac Ca channels to test whether Ca-mediated inactivation occurs universally across cells.

Two observations by Eckert and Tillotson (1981) are crucial to the hypothesis of Ca-mediated inactivation: (1) decay of Ca-channel current is slowed or absent when Ba or Sr replace extracellular Ca and (2) inactivation produced by a prepulse varies with entry of calcium during the prepulse. Voltage-mediated inactivation is characterized by (1) inactivation rates that increase monotonically with depolarization (and that can be significant at potentials too weak to activate Ca entry) and (2) a time course of inactivation that is not changed significantly by replacing extracellular Ca with Ba or Sr (Fox, 1981).

A.   Initial Evidence for Voltage-Dependent Inactivation

Inactivation of cardiac Ca-channel currents was perceived initially as a voltage-dependent process in experiments in multicellular preparations (Reuter, 1979; Coraboeuf, 1980). Experiments on Ca-dependent action potentials (slow responses) measured in partially depolarized Purkinje fiber bundles or in working myocardial muscle showed that this response inactivated over a voltage range more positive than that required to inactivate nerve sodium channels (Carmeliet, 1980; Reuter, 1979).

Voltage-clamp investigations in Purkinje fiber bundles (Reuter, 1967; Vitek and Trautwein, 1971) and other preparations (Rougier et al., 1969; Beeler and Reuter, 1970; New and Trautwein, 1972) soon confirmed the slow response experiments. Measurements of Ca-channel currents in these multicellular preparations were hampered by both nonuniformity of voltage along the preparation and overlap of several time-dependent membrane currents. The problem of nonuniformity of voltage is particularly troublesome for studies of nonlinear inward currents (such as Ca-channel currents); however, theoretical and experimental tests confirmed later that, in the calf Purkinje fiber particularly, inward currents the size of Ca-channel currents could be measured reliably (Kass et al., 1979; Kass and Bennett, 1984). The problem of ionic current separation has been largely overcome by recent experiments that showed that injection of quaternary ammonium ion compounds (Kass et al., 1982) or replacement of intracellular K by Cs (Marban, 1981) reduced greatly the overlapping outward currents that mask Ca-channel current.

Even before these advances, however, early work by Beeler and Reuter (1970) and Trautwein and his colleagues (New and Trautwein, 1972; McDonald and Trautwein, 1978) demonstrated a voltage-dependent, Ca-sensitive current that contributed to net membrane current records at voltages more positive than -40 mV. Using prepulse protocols based on sodium-channel current work in nerve, they found that the Ca-sensitive current became smaller when prepulses were made more positive. When normalized current was plotted against prepulse voltage, the data resembled the steady-state inactivation curve for nerve sodium-channel currents, except that the half-maximal voltage for the Ca-current inactivation curve was much more positive (near -20 mV).

Measurement of the time course of inactivation of Ca-channel current in these experiments was very difficult because of the contribution of time-dependent outward currents to the records. Nevertheless, several studies using the sucrose-gap voltage clamp found that the time constants for inactivation of Ca-channel current changed with membrane potential, increasing as voltages were made more positive (Reuter, 1979).

The interpretation of this work was that, as in nerve sodium channels, cardiac Ca channels inactivate as a function of membrane potential. That is, membrane potential causes the inactivation mechanism (gate) to change states. Depolarization results in a change from mostly open to mostly closed inactivation gates. Channels with closed inactivation gates are not available for ion conduction and are thus effectively blocked.

B. Inactivation Reevaluated: Evidence for Voltage- and Calcium-Mediated Mechanisms

Several groups have begun to reinvestigate the nature of Ca-channel inactivation in cardiac cells through improved techniques that have been introduced over the past five years: pharmacological separation of ionic currents (Kass *et al.*, 1982; Marban and Tsien, 1982) and enzymatic dispersion of cardiac myocytes (Lee and Tsien, 1982). Most of this work has been stimulated by observations of Ca-dependent inactivation in neuronal tissue (Eckert and Tillotson, 1981; Brown *et al.*, 1981). The next section reviews some of these observations.

Figure 1 shows the measurement of Ca-channel current in a multicellular calf Purkinje fiber preparation (Kass and Sanguinetti, 1984). Membrane current is measured during a series of voltage steps, and if time-dependent outward currents are not blocked (A), inward Ca-channel current is masked. In contrast, after blocking overlapping currents (B, left), time-dependent inward current is revealed. Leakage currents can be measured in the presence of a high concentration of a Ca-channel blocker (B, right) and subtracted to determine the voltage dependence of the Ca-channel current (C). The curve in (C) was determined by plotting peak, inward leak-subtracted current against test-pulse voltage. It is important to notice that this curve reaches a maximum near +5 mV, declines at more positive test voltages, and approaches 0 near +60 mV, the Ca-channel reversal potential in this experiment. Similar results for both the shape of the peak inward current–voltage relation and the Ca-channel reversal potential have been observed in isolated ventricular cells (Lee and Tsien, 1982; Isenberg and Klöckner, 1982).

Figure 2 illustrates one method of measuring the time course of inactivation of Ca-channel current. It shows leak-subtracted Ca currents measured during voltage steps to −8 mV (A) and +14 mV (B) recorded in a calf Purkinje fiber (Kass and Sanguinetti, 1984). In each case, current and its best fit by a two-exponential function are superimposed. In this multicellular Purkinje fiber preparation, the decay of inward current was fitted best consistently by functions with two exponential components. When Ca is the charge carrier, both time constants are fast ($\tau_1 \leqq 10$ msec; $\tau \leqq 100$ msec) and show little variation with test-pulse voltage. Similar results have been found in isolated ventricular cells (Isenberg and Klöckner, 1982).

Kass and Sanguinetti (1984) found that replacement of Ca by Ba or Sr (Fig. 3) slowed the time course of inactivation considerably, but certainly did not prevent

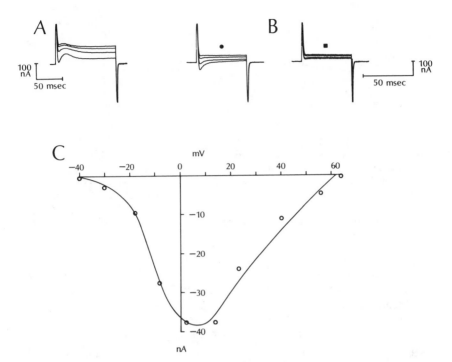

Fig. 1. Calcium channel reversal potential in Ca-containing solutions. (A) The transient outward current masks calcium current reversal potential in a calf Purkinje fiber that had not been injected with tetrabutylammonium (TBA). Currents are shown in response to voltage pulses to +10, +30, +55, and +68 mV from a −52 mV holding potential. Preparation 309-2. (B) Measurement of calcium current after TBS injection. Current traces are shown in response to pulses to −18, +2, +23, and +63 mV after outward currents were blocked by injections of TBA. Background currents measured in the presence of nisoldipine (10 μM, □) were subtracted from drug-free records (○) to obtain calcium-channel current. (C) Peak inward calcium-channel current is plotted against pulse voltage. Holding potential (HP) = −63 mV. Preparation 292-2. [Reproduced from Kass and Sanguinetti (1984) with permission.]

the decay of current through the Ca channel. When the inactivation rate for Sr and Ba currents was measured, however, over a wide voltage range, both time constants were found to be very voltage dependent (Fig. 4). This work showed that replacement of Ca by Ba or Sr altered the voltage dependence of the onset of inactivation (solid symbols, Fig. 4) markedly, but had little effect on recovery from inactivation (open symbols, Fig. 4). This observation raised the possibility that entry of Ca during depolarization might cause additional inactivation through a Ca-mediated process and account for the dramatic difference between the inactivation rates of Ca and Sr (or Ba) currents during depolarizing pulses.

Marban and Tsien (1981) were the first to suggest the possibility of Ca-

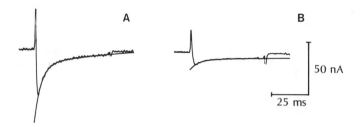

Fig. 2. Time course of calcium-current inactivation in a calf Purkinje fiber during depolarizing voltage pulses. The time dependence of membrane current was analyzed after subtracting background current measured in the presence of nisoldipine (10 μM). (A) Current in response to a voltage pulse to -8 mV. Time constants of best fit exponentials: $\tau_1 = 5$ msec, $\tau_2 = 60$ msec. (B) Current in response to a pulse to $+14$ mV. Time constants: $\tau_1 = 5$ msec, $\tau_2 = 47$ msec; 5.4 mM Ca; HP = -63 mV. Preparation 292-2. [Reproduced from Kass and Sanguinetti (1984) with permission.]

mediated inactivation in cardiac cells. Since their observation in nystatin-treated Purkinje fibers, others have also provided evidence that Ca-current inactivation in a variety of cardiac cells is mediated, at least in part, by Ca (Hume and Giles, 1982; Mentrard et al., 1984; Josephson et al., 1984; Kurachi, 1982). The principal evidence for this interpretation has come from the relationship between entry of Ca during a conditioning pulse and Ca-current inactivation during a subsequent test pulse, as first described in molluscan neurons by Tillotson (1979) and Eckert and Tillotson (1981). These workers found that as the prepulse voltage was made progressively more positive than $+10$ mV, the peak Ca current measured during the subsequent test pulse reached a minimum, but then became larger. This results in a U-shaped Ca-current-availability curve (Fig. 5) that is not predicted by previous voltage-dependent models for Ca-channel inactivation. Because entry of Ca decreases over this voltage range during the prepulse (see

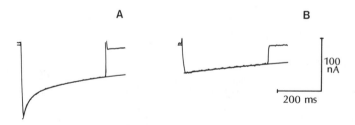

Fig. 3. Time course of Sr-current inactivation measured in a calf Purkinje fiber during depolarizing steps. Nisoldipine-sensitive current traces are shown superimposed on curves calculated by a fitting routine. (A) Pulse voltage = $+18$ mV. Time constants: $\tau_1 = 13$ msec, $\tau_2 = 155$ msec. (B) Pulse voltage = -11 mV. Time constants: $\tau_1 = 94$ msec, $\tau_2 = 744$ msec; HP = -50 mV. Preparation 301-1. 5.4 mM Sr-Tyrode solution. [Reproduced from Kass and Sanguinetti (1984) with permission.]

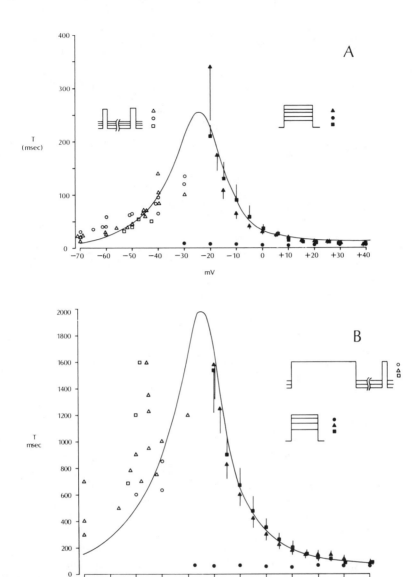

Fig. 4. Time course of inactivation in a calf Purkinje fiber: cumulative data. (A) Time constants for fast phase of inactivation. (B) Time constants for slower phase of inactivation. Time constants calculated from a fitting procedure are plotted for recovery from (open symbols) and onset of (solid symbols) inactivation. Data are shown for Ca ($\bigcirc$, $\bullet$, $n=10$), Sr ($\triangle$, $\blacktriangle$, $n=9$–10), and Ba ($\square$, $\blacksquare$, $n=7$) currents. Data for onset of inactivation are plotted as mean $\pm$ S.E.M. Individual time constants are plotted for recovery from inactivation. The theoretical curves plotted in the figure were generated using Eqs. (7) and (8) of Chiu (1977) with the following rate constants (msec^{-1}): $a_{10} = 0.00048$ $\exp(-(V+4)/12)$, $a_{10} = [0.0065]/[1 + \exp(-(V)/6)]$, $a_{12} = (0.0065)/[1 + \exp(-V/8)]$, and $a_{21} = 0.00008 \exp(-(V-5)/17)$. [Reproduced from Kass and Sanguinetti (1984) with permission.]

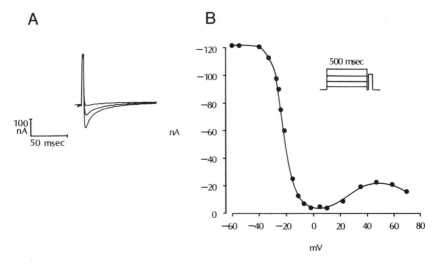

Fig. 5. Calcium current (500-msec) inactivation in a calf Purkinje fiber after prepulses to positive potentials. Pulse protocol (inset): current was measured during a test pulse to 0 mV that had been preceded by 500-msec conditioning prepulses. A 10-msec return to the holding potential (−63 mV) separated prepulse from test pulse. (A) Current traces recorded at 0 mV after prepulses to −55, −21, and +22 mV (bottom trace to top trace). (B) Plot of peak inward test current against conditioning pulse potential. 5.4 m*M* Ca-Tyrode solution. Preparation 227-1.

Fig. 1), the U-shaped inactivation curve is consistent with a Ca-mediated inactivation mechanism (Marban and Tsien, 1981).

The observation that the inactivation rate of Ca current is not current dependent argues against a purely Ca-mediated inactivation mechanism in calf Purkinje fibers. This can be inferred from the data in Figs. 1 and 4. During voltage steps more positive than +5 mV, the inactivation rates of Ca currents are fast but independent of the test potential, even though peak inward current decreases as the voltage becomes more positive.

Figure 6 shows that this is also the case in isolated ventricular cells. In this experiment (D. S. Krafte and R. S. Kass, unpublished data), the inactivation rate of Ca current remains very fast even at voltages more positive than the current's reversal potential. If inactivation of these channels were caused entirely by entry of Ca, the inactivation rates would be expected to become slower or nonexistent in this range of voltages.

The simplest interpretation of these results is that Ca-channel current in cardiac cells inactivates through mechanisms that are both voltage dependent and Ca dependent. The results obtained in Ba- or Sr-containing solutions may be explained if these divalent cations are unable to substitute for Ca in enhancing inactivation. In this view, Ba (or Sr) currents reflect a predominantly voltage-dependent process, whereas Ca currents reflect both voltage- and Ca-mediated mechanisms. If this is the case, then studies that focus on voltage-dependent inactivation of the Ca channel would be simplified if Ba or Sr were to replace Ca in the test solutions. This approach has already been taken in several investigations of Ca-channel modulation by organic compounds (Lee and Tsien, 1983; Sanguinetti and Kass, 1984a; Hess *et al.*, 1984).

C. Slow Inactivation

The time constants of the inactivation processes discussed above range from a few to hundreds of milliseconds (at 37°C). In addition to inactivation that occurs over these times, Kass and Scheuer (1982b) reported a very slow inactivating component of Ca-channel current in the calf Purkinje fiber. The time course of this process (at 37°C) is approximately several seconds and is independent of the species of divalent charge carrier. This suggests that slow inactivation is a voltage-mediated process and might be particularly important to drug-channel interactions with certain organic compounds. A very slow inactivation process

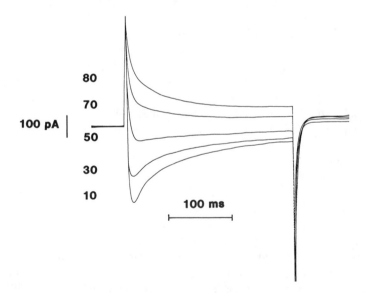

Fig. 6. Membrane current in response to 250-msec depolarizing voltage steps in an isolated, guinea-pig ventricular myocyte. Membrane potential was held at -50 mV and stepped to the indicated voltages. Peak current became less inward as the test potential became more positive; it reversed direction above $+50$ mV. Decaying currents for each test pulse were fitted by a biexponential function as in Fig. 3 with the following results: for $V_{test} = +10$ mV, $\tau_1 = 8.3$ msec and $\tau_2 = 89$ msec; for $V_{test} = +30$ mV, $\tau_1 = 14.3$ msec and $\tau_2 = 90$ msec; for $V_{test} = +70$ mV, $\tau_1 = 4.7$ msec and $\tau_2 = 42$ msec; for $V_{test} = +80$ mV, $\tau_1 = 4.3$ msec and $\tau_2 = 42$ msec.

has been observed also in isolated ventricular cells (D. S. Krafte and R. S. Kass, unpublished data).

Thus, cardiac Ca channels appear to resemble sodium channels in nerve (Chandler and Meves, 1970; Rudy, 1978) and Ca channels in *Aplysia* neurons (Adams and Gage, 1979), in that each of these channels has a very slow component of the inactivation process. In the discussions of drug-channel interactions that follow, it is important to remember the possible roles of this process.

III.   STATE-DEPENDENT MODULATION OF Ca-CHANNEL CURRENT

Pharmacological studies have provided considerable information about the molecular structure of ion channels in the membranes of excitable cells. For example, tetrodotoxin has been used to block, probe, and count Na channels in nerve and skeletal muscle. Quaternary ammonium compounds have proved to be very effective potassium-channel blockers and have been used to investigate the architecture of potassium channels in nerve and skeletal muscle preparations (Hille, 1977; Armstrong, 1969). More recently, organic compounds that block Ca channels in cardiac and smooth muscle cells have been used in electrophysiological and binding studies to probe the structure and function of these channels (Schwartz and Triggle, 1984). Advances in the characterization of Ca-channel current in recent years can be attributed, in large part, to the discovery of these organic compounds. Modulation of Ca-channel currents by these drugs seems to be affected strongly by the state of the channel (Sanguinetti and Kass, 1984a) and may even be caused by modification of the mode of channel gating (Hess *et al.,* 1984).

The remainder of this chapter reviews the proposed mechanisms of action of organic compounds that have been shown to modify Ca-channel currents in cardiac preparations. The review focuses on results from voltage-clamp studies of isolated cardiac tissue and single cardiac cells and emphasizes the actions of dihydropyridine derivatives (e.g., nifedipine and nisoldipine) and diarylalkylamine antagonists (e.g., verapamil, D600, and AQA39). More systematic reviews of the literature concerning the sites and mechanisms of action of Ca-channel inhibitors in smooth and cardiac muscle, including discussions of binding studies, can be found elsewhere (Schwartz and Triggle, 1984; Miller and Freedman, 1984: Janis and Scriabine, 1983).

A.   Mechanisms of Action of Ca-Channel Antagonists

Ca-channel currents are inhibited by metallic cations such as Mn^{2+}, Ni^{2+}, Co^{2+} (Kohlhardt *et al.,* 1973), Mg^{2+} (Chesnais *et al.,* 1975), and La^{3+} (Katzung *et al.*, 1973; Kass and Tsien, 1975), but this inhibition occurs at millimolar concentrations. In contrast, organic compounds that inhibit Ca-channel currents (Ca-channel antagonists) are effective in micromolar and even nanomolar concentrations. The effectiveness of these drugs depends on the conditions under which they are applied, specifically stimulation rate and cell resting potential. The mechanisms responsible for this sensitivity to experimental conditions are addressed in the following section.

Three chemically distinct groups of Ca-channel blockers have been defined by their clinical effectiveness in treating cardiovascular disorders (Singh *et al.*, 1983; Schwartz and Taira, 1983) as well as by distinct, high-affinity binding sites (Schwartz and Triggle, 1984; Janis and Scriabine, 1983). These groups are the diarylalkylamines such as verapamil and D600, the benzothiazepine derivatives typified by diltiazem, and the dihydropyridines such as nifedipine, nitrendipine, and nisoldipine (Fig. 7). In addition to having pharmacologically separable binding sites, these drugs, as shown in electrophysiological studies, differ also in their mechanisms of Ca-channel inhibition.

B. Frequency-Dependent Block

Thorough voltage-clamp investigations of the mechanisms of action of organic Ca-channel blockers have revealed that block of Ca current by all three classes of these compounds is strongly modulated by membrane potential. This phenomenon is responsible for their frequency (use) -dependent block of contractile activity and Ca current in cardiac tissue. In all cases, inhibition of Ca current is facilitated by depolarization, caused by either increasing the frequency of stimulation or, in the case of voltage-clamp studies, holding the membrane potential at depolarized levels. Conversely, hyperpolarization reverses Ca-current inhibition, presumably by causing a voltage-dependent decrease in the affinity of the drug for its receptor. An example of use-dependent effects of verapamil is illustrated in Fig. 8.

Frequency-dependent block of current results from a drug-induced prolongation of the time required for the channels to recover from inactivation. Ca channels normally recover in a biexponential manner, the time constants of which are dependent on voltage. D600 (Pelzer *et al.*, 1982), verapamil (Kohlhardt and Mnich, 1978), nisoldipine (Sanguinetti and Kass, 1984a), nitrendipine (Lee and Tsien, 1983), and diltiazem (Uehara and Hume, 1984) all prolong this recovery process. Those compounds that exhibit the greatest frequency-dependent block (e.g., D600, verapamil) slow this process to a greater extent than the dihydropyridines, which, under similar experimental conditions, exhibit use-dependent effects only at higher rates of stimulation.

How do Ca-channel antagonists retard the recovery from inactivation of Ca current, and why are some drugs more effective than others in this respect? A

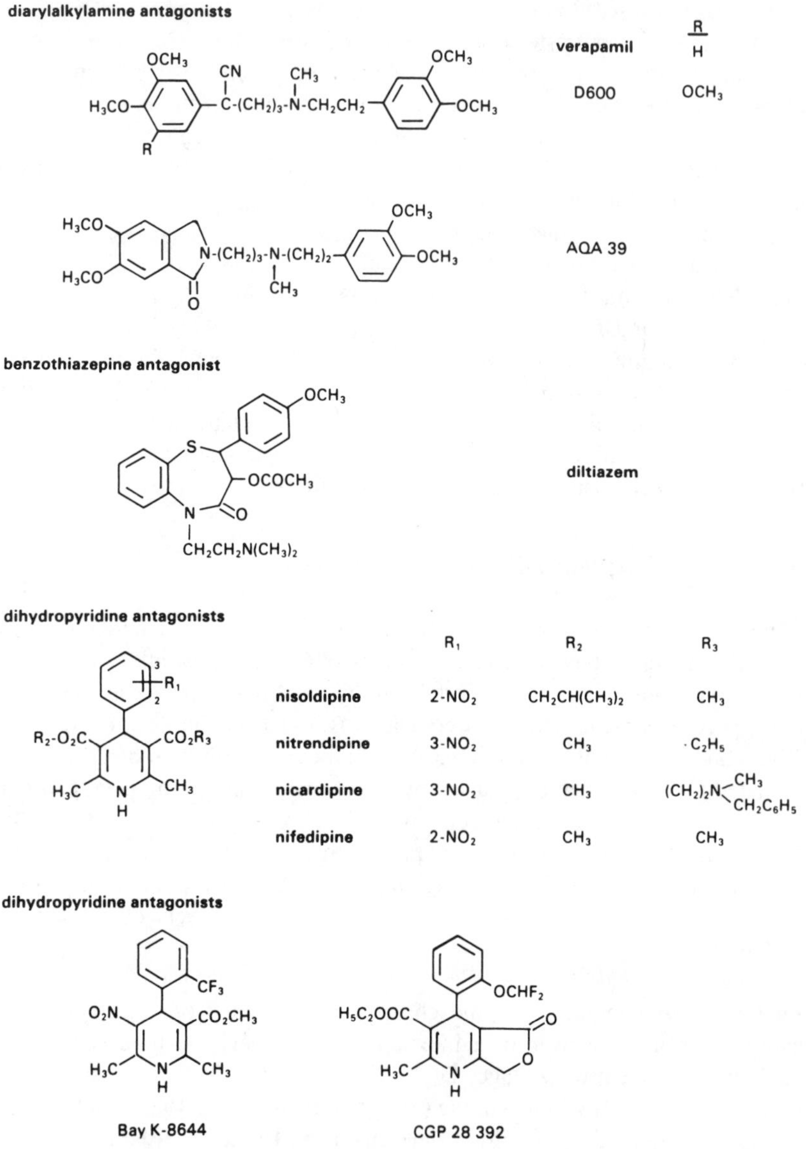

diarylalkylamine antagonists

	R
verapamil	H
D600	OCH$_3$

AQA 39

benzothiazepine antagonist

diltiazem

dihydropyridine antagonists

	R$_1$	R$_2$	R$_3$
nisoldipine	2-NO$_2$	CH$_2$CH(CH$_3$)$_2$	CH$_3$
nitrendipine	3-NO$_2$	CH$_3$	·C$_2$H$_5$
nicardipine	3-NO$_2$	CH$_3$	(CH$_2$)$_2$N$\big<^{CH_3}_{CH_2C_6H_5}$
nifedipine	2-NO$_2$	CH$_3$	CH$_3$

dihydropyridine antagonists

Bay K-8644   CGP 28 392

Fig. 7. Structural formulae of Ca-channel antagonists and agonists.

plausible explanation is provided by the modulated-receptor hypothesis (Hille, 1977; Hondeghem and Katzung, 1977). This hypothesis was proposed to account for the time and voltage dependence of drug interactions with ionic channels, originally for local anesthetic block of Na channels. The model proposes that local anesthetics bind to a site in or near the Na channel, and that the affinity for this site depends on the state of the channel (i.e., resting, open, or inactivated), which varies as a function of membrane potential. Furthermore, the model assumes the drug-bound channels do not conduct. This concept has been extended to explain the voltage-dependent interactions of organic Ca-entry blockers with

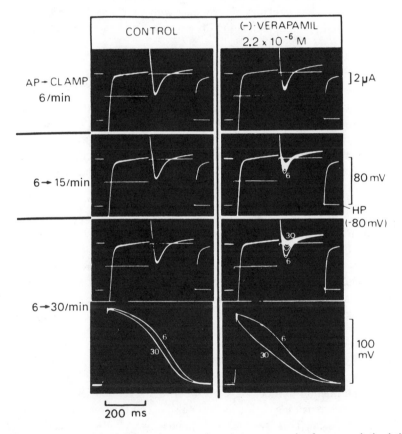

Fig. 8. Behavior of the slow inward current subsequent to a conversion from normal stimulation conditions (6/min) to voltage-clamp conditions. Superimposed traces of 12 consecutive clamp cycles recorded after application of voltage-clamp conditions. In the middle and lower panels, cycle frequency was increased after the first voltage-clamp cycle to 15/min and 30/min, respectively. The action potentials shown in the lower panel were recorded before frequency change and after voltage-clamp conditions were terminated. [Reproduced from Bayer *et al.* (1982) with permission.]

the Ca channel (Hondeghem and Katzung, 1984; McDonald *et al.*, 1984). The model predicts that ionized drugs can bind to the channel-associated receptor only when a hydrophilic pathway to this site is provided, that is, when the channels are open. Neutral drugs can reach this receptor through either this pathway or a hydrophobic pathway through the lipid membrane surrounding the channel. The degree of drug ionization can be calculated on the basis of the pKa of the compound and pH of the Tyrode solution. At physiological pH, the diarylalkylamines (verapamil, D600, AQA39; pKa = 8–9) are highly charged, whereas most dihydropyridines (nitrendipine, nisoldipine, nifedipine; pKa < 3) are almost exclusively neutral.

The results of voltage-clamp experiments with Ca-channel blockers support these generalized predictions relating drug ionization to mode of action.

1. Diarylalkylamine Antagonists

Exposure of cat ventricular trabeculae to D600 or AQA39 for 30 min without pulsing does not result in Ca-channel blockade, as assessed by a single depolarization applied after a pulse-free period (Pelzer *et al.*, 1982). Because no channels were opened during this pulse-free period (holding potential was −50 mV), neither D600 nor AQA39 could gain access to the channel-associated receptor. Block of Ca-channel current was observed only when a train of voltage pulses was imposed. Under this condition, a pulse-by-pulse decrease in current became evident. Similar voltage- and use-dependent block by D600 was observed in isolated guinea-pig ventricular cells (Lee and Tsien, 1983) and by verapamil in calf Purkinje fibers (Sanguinetti and Kass, 1984a). These results suggest that channels must open before the diarylalkylamine Ca-channel blockers can interact with a receptor and produce inhibition of Ca current.

Ca-channel block by AQA39 or D600 that has developed during a train of stimuli is readily reversed by hyperpolarizing the membrane potential to −90 mV for 90 sec (Pelzer *et al.*, 1982). This behavior was used to design a pulse protocol for further tests of whether activation of Ca channels is essential for block by D600 or AQA39 (Pelzer *et al.*, 1982). Removal of block by hyperpolarization was followed by five brief activating pulses to a variable conditioning potential (−50, −40, −20, or +5 mV) and then by a standard test pulse to +5 mV. The fraction of block developed during the five pulses was calculated from the current remaining during the test pulse in comparison to total Ca current available for block. This fraction corresponded well with the fraction of Ca channels opened (d_∞) during the five conditioning pulses. The relationship between block by D600 and the corresponding degree of Ca-channel activation (studied over a more complete voltage range) confirmed these results (Fig. 9 and McDonald *et al.*, 1984). Further evidence that D600 blocks activated Ca channels comes from experiments on isolated ventricular cells (Lee and Tsien, 1983).

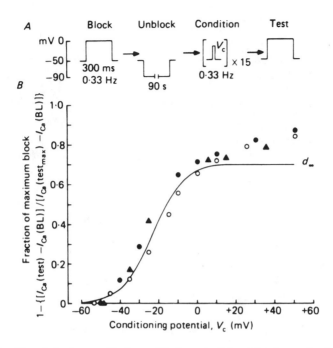

Fig. 9. The relation between block, conditioning potential, and the degree of activation of the Ca system. (A) Procedure. Muscles treated with 2 μM D600 for 60–90 min were stimulated at 0.33 Hz with 300-msec pulses from −50 to 0 mV (block). After unblock (90 sec at −90 mV, 20 sec at −50 mV), they were pulsed 15 times at 0.33 Hz with 30-msec steps to potentials V_c and then tested for block with a 300-msec pulse to 0 mV. (B) The fraction of maximum block versus the potential of the conditioning pulses (V_c). Maximum block refers to block achieved with the 300-msec pulses to 0 mV at 0.33 Hz. The effect of the conditioning pulses was determined by relating the amplitude of block-sensitive I_{Ca} after conditioning [$I_{Ca}(\text{test}) - I_{Ca}(\text{block})$] to maximum block-sensitive I_{Ca} [$I_{Ca}(\text{test}_{max}) - I_{Ca}(\text{block})$]; "test$_{max}$" was measured on test pulses immediately after unblock. Symbols represent determinations on three muscles. The continuous curve is the steady-state activation variable (d_∞) taken from Trautwein *et al.* (1975) and scaled in amplitude to fit the data between −50 and −10 mV. There is a noticeable divergence of the data from d_∞ at potentials positive at 0 mV. [Reproduced from McDonald *et al.* (1984) with permission.]

Although conclusive proof that these drugs bind preferentially to a specific channel state is lacking, it is clear that opening of Ca channels is a prerequisite for inhibition of Ca current by the diarylalkylamines. In fact it is conceivable that once these drugs gain access to the interior of the channel during activation they bind preferentially to the inactivated rather than the open configuration of the channel.

Both the rate of onset of Ca-channel block during a train of depolarizing pulses and the steady-state level of block achieved are increased when the duration of each pulse is prolonged. This characteristic has been observed in voltage-clamped ferret papillary muscle (Kanaya *et al.*, 1983) and calf Purkinje fibers (Sanguinetti and Kass, 1984a). If drug-bound channels undergo voltage- and time-dependent transitions of state, the end result of a prolonged depolarization (or repeated depolarizations of sufficient duration) should be stabilization of channels in the drug-bound inactivated state. The interaction of verapamil, D600, and AQA39 with the Ca channel can be visualized as occurring through the pathway R → O → O* → I* (McDonald *et al.*, 1984), shown below diagrammatically in a scheme first described by Hille (1977) for local anesthetic interaction with Na channels during a depolarizing event. In this scheme, R, O, and I represent Ca channels in the rested, open, and inactivated states, respectively, and R*, O*, and I* represent drug-bound channels. Support for such a mechanism comes from experiments with D600, which revealed a large drug-induced hyperpolarizing voltage shift in the availability of Ca current in isolated frog atrial cells (Uehara and Hume, 1984).

The effect of D600 on single Ca-channel activity was studied recently in cell-attached patch-clamp recordings from isolated guinea-pig ventricular cells (Pelzer *et al.*, 1984). D600 did not change single-channel conductance but did increase the probability of channel opening as well as the number of null sweeps (no channel openings during a prolonged depolarization). From these studies, Pelzer *et al.* (1984) concluded that D600 must reach its receptor from either the membrane or the cytoplasm. Their results confirmed the conclusions of earlier work that demonstrated the quaternary ammonium derivative of D600 blocks Ca current only when injected intracellularly (Hescheler *et al.*, 1982).

2. Dihydropyridine Antagonists

Initial voltage-clamp studies on nifedipine, nitrendipine, and nisoldipine demonstrated that these compounds were potent Ca-channel blockers, but were not characterized by significant use-dependent actions (Tung and Morad, 1983; Kass, 1982; Bayer and Ehara, 1978; Kohlhardt and Fleckenstein, 1977). Earlier

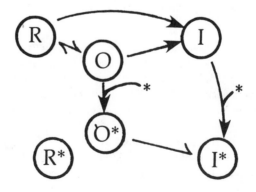

investigations concluded also that nifedipine did not alter the time course of recovery from inactivation (Kohlhardt and Fleckenstein, 1977). These results are consistent with a lack of use-dependent block and thus a channel state-independent mode of action. More recent investigations have made it clear, however, that these compounds *do* hinder recovery from inactivation and inhibit Ca-channel currents in a frequency-dependent manner (Lee and Tsien, 1983; Uehara and Hume, 1984; Sanguinetti and Kass, 1984a). Depending on experimental conditions, use-dependent block by the dihydropyridines can be described as mild (Lee and Tsien, 1983) or marked (Sanguinetti and Kass, 1984a). In the latter case, little or no block is caused by 0.2 μM nisoldipine when the holding potential is hyperpolarized (−70 mV) and the voltage pulses are brief (50 msec) and infrequent (0.2 Hz). Pulsing at high frequencies (5 Hz) results, however, in considerable (75%) block by the same concentration of nisoldipine.

The most dramatic difference between the actions of the diarylalkylamines and dihydropyridines is that membrane potential modulates block of Ca-channel currents by the dihydropyridines markedly, even in the absence of repetitive pulsing. For example, nisoldipine or nitrendipine (0.1 μM) inhibits Ca-channel current only slightly when the membrane potential is held at −70 mV for 2 min, but blocks the channels almost completely when the holding potential is changed to depolarized (−45 mV) levels (Sanguinetti and Kass, 1984b). As noted previously, in the presence of verapamil, no block develops simply by holding the membrane at −45 mV. This suggests that block of Ca channels by nisoldipine or nitrendipine can develop without the Ca channels being in the open state.

What causes the membrane potential to have such dramatic effects on Ca-channel inhibition by dihydropyridines? One possibility is that these drugs interact preferentially with channels that are inactivated.

To test this possibility, Sanginetti and Kass (1984a) measured the influence of a wide range of holding potentials on Ca-channel block by nisoldipine. They varied also how long the membrane was held at each of these conditioning potentials. These experiments revealed two important aspects of drug-channel interaction by this dihydropyridine: when the conditioning prepulses were brief (500 msec to 1 sec), the voltage dependence of Ca-channel availability was unchanged from drug-free conditions; however, when the prepulse durations were increased to 30 sec, nisoldipine caused a large (−19 mV), hyperpolarizing shift in the relationship between Ca-channel availability and membrane potential (Fig. 10). A drug-induced hyperpolarizing shift in the steady-state inactivation curve is consistent with an interaction between this drug and the inactivated state of the channel (Hille, 1977, 1978); however, the drug-induced shift occurs only if conditioning prepulses are sufficiently long. Thus, it is possible that this interaction is via the mechanism of slow inactivation of these channels.

Apparent dissociation constants for nisoldipine's binding to rested or inactivated channel conformations were calculated from the data shown in Fig. 10.

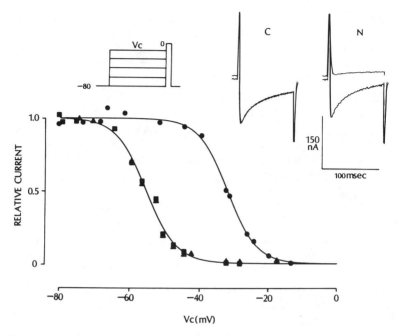

Fig. 10.   Effect of nisoldipine on voltage dependence of Ca-channel current availability in a calf Purkinje fiber. Prepulses (V_c), 30 sec in duration, were followed by a 100-msec test pulse (V_t) to 0 mV. Graph shows normalized plot of maximum inward current measured during V_t in the absence (●) and presence of nisoldipine (200 nM, ▲; 400 nM, ■) vs. V_c. Peak current in presence of nisoldipine was 87% (200 nM) and 77% (400 nM) of that recorded in control. Inset: pulse protocol and current traces in response to test pulse after 30-sec conditioning pulses to −44 and −74 mV, control (C), nisoldipine (N). Curve: best fit of function $(1 + \exp[(V − V_h)/k])^{-1}$ to data. Control: V_h = −32 mV, k = 4.1. Nisoldipine: V_h = −53.4 mV (200 nM), −55 mV (400 nM); k = 4.2 (200 nM), 4.4 (400 nM). 5.4 mM Sr^{2+}-Tyrode solution + 10 μM TTX. Preparation 339-1. [Reproduced from Sanguinetti and Kass (1984a) with permission.]

The results yielded dissociation constants of 1300 (resting channels) and 1 nM (inactivated channels). The calculations were made on the assumption that nisoldipine binds only to Ca channels in the resting or inactivated state. We used an equation (described by Bean *et al.*, 1983) that relates the shift in the steady-state availability curve, produced by a given drug concentration, to apparent dissociation constants for binding to inactivated or rested-state channels. In this computation, slow inactivation was not considered an additional state of the channel.

This 1000-fold difference in apparent binding constants (K_d) is the same as that reported previously for the discrepancy between the K_d for binding of [3H]nitrendipine to cardiac membranes (0.1–1.0 nM) and the concentration for 50% inhibition of contraction or of Ca current of cardiac tissues (Janis and

Scriabine, 1983; Ferry and Glossmann, 1982; Kass, 1982). Thus, the K_d for binding probably reflects the affinity of the drugs for depolarized membrane, perhaps specifically for channels that are in the inactivated state.

What causes the holding potential to modulate block by dihydropyridines but not that by diarylalkylamines? One possibility is the difference in the relative hydrophilicity of these compounds. Nisoldipine and nitrendipine respond almost identically to changes in membrane potential and, unlike verapamil or D600, both compounds are highly lipophilic. To determine whether the observed differences in blocking activity of these compounds are caused by differences in hydrophilicity or by structural dissimilarities, Sanguinetti and Kass (1984a) studied the influence of membrane potential on the blocking actions of nicardipine, a dihydropyridine (Fig. 7) that is ionized 28% at pH 7.4. These experiments showed that nicardipine exhibits an intermediate level of holding potential-dependent block of Ca-channel current. Thus, the dihydropyridines interact with Ca channels probably through pathway R → O → O* → I* or R → I → I* (Diagram 1), depending on the membrane voltage and hydrophilicity of a given compound.

C. Ca-Channel Agonists

Slight modifications in the structure of nifedipine have led to the discovery of dihydropyridines that *increase* smooth and cardiac muscle contractility (Schramm *et al.*, 1983). Subsequent studies have shown that one of these compounds, Bay K 8644, increases the magnitude of Ca-channel current (Cohen and Chung, 1984; Hess *et al.*, 1984; Sanguinetti and Kass, 1984b). In each study it was noted that the greatest increase in Ca-channel current occurred during weak depolarizations and that current measured during a pulse inactivated more rapidly in the presence of the drug. It was observed also that inward current tails measured after repolarization were larger and deactivated more slowly than under drug-free conditions.

Cell-attached patch recordings of single Ca-channel currents have revealed that Bay K 8644 increases the probability of and prolongs channel opening without altering the magnitude of single-channel current (Hess *et al.*, 1984). The long channel openings observed in the presence of Bay K 8644 are seen also in the absence of drug, but far less frequently. This and other findings prompted Hess *et al.* (1984) to propose that this mode of gating is intrinsic and merely enhanced by this drug. It was proposed further that dihydropyridine agonists and antagonists act at the same receptor to modulate different modes of Ca-channel gating. In this hypothesis, the antagonists act by promoting another gating mode that is characterized by a lack of channel openings upon depolarization. Binding studies support this interpretation by demonstrating that Bay K 8644 and nitrendipine share a common high-affinity binding site on isolated cardiac membranes

(Janis *et al.*, 1984). In rabbit cardiac membranes, the maximal number of binding sites is the same for both nitrendipine and Bay K 8644 (0.7 nmole/mg).

Bay K 8644 acts as only a partial agonist. Voltage-clamp studies have shown that it decreases both contractile force and Ca-channel current when holding potentials are sufficiently depolarized (more positive than −40 mV) (Sanguinetti and Kass, 1984b). The balance between its enhancement and block of Ca-channel current is determined by cell holding potential (Fig. 11). This is very important in predicting the activity of Bay K 8644 in cells that are not voltage-

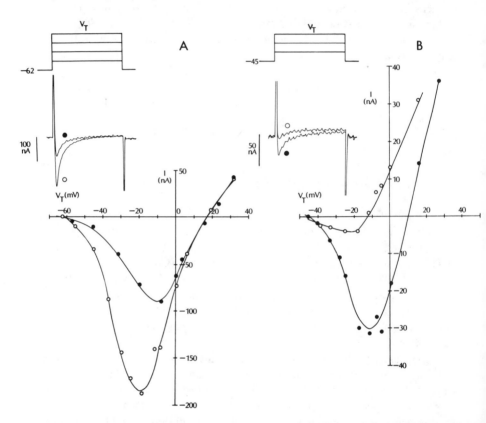

Fig. 11.   Influence of holding potential on the actions of Bay K 8644 (0.5 μ*M*) on membrane current in a calf Purkinje fiber. Membrane current was recorded in the presence of 10 μM TTX and in response to 100-msec test pulses (inset) applied from a holding potential of −62 mV (A) or −45 mV (B). The insets in both panels show current traces in response to voltage steps to −10 mV from each holding potential in the absence (●) or presence (○) of drug. The graphs show peak inward current plotted against test-pulse voltage in the absence (●) or presence (○) of drug, and the curves are hand drawn. The standard modified Tyrode solution consisted of (m*M*): 150 NaCl, 4 KCl, 5.4 $CaCl_2$, 0.5 $MgCl_2$, 5 glucose, and 10 Tris–HCl buffer (pH 7.4). Preparation 351-1. [Reproduced from Sanguinetti and Kass (1984b) with permission.]

clamped, because cells that are typically depolarized will respond to the drug much differently than those that have resting potentials near -80 mV.

Agonist-like effects also have been reported for the antagonist nitrendipine (Hess *et al.*, 1984). Records of single Ca-channel currents showed that nitrendipine increased the percentage of records containing openings of long duration, similar to those induced by Bay K 8644, but, as expected, reduced the number of records with detectable channel openings. In cultured neuroblastoma $\times$ glioma cells, another compound, CGP 28 392, produced effects similar to those of Bay K 8644 (Miller and Freedman, 1984).

It is tempting to speculate about the nature of the binding site for the dihydropyridine agonists/antagonists. Perhaps there is an indigenous ligand that can modulate Ca-channel gating by interacting with a receptor that also binds the dihydropyridines with great affinity (Schramm *et al.*, 1983; Hess *et al.*, 1984; see also Johnson *et al.*, Chapter 12).

IV. SUMMARY

In summary, dihydropyridine derivatives have been shown to markedly influence Ca-channel activity in excitable cells. In cardiac cells, antagonists have been shown to promote the inactivated state of Ca channel, and agonists have been shown to enhance mean channel open time. Future studies will be needed to determine if these two actions are interrelated and whether a single receptor regulates both actions. Furthermore, new work is needed to discover whether all Ca channels in all cell types respond identically to dihydropyridine derivatives.

REFERENCES

Adams, D. J., and Gage, P. W. (1979). Characteristics of sodium and calcium conductance changes produced by membrane depolarization in *Aplysia* neurone. *J. Physiol.* **291,** 467–481.

Armstrong, C. M. (1969). Inactivation of the potassium conductance and related phenomena caused by quaternary ammonium ion injection in squid axons. *J. Gen. Physiol.* **54,** 553–575.

Bayer, R., and Ehara, T. (1978). Comparative studies on calcium antagonists. *Prog. Pharmacol.* **2,** 31–37.

Bayer, R., Kaufmann, R., Mannhold, R., and Rodenkirchen, R. (1982). The action of specific Ca antagonists on cardiac electrical activity. *Prog. Pharmacol.* **5,** 53–85.

Bean, B. P., Cohen, C. J., and Tsien, R. W. (1983). Lidocaine block of cardiac sodium channels. *J. Gen. Physiol.* **81,** 613–642.

Beeler, G. W., Jr., and Reuter, H. (1970). Membrane calcium current in ventricular myocardial fibres. *J. Physiol.* **207,** 191–209.

Brown, A. M., Morimoto, K., Tsuda, Y., and Wilson, D. L. (1981). Calcium current-dependent and voltage-dependent inactivation in *Helix aspersa*. *J. Physiol.* **320,** 193–218.

Carmeliet, E. (1980). The slow inward current: Non-voltage-clamp studies. *In* "The Slow Inward Current and Cardiac Arrhythmias" (D. P. Zipes, J. C. Bailey, and V. Elharrar, eds.), pp. 97–110. Martinus Nijhoff, The Hague.

Chandler, W. K., and Meves, H. (1970). Slow changes in membrane permeability and long-lasting action potentials in axons perfused with fluoride solutions. *J. Physiol.* **211,** 707–728.

Chesnais, J. M., Coraboeuf, E., Sauviat, M. P., and Vassas, J. M. (1975). Sensitivity to H, Li, and Mg ions of the slow inward sodium current in frog atrial fibers. *J. Mol. Cell. Cardiol.* **7,** 627–642.

Chiu, S. Y. (1977). Inactivation of sodium channels: Second order kinetics in myelinated nerve. *J. Physiol.* **273,** 573–596.

Cohen, C. J., and Chung, M. (1984). A nifedipine derivative (Bay K 8644) that increases Ca currents in myocardial cells: A novel positive inotropic agent. *Biophys. J.* **45,** 394a.

Coraboeuf, E. (1980). Voltage clamp studies of the slow inward current. *In* "The Slow Inward Current and Cardiac Arrhythmias" (D. P. Zipes, J. C. Bailey, and V. Elharrar, eds.), pp. 25–95. Martinus Nijhoff, The Hague.

Cranefield, P. F. (1977). Action potentials, afterpotentials, and arrhythmias. *Circ. Res.* **41,** 415–423.

Eckert, R., and Tillotson, D. L. (1981). Calcium-mediated inactivation of the calcium conductance in caesium-loaded giant neurones of *Apylsia californica. J. Physiol.* **314,** 265–280.

Ferry, D. R., and Glossmann, H. (1982). Evidence for multiple receptor sites within the putative calcium channel. *Naunyn-Schmied. Arch. Pharmacol.* **321,** 80–83.

Fox, A. P. (1981). Voltage-dependent inactivation of a calcium channel. *Proc. Natl. Acad. Sci.* **78,** 953–956.

Hagiwara, S., and Byerly, L. (1981). Calcium channel. *Ann. Rev. Neurosci.* **4,** 69–125.

Hescheler, J., Pelzer, D., Trube, G., and Trautwein, W. (1982). Does the organic calcium channel blocker D600 act from inside or outside on the cardiac membrane? *Pflügers Arch.* **393,** 287–291.

Hess, P., Lansmann, J. B., and Tsien, R. W. (1984). Modulation of single calcium channels by the calcium agonist Bay K 8644. *Biophys. J.* **45,** 394a.

Hille, B. (1977). Local anesthetics: Hydrophilic and hydrophobic pathways for the drug–receptor reaction. *J. Gen. Physiol.* **69,** 497–515.

Hille, B. (1978). Local anesthetic action on inactivation of the Na channel in nerve and skeletal muscle. Possible mechanisms for antiarrhythmic agents. *In* "Biophysical Aspects of Cardiac Muscle" (M. Morad, ed.), pp. 55–74. Academic Press, New York.

Hodgkin, A. L., and Huxley, A. F. (1952). A quantitative description of membrane current and its application to conduction and excitation in nerve. *J. Physiol.* **117,** 500–544.

Hoffman, B. F., and Rosen, M. R. (1981). Cellular mechanisms for cardiac arrhythmias. *Circ. Res.* **49,** 1–15.

Hondeghem, L. M., and Katzung, B. G. (1977). Time- and voltage-dependent interactions of antiarrhythmic drugs with cardiac sodium channels. *Biochim. Biophys. Acta* **472,** 373–398.

Hondeghem, L. M., and Katzung, B. G. (1984). Antiarrhythmic agents: the modulated receptor mechanism of action of sodium and Ca channel blocking drugs. *Ann. Rev. Pharmacol. Toxicol.* **24,** 387–423.

Hume, J. R., and Giles, W. (1982). Turn-off of a TTX-resistant inward current "i_{Ca}" in single bullfrog atrial cells. *Biophys. J.* **37,** 240a.

Isenberg, G., and Klöckner, U. (1982). Calcium currents of isolated bovine ventricular myocytes are fast and of large amplitude. *Pflügers Arch.* **395,** 30–41.

Janis, R. A., and Scriabine, A. (1983). Sites of action of Ca^{2+} channel inhibitors. *Biochem. Pharmacol.* **32,** 3499–3507.

Janis, R. A., and Scriabine, A. (1983). New developments in Ca^{2+} channel antagonists. *J. Med. Chem.* **26,** 775–785.

Janis, R. A., Rampe, D., Sarmiento, J. G., and Triggle, D. J. (1984). Specific binding of a calcium channel activator, [³H] Bay K 8644, to membranes from cardiac muscle and brain. *Biochem. Biophys. Res. Comm.* **121,** 317–323.

Josephson, I. R., Sanchez-Chapula, J., and Brown, A. M. (1984). A comparison of calcium currents in rat and guinea pig single ventricular cells. *Circ. Res.* **54,** 144–156.

Kanaya, S., Arlock, P., Katzung, B., and Hondeghem, L. M. (1983). Diltiazem and verapamil preferentially block inactivated cardiac calcium channels. *J. Mol. Cell. Cardiol.* **15,** 145–148.

Kass, R. S. (1982). Nisoldipine: A new, more selective calcium current blocker in cardiac Purkinje fibers. *J. Pharm. Exp. Ther.* **223,** 446–456.

Kass, R. S., and Bennett, P. B. (1984). Microelectrode voltage clamp: the cardiac Purkinje fiber. *In* "Voltage and Patch Clamping with Microelectrodes" (T. G. Smith, Jr., H. Lecar, S. J. Redman, and P. W. Gage, eds.), pp. 171–189. American Physiological Society, Bethesda, Maryland.

Kass, R. S., and Sanguinetti, M. C. (1984). Inactivation of Ca channel current in the calf cardiac Purkinje fiber: Evidence for voltage and Ca-mediated mechanisms. *J. Gen. Physiol.* **84,** 705–726.

Kass, R. S., and Scheuer, T. (1982a). Calcium ions and cardiac electrophysiology. *In* "Calcium Blockers: Mechanisms of Action and Clinical Applications" (S. F. Flaim and R. Zelis, eds.), pp. 3–19. Urban and Schwarzenberg, Baltimore.

Kass, R. S., and Scheuer, T. (1982b). Slow inactivation of calcium channels in the cardiac Purkinje fiber. *J. Mol. Cell. Cardiol.* **14,** 615–618.

Kass, R. S., and Tsien, R. W. (1975). Multiple effects of calcium antagonists on plateau currents in cardiac Purkinje fibers. *J. Gen. Physiol.* **66,** 169–192.

Kass, R. S., Siegelbaum, S., and Tsien, R. W. (1976). Incomplete inactivation of the slow inward current in cardiac Purkinje fibres. *J. Physiol.* **263,** 127–128P.

Kass, R. S., Siegelbaum, S. A., and Tsien, R. W. (1979). Three-micro-electrode clamp experiments in calf cardiac Purkinje fibers: Is slow inward current adequately measured? *J. Physiol.* **290,** 201–225.

Kass, R. S., Scheuer, T., and Malloy, K. J. (1982). Block of outward current in cardiac Purkinje fibers by injection of quaternary ammonium ions. *J. Gen. Physiol.* **79,** 1041–1063.

Katzung, B. G., Reuter, H., and Porzig, H. (1973). Lanthanum inhibits Ca-inward current but not Na–Ca exchange in cardiac muscle. *Experientia* **29,** 1073–1075.

Kohlhardt, M., and Fleckenstein, A. (1977). Inhibition of the slow inward current by nifedipine in mammalian ventricular myocardium. *Naunyn-Schmiedeberg's Arch. Pharmacol.* **298,** 267–272.

Kohlhardt, M., and Mnich, Z. (1978). Studies on the inhibitory effect of verapamil on the slow inward current in mammalian ventricular myocardium. *J. Mol. Cell. Cardiol.* **10,** 1037–1052.

Kohlhardt, M., Bauer, B., Krause, H., and Fleckenstein, A. (1973). Selective inhibition of transmembrane Ca conductivity of mammalian myocardial fibres by Ni, Co, and Mn ions. *Pflügers Arch.* **338,** 115–123.

Kurachi, Y. (1982). The effects of intracellular protons on the electrical activity of single ventricular cells. *Pflügers Arch.* **394,** 264–270.

Lee, K. S., and Tsien, R. W. (1982). Reversal of current through calcium channels in dialyzed single heart cells. *Nature* **297,** 498–501.

Lee, K. S., and Tsien, R. W. (1983). Mechanism of calcium channel block by verapamil, D600, diltiazem, and nitrendipine in single dialyzed heart cells. *Nature* **302,** 790–794.

McDonald, T. F., and Trautwein, W. (1978). Membrane currents in cat myocardium: Separation of inward and outward components. *J. Physiol.* **274,** 193–216.

McDonald, T. F., Pelzer, D., and Trautwein, W. (1984). Cat ventricular muscle treated with D600: Characteristics of calcium channel block and unblock. *J. Physiol.* **352,** 217–241.

52   Robert S. Kass *et al.*

Marban, E. (1981). Inhibition of transient outward current by intracellular ion substitution unmasks slow inward current in cardiac Purkinje fibers. *Pflügers Arch.* **390**, 102–106.

Marban, E., and Tsien, R. W. (1981). Is the slow inward calcium current of heart muscle inactivated by calcium? *Biophys. J.* **33**, 143a.

Marban, E., and Tsien, R. W. (1982). Effects of nystatin-mediated intracellular ion substitution on membrane currents in calf Purkinje fibres. *J. Physiol.* **329**, 569–587.

Matteson, D. R., and Armstrong, C. M. (1984). Na and Ca channels in a transformed line of anterior pituitary cells. *J. Gen. Physiol.* **83**, 371–394.

Mentrard, D., Vassort, G., and Fischmeister, R. (1984). Calcium-mediated inactivation of the calcium conductance in cesium-loaded frog heart cells. *J. Gen. Physiol.* **85**, 105–131.

Miller, R. J., and Freedman, S. G. (1984). Are dihydropyridine binding sites voltage sensitive calcium channels? *Life Sci.* **34**, 1205–1221.

New, W., and Trautwein, W. (1972). Inward membrane currents in mammalian myocardium. *Pflügers Arch.* **334**, 1–23.

Pelzer, D., Trautwein, W., and McDonald, T. F. (1982). Calcium channel block and recovery from block in mammalian ventricular muscle treated with organic channel inhibitors. *Pflügers Arch.* **394**, 97–105.

Pelzer, D., Cavalié, A., and Trautwein, W. (1984). Modulation of single Ca channel gating by D600 in cardiac myocytes. *Pflügers Arch.* **400** (Suppl.), R29.

Reuter, H. (1967). The dependence of slow inward current in Purkinje fibres on the extracellular calcium concentration. *J. Physiol.* **192**, 479–492.

Reuter, H. (1979). Properties of two inward membrane currents in the heart. *Ann. Rev. Physiol.* **41**, 413–424.

Rougier, O., Vassort, G., Garnier, D., Gargouil, Y. M., and Coraboeuf, E. (1969). Existence and role of a slow inward current during the frog atrial action potential. *Pflügers Arch.* **308**, 91–110.

Rudy, B. (1978). Slow inactivation of the sodium conductance in squid giant axons. Pronase resistance. *J. Physiol.* **283**, 1–21.

Sanguinetti, M. C., and Kass, R. S. (1984a). Voltage-dependent block of calcium channel current in the calf cardiac Purkinje fiber by dihydropyrine Ca channel antagonists. *Circ. Res.* **55**, 336–348.

Sanguinetti, M. C., and Kass, R. S. (1984b). Regulation of cardiac calcium channel current and contractile activity by the dihydropyridine Bay K 8644 is voltage-dependent. *J. Mol. Cell. Cardiol.* **16**, 667–670.

Schramm, M., Thomas, G., Towart, R., and Frankowiak, G. (1983). Novel dihydropyridines with positive inotropic action through activation of Ca^{2+} channels. *Nature* **303**, 535–537.

Schwartz, A., and Taira, N. (eds.) (1983). Symposium on calcium channel blocking drugs: A novel intervention for the treatment of cardiac disease. *Circ. Res.* **52** (Part II, Suppl.), 181 pp.

Schwartz, A., and Triggle, D. J. (1984). Cellular action of calcium channel blocking drugs. *Ann. Rev. Med.* **35**, 325–339.

Singh, B. N., Nademanee, K., and Baky, S. H. (1983). Calcium antagonists. Clinical use in the treatment of arrhythmias. *Drugs* **25**, 125–153.

Tillotson, D. (1979). Inactivation of Ca conductance dependent on entry of Ca ions in molluscan neurons. *Proc. Natl. Acad. Sci.* **76**, 1497–1500.

Trautwein, W., McDonald, T. F., and Tripathi, O. (1975). Calcium conductance and tension in mammalian ventricular muscle. *Pflügers Arch.* **354**, 55–74.

Tsien, R. W. (1983). Calcium channels in excitable cell membranes. *Ann. Rev. Physiol.* **45**, 341–358.

Tung, L., and Morad, M. (1983). Electrophysiological studies with Ca^{2+} entry blockers. *In* "Ca^{2+} Entry Blockers, Adenosine, and Neurohumors" (G. F. Merrill and H. R. Weiss, eds.), pp. 19–38. Urban and Schwarzenberg, Baltimore.

Uehara, A., and Hume, J. R. (1984). Interactions of organic Ca channel antagonists with Ca channels in isolated frog atrial cells: Test of a modulated receptor hypothesis. *Biophys. J.* **45,** 50a.

Vitek, M., and Trautwein, W. (1971). Slow inward current and action potential in cardiac Purkinje fibres. The effect of Mn ions. *Pflügers Arch.* **323,** 204–218.

3

Negative Surface Charge: Its Identification and Regulation of Cardiac Electrogenesis

Richard D. Nathan

I. INTRODUCTION

Although it is well known that most ion channels in cardiac cell membranes are gated by the transmembrane potential (Reuter, 1984), it is often not appreciated that this potential (V_m) comprises three distinct components: an external surface potential (ψ_o) induced by fixed charges lining the outer surface of the sarcolemma, an internal surface potential (ψ_i) induced by fixed charges lining the inner surface of the sarcolemma, and the potential difference measured between the bulk intracellular and extracellular compartments (V). Because the usual convention is to express the internal potential with respect to the external potential, the transmembrane potential can be written

$$V_m = V + \psi_i - \psi_o \qquad (1)$$

Figure 1 illustrates how fixed negative charges on both the inner and outer faces of the sarcolemma can modify V_m and the electric field (slope of the potential profile) sensed by channel gating structures within the membrane. Thus, internal and external surface potentials can contribute significantly to the movement of ions through membrane channels.

Another way in which these surface potentials can modulate ion fluxes is by concentrating cations at the mouth of the pore. Because of the electrostatic attraction by negative surface charge, the concentration of cations at the membrane's surface (C^*) will be greater than that in the bulk phase (C). The rela-

CARDIAC MUSCLE:
THE REGULATION OF EXCITATION AND CONTRACTION

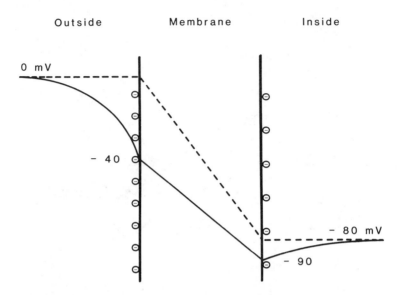

Fig. 1. Comparison of the transmembrane potential (V_m) in the absence (dashed line) and presence (solid line) of fixed negative surface charge. The actual electric field across the membrane (the slope of the potential profile) is less than that induced by the bulk potential difference. $V_m =$ −80 mV without and −50 mV with the surface charge. Note that the diagram is not to scale.

tionship between the two concentrations can be determined from the Boltzmann distribution:

$$C^* = C \exp(-ZF\psi/RT) \tag{2}$$

where ψ is either the external or internal surface potential, Z is the valence of the cation, $F = 96,500$ coul/mole, $R = 8.314$ J/°K•mole, and T is the absolute temperature in °K. Note that at the same surface potential, divalent cations will be much more concentrated than monovalent cations. Because the effective permeability of *open* channels depends on both the electrical driving force across the channel and the *local* concentrations of permeant ions on either side of the pore, that permeability (as well as the channel's ion selectivity, defined by ratios of ion permeabilities) can also be affected by surface potentials. For example, in the absence of such potentials, the expression for the sodium permeability (P_{Na}) can be obtained from the constant-field equation (Goldman, 1943; Hodgkin and Katz, 1949):

$$I_{Na} = \frac{P_{Na} V_m F^2}{RT} \frac{\{[Na]_o^* - [Na]_i^* \exp(V_m F/RT)\}}{1 - \exp(V_m F/RT)} \tag{3}$$

Now if surface potentials are included (Frankenhaeuser, 1960), Eq. (2) can be written specifically for sodium ions as

$$[Na]_o^* = [Na]_o \exp(-F\psi_o/RT) \tag{4}$$

and

$$[Na]_i^* = [Na]_i \exp(-F\psi_i/RT) \tag{5}$$

If Eqs. (1), (3), (4), and (5) are combined, the sodium current, as modified by external and internal surface potentials, can be written

$$I_{Na} = \frac{P_{Na}F^2}{RT} (V + \psi_i - \psi_o) \exp(-F\psi_o/RT) \frac{\{[Na]_o - [Na]_i \exp(VF/RT)\}}{\{1 - \exp[(V + \psi_i - \psi_o)F/RT]\}} \tag{6}$$

In addition to concentrating inorganic cations, negative surface charge also can concentrate organic cations to varying degrees, depending on their valence and the surface potential. For example, tubocurarine, a divalent antagonist of acetylcholine, would be concentrated 100-fold at the neuromuscular junction (for a -60-mV surface potential), whereas acetylcholine, a monovalent cation, would be concentrated only 10-fold by the same potential. Thus, modification of the surface potential by divalent cations such as Ca^{2+} or Mg^{2+} would be expected to affect the binding and, therefore, action of curare much more than that of acetylcholine (Van der Kloot and Cohen, 1979). A similar argument could be made for calcium antagonists such as verapamil (or D600), a monovalent cation, and dihydropyridines such as nisoldipine, which are uncharged at physiological pH; however, because these drugs appear to act from the cytoplasmic side of the calcium channel (Hescheler et al., 1982), their lipid solubility might be an even more important factor (see also Kass et al., Chapter 2).

This chapter reviews the evidence for fixed negative charges on the surface of cardiac myocytes and describes some of the attempts to identify these anionic moieties.

II. FIXED NEGATIVE CHARGES ON THE SURFACE OF CARDIAC MYOCYTES

A. Theory

It is well known that calcium and other divalent cations exert a stabilizing effect on excitable membranes. Frankenhaeuser and Hodgkin (1957) were first to show that these effects are mediated by shifts of conductance–voltage curves along the voltage axis. Such shifts were first explained by A. F. Huxley, who suggested that Ca^{2+} might adsorb (bind) to fixed negative charges on the external surface and thereby alter the electric field across the membrane but not the potential difference in the bulk phase (Frankenhaeuser and Hodgkin, 1957). In squid giant axons, a layer of negative fixed charges lining the *inner* surface of the membrane was proposed to account for the effect of internal ionic strength on sodium inactivation (Chandler *et al.*, 1965). Similar experiments need to be performed with internally perfused cardiac myocytes.

In general, the distribution of surface charge on excitable cells has been modeled by two types of theories, the "diffuse double-layer theory" of Gouy and Chapman (Grahame, 1947; Delahay, 1965), which assumes a *uniformly* smeared surface charge, and discrete-charge theories that assume specific geometries and separations of the charge (Cole, 1969; Brown, 1974). Although the relative merits of both approaches have been discussed (Brown, 1974; Sauvé and Ohki, 1979), the former theory has been used almost exclusively in calculating surface potentials, surface charge densities, and cation–membrane binding constants.

Such parameters can be determined from experiments in which monovalent or multivalent cations bind and/or screen the negative surface charge, thereby altering the surface potential and the voltage dependence of channel gating. Binding can be defined as the chemical adsorption of a cation with the negatively charged site, an effect that depends on the particular cation species and is dictated by the size and electron structure of the ion. In contrast, screening is the reduction in negative surface potential produced by electrostatic *attraction* of a cation to the negatively charged site. Because the cation is treated as a point charge, the latter effect depends only on its valence. Although both screening and binding can reduce the negative surface potential, one can distinguish the two simply by testing how well the experimental results are fitted by theoretical curves relating surface potential and cation concentration for the two situations (McLaughlin *et al.*, 1971). The following equation (Grahame, 1947) can be used to determine the external surface charge density (σ) when *only screening* occurs:

$$\sigma = \frac{1}{G} \left\{ \sum_{i=1}^{n} C_i \left[\exp(-Z_i F\psi_o/RT) - 1\right]\right\}^{1/2} \tag{7}$$

where

$$G = \frac{F}{N} \left[\frac{2\pi}{RT\epsilon\epsilon_o} \right]^{1/2} \tag{8}$$

and C_i is the concentration in the external bulk solution of ionic species (i), n is the number of ionic species, Z_i is the valence of ionic species (i), N is Avogadro's number (6.02×10^{23} electrons/mole), ϵ is the dielectric constant of water (74.1 at 37°C), and ϵ_o is the permittivity of free space [$(4\pi)(8.85 \times 10^{-12}$

coul^2/newt·m^2)]. At 37°C, $G = 276$ in units of (Å^2/electronic charge)·(mole/liter)$^{1/2}$. For the constraint that

$$[C^-]_o = [C^+]_o + 2[C^{2+}]_o \tag{9}$$

where $[C^-]_o$ is the concentration of monovalent anions, $[C^+]_o$ is the concentration of monovalent cations, and $[C^{2+}]_o$ is the concentration of divalent cations in the bulk solution, Eq. (7) can be written (Schauf, 1975; Cohen and Van der Kloot, 1978)

$$\sigma = \frac{1}{G} \{[C^+]_o [\exp(F\psi_o/RT) + \exp(-F\psi_o/RT) - 2] + [C^{2+}]_o [2 \exp(F\psi_o/RT)$$
$$+ \exp(-2F\psi_o/RT) - 3]\}^{1/2} \tag{10}$$

In most experiments, $[C^+]_o$ is not modified. Thus, by measuring the effective change in surface potential ($\Delta\psi_o$) for a known alteration in $[C^{2+}]_o$, one can solve a pair of simultaneous equations for ψ_o and then use this value in Eq. (10) to estimate the surface charge density. Experimentally, $\Delta\psi_o$ is taken to be the shift in voltage dependence of a particular channel-gating parameter such as steady-state inactivation. A best fit of data obtained at several different concentrations can then be obtained by determining those values of ψ_o that satisfy Eq. (10). If *minimal* binding has occurred between the divalent cation and negative surface charge, there should be good correspondence between these experimental and theoretical curves. Those inorganic cations that meet this criterion and are *least* effective in producing voltage shifts are Ba^{2+}, Sr^{2+}, and Mg^{2+} (McLaughlin *et al.*, 1971; Hille *et al.*, 1975; Ohmori and Yoshii, 1977; Kostyuk *et al.*, 1982). McLaughlin *et al.* (1983) have synthesized an organic divalent cation called dimethonium (ethane-bis-trimethylammonium), which exerts *only* a screening effect on negatively charged phospholipid bilayers. It will be interesting to see if this cation also fails to bind to *intact* cell membranes.

For other divalent cations such as Ca^{2+}, Co^{2+}, Mn^{2+}, Ni^{2+}, and Zn^{2+} and trivalent cations such as La^{3+}, both screening and binding must be taken into account. In such cases, the Gouy–Chapman equation for screening (Eq.(7)) should be modified to include the factor $f(M, K, \psi_o)$ (Gilbert and Ehrenstein, 1969; Gilbert, 1971):

$$\sigma = \frac{1}{G} \left\{ \sum_{i=1}^{n} C_i [\exp(-Z_iF\psi_o/RT) - 1] \right\}^{1/2} \cdot f(M,K,\psi_o) \tag{11}$$

where

$$f(M,K,\psi_o) = MK \exp(-ZF\psi_o/RT) + 1 \tag{12}$$

M is the concentration of divalent or trivalent cations in the bulk solution, and K is the equilibrium constant for binding of the cation to negatively charged sites on the membrane.

To solve Eq. (11), *two* parameters, the external surface potential and the intrinsic cation–membrane binding constant, must be adjusted to fit the experimental data. This presents a dilemma because shifts in conductance–voltage curves upon addition of, for example, Ca^{2+} could be caused by either a small ψ_o and a large K_{Ca} or a large ψ_o and a small K_{Ca}. In fact Hille *et al.* (1975) were able to obtain satisfactory fits of their Ca^{2+} and Ba^{2+} data from frog myelinated nerve by using either combination of parameters (see their Table 2). One approach to this problem is to find a divalent cation that does not bind to biological membranes. In that case, $K = 0$, $f(M,K,\psi_o) = 1$, and Eq. (11) simplifies to Eq. (7). As discussed above, this equation can be solved explicitly for ψ_o and then for σ. Thus once these two variables are known, Eq. (11) can be solved for K, the cation–membrane intrinsic binding constant. Utilizing isolated cardiac myocytes, we have begun to determine the suitability of dimethonium (McLaughlin *et al.*, 1983) as such a screening cation (see below).

Although the diffuse double-layer theory of Gouy and Chapman has been adequate to describe most of the experimental data derived from cardiac cells, the theory fails to take account of the molecular nature and discreteness of the added ions and solvent or the membrane's fixed charges. The assumption of a charge density smeared uniformly across an impenetrable plane surface ignores the structured specificity and heterogeneity of the sarcolemma as well as the presence of oriented dipoles on the membrane interface. Because dipoles such as phospholipid head groups tend to be oriented with their positive charge toward the membrane and negative charge toward the bathing medium, the dipole field tends to augment that of the fixed negative charge. With regard to ion channels, it is important to note the following: (a) the surface charge density associated with one type of channel (e.g., delayed rectifier) may not necessarily be the same as that associated with other types of channels; (b) because of their different locations within the membrane, gating and permeation (selectivity) structures associated with a given type of channel may not experience the same electric field strength from the surface charge; (c) because of their different locations, distinct gating processes (such as activation and inactivation) associated with a given channel may not experience the same field strength either; and (d) forward and backward rate constants for such processes may respond differently to alterations in the surface potential if the electric field strength is not uniform across the width of the membrane (Tsien, 1974a), as would be expected for a *discrete* distribution of surface charge.

B. Experiments

1. Sodium Channels

Weidmann (1955) was first to investigate the stabilizing effects of Ca^{2+} on cardiac tissue. Using the maximum upstroke velocity ($\dot{V}_{max}$) of the action potential as an indicator of sodium current (i_{Na}) and a voltage-clamp circuit to control the membrane potential, he found that increasing $[Ca^{2+}]_o$ from 2.6 to 10.4 mM shifted the S-shaped $\dot{V}_{max}(V)$ curve to more positive potentials by 5.6 ± 1.6 mV (mean ± S.E.M., $n = 7$) in calf and sheep Purkinje fibers. In agreement with these results, when $[Ca^{2+}]_o$ was increased from 2 to 8 mM, canine Purkinje fibers exhibited a (significant) 7.4-mV depolarization of the voltage at which $\dot{V}_{max}$ was half inactivated (V_h) (Pressler et al., 1982). The slope factor (k) used to model the $\dot{V}_{max}(V)$ relationship was increased significantly (from 4.9 ± 0.2 to 6.4 ± 0.3, $n = 5$) in the latter investigation, suggesting that Ca^{2+} may have had effects in addition to reducing the external surface potential. Because $\dot{V}_{max}$ is not a precise measure of i_{Na} (Cohen et al., 1981), the results described above are useful only in suggesting the *direction* of Ca^{2+}-induced shifts of i_{Na} gating parameters.

Although i_{Na} was not well controlled, Beeler and Reuter (1970) used the double-pulse voltage-clamp technique of Hodgkin and Huxley (1952) to obtain i_{Na} steady-state inactivation–voltage [$h_\infty(V)$] curves for canine ventricular trabeculae in the presence of 0.2, 1.8, and 7.2 mM $[Ca^{2+}]_o$. In one experiment, V_h was −64, −58, and −54 mV, respectively; k was approximately 3.0 mV for each of the three curves. Moreover, Beeler and Reuter determined that uncompensated series resistance and lack of voltage control had shifted the $h_\infty(V)$ curves by approximately +3 mV. In another study in which i_{Na} was poorly controlled, the threshold potential for the current's onset (derived from an extremely steep negative-slope region of the $I–V$ curve) was employed as an index of the position of activation and inactivation relationships along the voltage axis (Brown, 1974; Brown and Noble, 1978). In both sheep Purkinje fibers and frog atrial muscle, Brown and Noble observed a 5- or 6-mV shift in threshold per fourfold increase or decline in $[Ca^{2+}]_o$. Using Eq. (11) above, but considering that *hydrogen ions* can also bind to divalent surface charge, they found that their data were best fitted when they assumed that for both the Purkinje fiber and atrium, $\sigma = 1$ electronic charge/6.25 nm^2 and $K_{Ca} = 0.005$ mM^{-1}, whereas $pK_H = 5.3$ for the Purkinje fiber and 4.3 for the atrium. These values predict a surface potential of −18 mV for both cardiac preparations when pH = 7.4, when the Purkinje fibers are in 1.8 mM Ca^{2+} and when the atrial muscles are in 1.1 mM Ca^{2+}. They suggest also that Ca^{2+} and H^+ titrate the same negatively charged sites near the sodium channel. Interestingly, the relationships between the shift in threshold and $[Ca^{2+}]_o$ or $[H^+]_o$ were less well fitted by a discrete surface-charge model (Brown, 1974) than by the uniform model described above.

In cardiac Purkinje fibers, the effect of pH on i_{Na} threshold was strongly dependent on the *direction* of the pH change. An increase in pH from 7.4 to 9.0 produced essentially no change (Brown and Noble, 1978; van Bogaert et al., 1978), whereas a reduction to pH 4.1 or 4.2 shifted the threshold by +15 mV (Brown and Noble, 1978). The mechanism for such a shift could not be investigated in these early studies because of the inability to record i_{Na} accurately in multicellular preparations. More recently, however, the effects of extracellular pH on i_{Na}, itself, have been determined in single, isolated rat ventricular cells (Yatani *et al.*, 1984), a preparation that is much more suitable for accurate recording of i_{Na} (Brown *et al.*, 1981). In this study, activation, as approximated by the peak $I_{Na}(V)$ curve, was shifted -5.0 ± 3.3 mV at pH 9.5 but $+16.9 \pm 5.5$ mV ($n = 7$) at pH 5.0. These shifts, as well as depolarizing shifts in the $h_\infty(V)$ curve (16.0 ± 6.5 mV, $n = 8$) and inactivation time constant–voltage curve (20 mV) at pH 5.0, were attributed to screening and/or binding of hydrogen ions to fixed negative charges on the sarcolemma. On the other hand, a concentration-dependent reduction of i_{Na} by H^+ was ascribed to protonation of an acidic group ($pK_a = 5.4$) within the sodium channel. No changes in the reversal potential for i_{Na} were observed under either acidic or alkaline pH conditions.

2. Calcium Channels

Very little information is available on the existence of negative surface charge associated with calcium channels. In rabbit sinoatrial node cells, the sigmoid relationship for $\dot{V}_{max}(V)$ was shifted -4.2 mV (average of five experiments) by a reduction of $[Ca^{2+}]_o$ from 1.8 mM to (nominal) zero, but was shifted $+9.0$ mV (average of four experiments) by an increase of $[Ca^{2+}]_o$ from 1.8 to 10.0 mM (Noma and Irisawa, 1976).

In agreement with the finding that Ba^{2+} exhibits equal screening but less binding that Ca^{2+} (Hille *et al.*, 1975; Ohmori and Yoshii, 1977), the addition of 10 mM Ba^{2+} shifted the steady-state inactivation curve for the slow inward current (i_{si}) only 3–4 mV in the positive direction (Osterrieder *et al.*, 1982). Using bovine ventricular trabeculae, Reuter and Scholz (1977) observed 4- and 7-mV depolarizing shifts in the steady-state activation–voltage curve for i_{si} when $[Ca^{2+}]_o$ was increased from 1.8 to 5.4 and 7.2 mM, respectively. Although these investigators were careful to take account of the external surface potential in their calculations of ionic current (Eq. (6)) and permeability (selectivity) ratios for the calcium channel, they failed to use their own experimental data to calculate the surface potential. Such information, already obtained for neuronal (Wilson *et al.*, 1983) and egg cell (Ohmori and Yoshii, 1977) membranes, is necessary for a complete functional description of cardiac calcium channels.

In an attempt to initiate such a description in single cells from the sinoatrial node, we have made a qualitative assessment of the negative surface potential by comparing i_{Ca} steady-state inactivation curves derived from single cultured pacemaker cells with those obtained from small multicellular sinoatrial-node preparations (Irisawa and Yanagihara, 1980). The similarity of the two curves in Fig. 2, the relative agreement of their half-inactivation potentials (-36.5 and

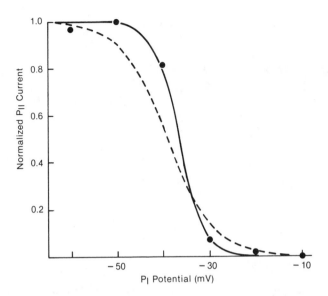

Fig. 2. Slow inward current steady-state inactivation curves for a small multicellular preparation (dashed curve redrawn from Fig. 15, Irisawa and Yanagihara (1980), with the permission of Martinus-Nijhoff Publishers) and a single myocyte after 2 days in culture (solid curve; Nathan and Roberts, unpublished results), both isolated from rabbit sinoatrial node. The latter experiment used a double-pulse protocol in which the prepulse was of variable amplitude and 300 msec in duration. The test pulse, to -30 mV, followed a 10-msec delay at the holding potential (-60 mV). Data were fit by the equation $[1 + \exp[(V - V_{1/2})/k]]^{-1}$ (Hodgkin and Huxley, 1952), where $V_{1/2}$ is the half-inactivation potential and k is a slope factor. $V_{1/2} = -36.6$ mV and $k = 2.6$ mV for the solid curve. Temperature 37°C.

-40 mV, respectively), and the (5- to 10-mV) positive shifts of V_h following the addition of 10 mM CaCl$_2$ suggest that fixed negative charges on the isolated myocytes were not altered markedly by the isolation and culture procedures (Nathan, 1986). Because channel gating and permeation are influenced strongly by the surface potential, such alterations could be a significant problem in studies that employ single myocytes. Although changes in surface charge directly associated with ion channels have yet to be documented, partial or complete loss of the glycocalyx has been reported in some *freshly isolated* rat ventricular myocytes (Desilets and Horackova, 1982; Isenberg and Klöckner, 1980). In contrast, the same type of cells exhibit a coherent glycocalyx after several days in culture (Piper *et al.*, 1982). Thus, it appears that some time is needed for complete regeneration of the glycocalyx; however, it remains to be seen whether such a process is required for the fixed charges that influence gating and permeation of specific ion channels directly.

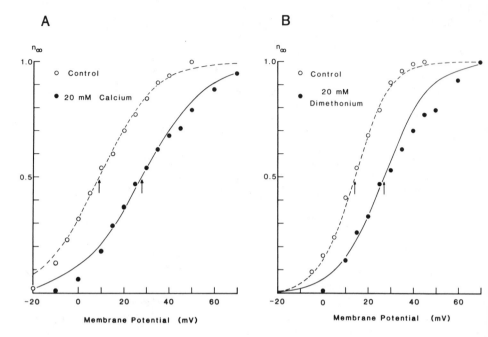

Fig. 3. Steady-state activation of delayed rectifier current recorded in two cells (isolated from 7-day embryonic chick ventricle) after 2 days in culture. Outward current tails (after a 10-sec step to the potentials indicated) were measured with respect to the holding current at −50 mV and then normalized to their maximum value. The normalized data (n_∞) were fit by the equation $1 - |1 + \exp[V - V_{1/2})/k]|^{-1}$, where $V_{1/2}$ = half-activation potential (arrows) and k is a slope factor (Hodgkin and Huxley, 1952). (A) Control: $V_{1/2}$ = +9 mV, k = 12 mV. After 5–30 min in 20 mM CaCl$_2$: $V_{1/2}$ = +28 mV, k = 14 mV. (B) Control: $V_{1/2}$ = +14 mV, k = 7.7 mV. After 5–16 min in 20 mM dimethonium bromide: $V_{1/2}$ = +27 mV, k = 10 mV. Temperature = 24°C.

3. Delayed Rectifier Channels

Kass and Tsien (1975) observed a marked reduction in delayed rectifier (i_x) tails when calf Purkinje fibers were exposed to 3 mM Mn^{2+}, 0.5 mM La^{3+}, or 5 × 10^{-7} gm/ml D600. The current tails (elicited at −40 mV) followed 1- to 10-sec voltage steps, during which i_x was activated increasingly at potentials between −40 and +10 mV. Similar effects were seen with Ca^{2+}: a 6.4-mV positive shift (mean of five preparations) of the isochronal activation curve occurred as [Ca^{2+}]$_o$ was increased from 1.8 to 7.2 mM. In preliminary experiments with single myocytes isolated from 7-day embryonic chick ventricle (R. D. Nathan, unpublished results), addition of 20 mM Ca^{2+} shifted the i_x (10-sec) isochronal activation curve by +19 mV (Fig. 3A). Such a large shift is, most likely, a reflection of *both* screening and binding of Ca^{2+} to the negative external surface charge. On the other hand, the smaller shift ($+13$ mV) induced by dimethonium (Fig. 3B) raises the possibility that dimethonium may not bind to the surface charge. Additional experiments are necessary to confirm this hypothesis.

A more complete analysis of surface charge associated with the delayed rectifier has been undertaken by DiFrancesco and McNaughton (1979) in sheep Purkinje fibers. They observed an 8- to 10-mV positive shift in the i_{x1} steady-state activation curve when $[Ca^{2+}]_o$ was increased from 2 to 8 mM, but a 15- to 19-mV negative shift when $[Ca^{2+}]_o$ was reduced to 0.1 mM. Figure 4 illustrates a best fit of their data. The solid curve was derived from Eq. (11) with $K_{Ca} = 0.0126$ mM^{-1}, $\sigma = 0.38$ electronic charges·nm^{-2}, and $\psi_o = -26.9$ mV in normal Tyrode solution. DiFrancesco and McNaughton investigated the effect of Ca^{2+} on the rectifier ratio (Noble and Tsien, 1968) for i_{x1}, also:

$$\bar{i}_{x1}(V) = \frac{\Delta i_{x1}}{\Delta_{x1}} \tag{13}$$

where Δi_{x1} is the steady-state amplitude of plateau current at the potential (V) and Δ_{x1} is the initial amplitude of current tails elicited upon changing the poten-

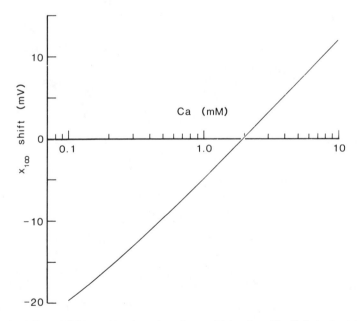

Fig. 4. Effect of Ca^{2+} on the voltage dependence of delayed rectifier (i_{x1}) steady-state activation in sheep cardiac Purkinje fibers. The curve was calculated from Eq. (11) with $K_{Ca} = 0.0126$ mM^{-1}, $\sigma = 0.38$ electronic charges·nm^{-2}, and $\psi_o = -26.9$ mV. [Redrawn from Fig. 5, DiFrancesco and McNaughton (1979), with the permission of the Physiological Society.]

tial from V to the holding potential. They found that 8 mM [Ca^{2+}]$_o$ reduced $\bar{i}_{x1}$ at $\bar{i}_{x1}$(V) potentials positive to the reversal potential (E_{x1}) but increased $\bar{i}_{x1}$ at potentials negative to E_{x1}; i.e., Ca^{2+} produced an asymmetric positive shift in the $\bar{i}_{x1}$ (V) relationship. Such a shift would be unlikely from the standpoint of calcium's effect on the external surface potential, because a decline in ψ_o would tend to reduce the surface concentrations of both K$^+$ and Na$^+$ and would, therefore, shift the curve to more *negative* potentials. Because increased [K$^+$]$_o$ mimicked the effect of [Ca^{2+}]$_o$, they proposed that increased [Ca^{2+}]$_o$ might somehow raise the concentration of K$^+$ in the restricted space just outside the membrane.

In single cells isolated from bullfrog atrium, where such a restricted space is absent, the existence of fixed negative charge on the sarcolemma has been investigated by observing the effect of La^{3+} on the voltage dependence of delayed rectifier (i_K) steady-state activation [$n_\infty(V)$] and rate constants ($1/\tau_n$) for activation and deactivation of i_K (Nathan *et al.*, 1986). As illustrated in Fig. 5A, 5×10^{-6} M La^{3+} had no significant effect on $n_\infty(V)$, whereas 5×10^{-4} M reduced i_K tails significantly at each potential and shifted the half-activation potential by +13.5 mV. A lower concentration ($10^{-5}M$) had no significant effect on the rate constants (Fig. 5B); however, 5×10^{-4} M LaCl$_3$ slowed the activation of i_K significantly at +30 and +40 mV ($P < 0.02$ and $P < 0.01$, respectively) but not at more negative potentials. Such an asymmetric shift has been observed previously for the pacemaker current when calf Purkinje fibers were exposed to epinephrine (Tsien, 1974a). The asymmetry arose from a great-er shift of the deactivation rate coefficient (β) than the activation rate coefficient (α), and such differences were attributed to the possibility that *discrete* surface charges might produce an electric field that was not constant throughout the membrane (Tsien, 1974a). Thus, a charged gating particle could experience one field strength as it moved in one direction but another field strength as it moved in the opposite direction.

4. Pacemaker Channels

As yet, investigations of membrane surface charge have focused on cardiac Purkinje fibers but not pacemaker cells of the sinoatrial node. Because these studies were performed before reinterpretation of the pacemaker potassium cur-rent (i_{K2}) (Noble and Tsien, 1968) as an *inward* current activated by hyper-polarization (DiFrancesco, 1981), I use the older terminology in this section and describe the actions of Ca^{2+}, H$^+$, epinephrine, and salicylate ions on gating and permeation of the pacemaker channel.

Kass and Tsien (1976) observed a 4-mV positive shift in the steady-state activation curve for i_{K2}, $s_\infty(V)$, in calf Purkinje fibers when [Ca^{2+}]$_o$ was in-creased from 1.8 to 7.2 mM. A much greater positive shift (10 mV) was found for sheep Purkinje fibers with the same change in [Ca^{2+}]$_o$, as well as a 4-mV

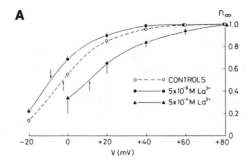

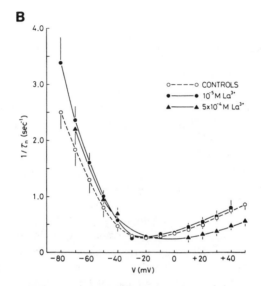

Fig. 5. Effect of La^{3+} on voltage-dependent gating of delayed rectifier current (i_K) in single myocytes isolated from bullfrog atrium. (A) Steady-state activation curves for i_K were calculated from tail currents (at -60 mV) immediately after a 10-sec prepulse. Smooth curves were calculated as in Fig. 3. The arrows indicate half-activation potentials (-8, -2.5, and $+11$ mV). (B) Rate constants for activation (-30 to $+50$ mV) and decay (-80 to -40 mV) of i_K. Smooth curves were fitted by eye to the mean values.

negative shift when $[Ca^{2+}]_o$ was reduced from 2 to 0.5 mM (DiFrancesco and McNaughton, 1979). A comparison of voltage shifts induced by Ca^{2+} and Mg^{2+} is illustrated in Fig. 6. Both curves were calculated from Eq. (11) with $K_{Ca} = 0.003\ M^{-1}$, $\sigma = 0.51$ electronic charges·nm^{-2}, and $\psi_o = -63.7$ mV in normal Tyrode solution. A best fit of the Mg^{2+} data was obtained by assuming that Mg^{2+} does not bind to the negatively charged sites. Note that Ca^{2+}, which screens and binds to negative surface charge, had a greater effect than Mg^{2+}, which screens but binds only weakly to the surface charge. It is also interesting to compare the effects of Ca^{2+} on the delayed rectifier (Fig. 4) and the pacemaker

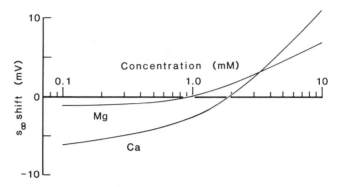

Fig. 6.   Effect of Ca^{2+} and Mg^{2+} on the voltage dependence of pacemaker current (i_{K2}) steady-state activation in sheep cardiac Purkinje fibers. The curves were calculated from Eq. (11) with K_{Ca} = 0.003 M^{-1}, K_{Mg} = 0, σ = 0.51 electronic charges·nm^{-2}, and ψ_o = −63.7 mV. [Redrawn from Fig. 5, DiFrancesco and McNaughton (1979), with the permission of the Physiological Society.]

channel (Fig. 6). One explanation for their difference, as proposed by DiFrancesco and McNaughton (1979), is that negatively charged groups near each type of channel might have very different affinities for Ca^{2+}. Also using sheep Purkinje fibers, Brown and Noble (1978) observed an 8-mV shift of $s_\infty(V)$ for a fourfold change in $[Ca^{2+}]_o$. They were able to fit their data by assuming that K_{Ca} = 0.3 mM^{-1}, σ = 0.31 electronic charges·nm^{-2}, and ψ_o = −16 mV in normal Tyrode solution. By comparing the two sets of values for K_{Ca} and ψ_o above (both calculated from experiments employing the same cardiac preparation), one can appreciate that solutions of Eq. (11) are not unique. In evaluating possible surface-charge effects of Ca^{2+} on pacemaker-channel permeation, only DiFrancesco and McNaughton (1979) found a change in $\bar{i}_{K2}$, the rectifier ratio. The small *increase* in $\bar{i}_{K2}$ that they did observe (in the presence of 8 mM Ca^{2+}) could not be explained, however, by a reduction of $[K^+]_o$ at the mouth of the channel, because the reversal potential for i_{K2} was shifted to more *positive* potentials. Instead, they proposed that elevation of $[Ca^{2+}]_o$ caused an increase in $[K^+]$ in the restricted space outside the cells, possibly because of partial inhibition of the Na–K pump by Ca^{2+}.

The influence of $[H^+]_o$ on i_{K2} has been reported to be variable for acid pH (Brown and Noble, 1978) and in a direction opposite to that expected for alkaline pH (van Bogaert *et al.*, 1978). In the former study $s_\infty(V)$ was unaffected by pH 5.5 in one trial, shifted −8 mV in two trials, and shifted +17 mV in another trial. In the latter study at pH 9.5, $s_\infty(V)$ was shifted +5.9 ± 0.5 mV (n = 8), and the time constant for activation (τ_s) was shifted +6.4 ± 0.9 mV. If external pH affects only the external surface potential, increased pH should increase ψ_o and thereby shift the gating parameters to more *negative* potentials. Because increasing the *intracellular* pH also shifted $s_\infty(V)$ to the right (by 10 mV), van

Bogaert *et al.* suggested that the effects seen with external pH = 9.5 were mediated by intracellular alkalinization. In that case, acidic groups on the inner side of the membrane (which must exhibit a lower apparent pK) would have been deprotonated, thereby producing a more negative internal surface potential and a positive shift in the gating variables. Brown and Noble (1978) also proposed that H^+ might influence internal as well as external surface charge and that the net effect would depend on which titration predominates. This hypothesis has been confirmed recently (van Bogaert, 1985) by experiments in which intracellular acidosis (pH_i = 6.9), at constant extracellular pH, shifted the half-activation potential for pacemaker current (i_f) by -8.4 ± 1.9 mV (n = 6). In addition to these actions on gating, the fully activated current–voltage relationship for i_{K2} was reduced by acid pH (Brown and Noble, 1978), but increased by alkaline pH (van Bogaert *et al.*, 1978). Because the reversal potential for i_{K2} was shifted by at least 20 mV to more positive potentials when the pH was reduced from 7.2 to 7.0 (Brown *et al.*, 1978), the reduction of $\bar{i}_{K2}$ was attributed to an increase in cleft $[K^+]$, possibly because of blockade of the Na–K pump by hydrogen ions.

The *internal* surface potential might also play a role in the adrenaline-induced acceleration of the Purkinje fiber pacemaker potential, which has been attributed to positive shifts of the $s_\infty(V)$ and $\tau_s(V)$ relationships (Hauswirth *et al.*, 1968; Tsien, 1974a). McNaughton and Noble (1973) proposed that a reduction of intracellular Ca^{2+} can mediate these effects by minimizing this cation's screening and binding of internal, negative surface charge, thereby increasing ψ_i. To support this hypothesis, they showed that adrenaline induced an 8-mV depolarizing shift of $s_\infty(V)$ when EGTA was present with KCl in the current pools of a sucrose-gap voltage clamp, but no shift was seen when the current pools contained 20 mM $CaCl_2$. In a more detailed study, Tsien (1974a) found that in addition to effecting positive shifts of $s_\infty(V)$ and $\tau_s(V)$, epinephrine (a) changed the slope of $s_\infty(V)$, (b) increased the maximum τ_s and altered the shape of the $\tau_s(V)$ curve, (c) shifted $\tau_s(V)$ asymmetrically (the activation rate coefficient (α_s) was shifted more than the deactivation rate coefficient (β_s)) and (d) steepened the $\alpha_s(V)$ curve. On the other hand, $\bar{i}_{K2}(V)$ was unaffected, suggesting that the gating and permeation structures of the pacemaker channel are not influenced by the same surface potential. Because of unequal shifts in $\alpha_s(V)$ and $\beta_s(V)$, as well as the absence of an effect of epinephrine on the threshold potential for i_{Na}, Tsien proposed also that the surface charge associated with the pacemaker channel must be *discrete* rather than smeared uniformly across the surface of the sarcolemma (see Section II,A for further discussion).

Tsien (1974b) was able to prove that epinephrine does not affect i_{K2} by adding its own positive charge to the outside of the membrane near the pacemaker channel, as proposed by Hauswirth *et al.* (1968). To refute that hypothesis, he showed that theophylline and R07-2956, two inhibitors of phosphodiesterase that are uncharged at physiological pH, mimicked or occluded epinephrine's actions, whereas 0.5 mM La^{3+} shifted $s_\infty(V)$ by $+8$ to $+10$ mV, but failed to occlude epinephrine's actions. As an alternative, Tsien suggested two ways in which increased [cAMP]$_i$ might result in a more negative internal surface potential: (a) cAMP could activate a protein kinase that would bring about phosphorylation of sarcolemmal groups near the pacemaker channel or (b) cAMP could promote the phosphorylation of sarcoplasmic reticulum (SR) membrane, thereby enhancing uptake of Ca^{2+} by the SR and, as proposed by McNaughton and Noble (1973), removal of Ca^{2+} from specific binding sites near the pacemaker channel.

Finally, Cohen et al. (1979) have investigated the actions of salicylate, a monovalent anion, on i_{K2} to determine the effects of an *increased* negative surface potential. Although values for σ, ψ_o, and K$_{salicylate}$ were not calculated, they observed a -22-mV shift of $s_\infty(V)$ for a fivefold change in [Na salicylate]$_o$, and a -10-mV shift of $\tau_s(V)$ with the application of 10 mM salicylate. In some experiments, the hyperpolarizing shifts were accompanied by changes in the shape of both $s_\infty(V)$ and $\tau_s(V)$ curves; however, such shape changes do not necessarily imply that a simple alteration of the surface potential did not take place. In fact, Attwell and Eisner (1978) have shown that if one considers incomplete titration of *discrete* surface charge in the vicinity of a channel as well as fluctuations in the occupancy of these sites, the shapes of activation or time-constant curves do indeed change, depending on the fraction of time the sites are titrated.

When 10 mM salicylate was added in the presence of 2.7 mM [K$^+$]$_o$, Cohen et al. recorded a negative shift of nearly 20 mV in the reversal potential for i_{K2}, but only a negligible shift when [K$^+$]$_o$ was 8 mM. They attributed these results, as well as an increase in $\bar{i}_{K2}$ after the addition of salicylate, to a decline in cleft [K$^+$]. They speculated that the more negative surface potential induced by salicylate could increase the surface activity of K$^+$, which, in turn, might stimulate the Na–K pump, thereby depleting K$^+$ in the clefts. In 8 mM [K$^+$]$_o$, the pump sites would be saturated, and salicylate would be expected to have little or no effect.

5. Summary

Tables I and II summarize the data available for the surface charge/surface potential properties of voltage-gated ion channels in cardiac myocytes. As confirmed by significant voltage shifts of activation, inactivation, or time constant–voltage curves after the addition of divalent or multivalent cations, fixed negative charges are indeed located close to the gating structure(s) of each type of channel. On the other hand, because changes in reversal potentials and the amplitude of current through open channels were opposite to those expected from a simple modification of surface potential, it is unlikely that *permeation* of these channels is influenced by the same charges. Particularly apparent from Tables I

TABLE I

Surface-Charge Properties of Cardiac Myocytes and Effect of Divalent/Trivalent Cations[a]

Channel type	Preparation	Gating parameter	Shift (mV)/fourfold $\Delta[\text{Ca}^{2+}]_\text{o}$	σ ($e^- \cdot$ nm^{-2})	ψ_o (mV)	K_Ca (mM^{-1})	Reference
Sodium	PF	$\dot{V}_\text{max}$	5.6 ± 1.6				Weidmann (1955)
	PF	$\dot{V}_\text{max}$	7.4				Pressler et al. (1982)
	PF	i_Na thr.	5 or 6	0.16	−18	0.05	Brown and Noble (1978)
	Atrium	i_Na thr.	5 or 6	0.16	−18	0.05	Brown and Noble (1978)
	Ventr.	$h_\infty(V)$	4				Beeler and Reuter (1970)
Calcium	SA node	$\dot{V}_\text{max}$	6.5				Noma and Irisawa (1976)
	SA node	i_si act.	3–4 (10 mM Ba^{2+})				Osterrieder et al. (1982)
	SA node	$f_\infty(V)$	3–6				Nathan (unpublished)
	Ventr.	i_si act.	7				Reuter and Scholz (1977)
Delayed rectifier	PF	i_x act.	6.4				Kass and Tsien (1975)
	PF	i_x1 act.	8–10	0.38	−26.9	0.013	DiFrancesco and McNaughton (1979)
	Atrium	i_K act.	13.5 (0.5 mM La^{3+})				Nathan et al. (1986)
	Ventricle	i_K act.	6.3				Nathan (unpublished)
Pacemaker	PF	$s_\infty(V)$	4				Kass and Tsien (1976)
	PF	$s_\infty(V)$	10	0.51	−63.7	3×10^{-6}	DiFrancesco and McNaughton (1979)
	PF	$s_\infty(V)$	8	0.31	−16	0.30	Brown and Noble (1978)
	PF	$s_\infty(V)$	8–10 (0.5 mM La^{3+})				Tsien (1974b)

[a] Abbreviations: σ = surface charge density; ψ_o = external surface potential; K_Ca = equilibrium binding constant; PF = Purkinje fiber; $\dot{V}_\text{max}$ = maximum upstroke velocity of the action potential; $h_\infty(V)$ = i_Na steady-state inactivation (fraction of channels available for activation); $s_\infty(V)$ = steady-state activation of i_K2; $f_\infty(V)$ = steady-state inactivation of i_Ca.

TABLE II

Surface-Charge Properties of Cardiac Myocytes and Effect of Extracellular pH[a]

Channel type	Preparation	Gating parameter	Shift (mV) and (pH)	pK_H	Reference
Sodium	PF	i_{Na} thr.	+15 (4.2)	5.1	Brown and Noble (1978)
	Ventr.	$h_\infty(V)$	+16 ± 6.5 (5.0)		Yatani et al. (1984)
		$\tau_h(V)$	+20 (5.0)		
		$i_{Na}(V)$	+16.9 ± 5.5 (5.0)	5.4	
			−5.0 ± 3.3 (9.5)		
Pacemaker	PF	$s_\infty(V)$	+5.9 ± 0.5 (9.5)		van Bogaert et al.
			+6.4 ± 0.9 (9.5)		(1978)
		$Y_\infty(V)$	−8.4 ± 1.9 (6.9)[b]		van Bogaert (1985)

[a] Abbreviations: $\tau_h(V)$ = time constant–voltage relationship for inactivation of i_{Na}; $Y_\infty(V)$ = steady-state activation factor for pacemaker current (i_f) activated by hyperpolarization.

[b] Intracellular pH.

and II is that more studies are needed to compare calculated values of surface-charge densities, surface potentials, and Ca^{2+} binding constants among different types of channels as well as among different types of cardiac cells.

III. IDENTIFICATION OF THE NEGATIVE SURFACE CHARGE

In theory, fixed negative charges that influence the gating properties of sodium, calcium, delayed-rectifier, and pacemaker channels could arise from (a) the phosphate groups of phospholipids, (b) negatively charged groups of anionic phospholipids such as phosphatidylserine and phosphatidylinositol, (c) acidic carbohydrates, such as sialic acids, which constitute glycoproteins and glycolipids, and (d) the anionic side chains or carboxy-terminal end of proteins. This section will discuss the evidence available for each of these potential binding sites.

A. Histochemical and Biochemical Evidence

Qualitative confirmation of anionic moieties on the surface of cardiac myocytes has been obtained by electron-microscopic histochemical techniques used to verify a reduction of cationic staining after treatment with substrate-specific enzymes. For example, we and others have found that phospholipase C removes much of the polycationic ferritin (PCF), or lanthanum-staining material, from embryonic chick ventricular myocytes (Barron *et al.*, 1982; Lesseps, 1967), as well as the colloidal iron-staining material from isolated rat heart sarcolemma (Matsukubo *et al.*, 1981). Similarly, neuraminidase, an enzyme that specifically cleaves the glycosidic linkage of sialic acids in glycoproteins and glycolipids (Drzeniek, 1973), reduces (a) PCF staining of embryonic chick ventricular myocytes (Nathan *et al.*, 1980; Barron *et al.*, 1982), (b) colloidal iron staining of neonatal rat heart cells (Frank *et al.*, 1977) and isolated rat heart sarcolemma (Matsukubo *et al.*, 1981), (c) lanthanum staining of neonatal rat heart cells (Frank *et al.*, 1977) and guinea pig atria (Harding and Halliday, 1980), and (d) ruthenium red staining of cell clusters from canine sinoatrial node, atrial myocytes, and ventricular myocytes but not Purkinje fibers (Woods *et al.*, 1982). Additional evidence of the presence of sialic acid residues has been obtained from the binding of colloidal thorium to adult mouse myocardial cells at pH 2.6 (Gros and Challice, 1975), binding of colloidal iron to adult rabbit and neonatal rat myocytes at pH 1.8 (Frank *et al.*, 1977), and binding of PCF to embryonic chick ventricular myocytes at pH 3.4 (Barron *et al.*, 1982); only sulfate and carboxyl groups (sialic acid) are ionized at these pH's. Colloidal iron staining of isolated rat heart sarcolemma was reduced also by pretreatment with trypsin, a proteolytic enzyme (Matsukubo *et al.*, 1981). As a whole, these results suggest that the negative surface charge is not caused by any single component but rather by a combination of phospholipids, sialic acids, and proteins.

Tables III and IV list, respectively, the phospholipid composition and sialic acid content of isolated and intact cardiac sarcolemma from various animal species. Note that the acidic phospholipids (designated by asterisks) make up less than 20% of the total composition and that most of the values are relatively constant among species. In Table IV there is surprisingly good agreement for sialic acid content among various heart tissues and animal species. It is probable that the greater sialic acid content of isolated sarcolemma reflects the smaller protein content of that preparation in comparison to the whole cell.

There is now evidence that the phospholipid composition and/or sialic acid content of the cardiac sarcolemma may be altered by pathological conditions. For example, ventricular sarcolemma isolated from streptozotocin-induced diabetic rats exhibited a significant decline in phosphatidylserine and diphosphatidyl-glycerol but a significant rise in lysophosphatidylcholine. Sialic acid content was reduced by 28%, but was restored to normal levels (35.2 ± 2.8 nmole/mg protein) when the diabetic rats received insulin. ATP-independent Ca^{2+} binding to isolated sarcolemma was depressed by 55%, but could also be restored to normal (193.4 ± 16.7 nmole/mg protein in 1.25 mM Ca^{2+}) with insulin (Pierce *et al.*, 1983). In canine myocardium after 1 hr of ischemia (ligation of the left, anterior descending artery), the content of phosphatidylcholine was reduced significantly ($5.2 \pm 1.2\%$, $n = 5$); after 3 hr of ischemia, both phos-

TABLE III

Phospholipid Composition of Isolated Cardiac (Ventricle) Sarcolemmal Membranes

	Percentage of total[a]		
Phospholipid	Rabbit $(n=4)$[b]	Dog $(n=4)$[c]	Rat $(n=3)$[d]
Phosphatidylcholine	39.2 ± 3.2	44.3 ± 0.5	38.5 ± 3.5
Phosphatidylethanolamine	29.8 ± 3.3	27.9 ± 1.1	38.0 ± 0.9
Phosphatidylinositol*	7.4 ± 2.0	13.5 ± 0.5[e]	2.7 ± 0.5
Phosphatidylserine*	5.6 ± 2.2		5.9 ± 1.5
Diphosphatidylglycerol*	0.6 ± 0.2		9.1 ± 0.5
Sphingomyelin	11.5 ± 0.7	8.8 ± 1.5	5.3 ± 1.4
Lysophosphatidylcholine	1.9 ± 1.0		0.5 ± 0.3

[a] Values are mean ± S.E.M.
[b] Philipson et al. (1980).
[c] Philipson et al. (1983).
[d] Pierce et al. (1983).
[e] Total content of phosphatidylinositol and phosphatidylserine.
*Anionic phospholipids.

TABLE IV

Sialic Acid Content of Myocardium and Isolated Sarcolemma

Preparation	Content[a] (nmole/mg protein)	Reference
Intact cells		
Neonatal rat heart	15.4 ± 1.3 $(n=5)$	Langer et al. (1981)
Embryonic chick ventricle	14.2 ± 3.2 $(n=6)$	Nathan et al. (1980)
Guinea pig atrium	16.4 ± 1.2[b] $(n=6)$	Harding and Halliday (1980)
Guinea pig ventricle	14.9 ± 1.4[b] $(n=4)$	Harding and Halliday (1980)
Canine Purkinje fibers	12.6 ± 1.2[b] $(n=10)$	Kimura et al. (1984)
	11.5 ± 0.7 $(n=9)$	Nathan and Shelton (unpublished)
Isolated sarcolemma		
Rabbit ventricle	81.3 ± 14.2 $(n=6)$	Philipson et al. (1980)
Neonatal rat heart	111 ± 19	Langer and Nudd (1983)
Adult rat ventricle	40.4 ± 3.1	Matsukubo et al. (1981)
Canine ventricle	73.4 ± 10.6 $(n=6)$	Frank et al. (1984)
	80.2 ± 15.0 $(n=4)$	Takahashi and Kako (1984)

[a] Sialic acid content, expressed as mean ± S.E.M., was determined by the thiobarbituric acid assay (Warren, 1959) in each case except for Nathan and Shelton, who used a more sensitive fluorometric procedure (Hammond and Papermaster, 1976).
[b] Content was estimated assuming that protein was 10% of wet weight.

phatidylcholine and phosphatidylethanolamine were reduced significantly (11.6 ± 0.9%, $n = 4$) (Chien et al., 1981). Similar but greater changes were observed in sarcolemmal preparations isolated from canine left ventricle after 1.5 hr of coronary occlusion and 3 hr of reflow (Takahashi and Kako, 1984). Phosphatidylcholine and phosphatidylethanolamine were reduced by approximately 43%; the acidic phospholipids decreased, too, but not significantly. In contrast, the sarcolemmal content of sialic acid *increased* significantly (by 97%). In preliminary investigations of how hypoxia and reoxygenation affect the sialic acid content of canine ventricular muscle *in vitro* (R. D. Nathan and V. L. Shelton, unpublished results), we found that a 2-hr (but not a 1-hr) period of hypoxia followed by a half hour of reoxygenation increased the amount of sialic acid released into the bathing medium significantly, i.e., from 0.31 ± 0.16 nmole/mg protein during O_2 ($n = 8$) to 1.18 ± 0.32 nmole/mg protein during N_2 ($n = 6$). Because ventricular tissue contains other cell types besides myocytes, it would be inappropriate to conclude that only *myocyte* sialic acid was released in these experiments. Additional studies are necessary to determine whether pathological alterations in sialic acid content or phospholipid composition have any effect on the surface potential or permeability of voltage-gated ion channels, i.e., whether such structural alterations are functionally important.

B. Evidence from Studies of Calcium Binding

Both phosphatidylserine in lipid bilayer membranes and *N*-acetylneuraminic acid (NANA, sialic acid) in solution bind calcium ions. The intrinsic (1 : 1) association constants are 12 M^{-1} (McLaughlin et al., 1981) and 121 ± 5 M^{-1} (Jaques et al., 1977), respectively. To determine which of these potential binding sites is more important in intact membranes, investigators have altered the phospholipid composition or sialic acid content and measured the resulting changes in Ca^{2+} binding. For example, neuraminidase reduced Ca^{2+} binding by 42.7% (Matsukubo et al., 1981) or 8.2% (Limas, 1977) in rat, by 13% in rabbit (Philipson et al., 1980), by 10% in neonatal rat (Langer and Nudd, 1983), and by an insignificant amount in canine (ventricle) sarcolemmal membranes (Pang, 1980). The wide disparity in these results might be explained, in part, by the following: (a) how much sialic acid was removed in preparing the sarcolemma, (b) how many sarcolemmal vesicles were inside-out and thus contained sialic acid residues inaccessible to Ca^{2+}, (c) how much sialic acid was removed by neuraminidase, (d) differences in the measurement of Ca^{2+} binding, and (e) species differences in Ca^{2+} binding. The first two possibilities are likely to be the most important because sialic acid content can be as much as 40-fold greater in vesicles prepared by the hypotonic shock–LiBr procedure than in those prepared by the sucrose density-gradient method (Moffat et al., 1983) and because as many as 40% of the sarcolemmal vesicles prepared from dog or rabbit hearts by the latter method can be inside-out (Frank *et al.*, 1984).

Even though Limas (1977) and Matsukubo *et al.* (1981) both used the LiBr method of isolation, Limas observed only a 3% reduction in ^{45}Ca binding, whereas the latter group found a 32% reduction after treating rat heart sarcolemma with phospholipase C. Both groups observed a 49% reduction with trypsin. Employing the sucrose density-gradient technique, Philipson *et al.* (1980) measured 75–80% less binding of Ca^{2+} to rabbit sarcolemmal vesicles that had been treated with phospholipase C. By manufacturing vesicles from pure phospholipids, they were also able to demonstrate the relative binding sequence of Ca^{2+} to phospholipids: diphosphatidylglycerol (cardiolipin) > phosphatidylserine > phosphatidylinositol > phosphatidylethanolamine. As expected, the acidic phospholipids had the greatest affinity for Ca^{2+}. Finally, Langer and Nudd (1983) employed a novel gas dissection technique to isolate sarcolemmal membranes from neonatal rat ventricles, but found no significant effect of *Bacillus cereus* phospholipase C on lanthanum-displaceable ^{45}Ca. Nevertheless, Langer has obtained other evidence for Ca^{2+} binding to phospholipids (see Chapter 10).

Taken together, these results do not rule out the possibility that Ca^{2+} binds to many different sarcolemmal sites, including phospholipids, sialic acids, and proteins, in intact cardiac cells. On the other hand, because of the technical difficulties mentioned above, it is extremely difficult to predict which anionic moieties are more likely to bind Ca^{2+}. To rectify this problem, Ca^{2+}-binding experiments need to be performed with a highly purified preparation of *intact myocytes* (in the absence of other cell types) in which the phospholipid composition and sialic acid content are known both before and after the addition of phospholipase or neuraminidase. Even with this information, it will be extremely difficult to say whether the anionic sites that bind Ca^{2+} are the same ones that modulate gating of ion channels.

C.   Evidence from Studies of Calcium Exchange

Studies employing neuraminidase or phospholipase have obtained evidence to support the hypothesis that both sialic acids and phospholipids play a role in regulating calcium exchange across the sarcolemma. Pretreatment of cultured neonatal rat heart cells with neuraminidase (0.25 U/ml for 15 min) increased the rate of ^{45}Ca uptake by five- to sixfold (Frank *et al.*, 1977). Asymptotic labeling was reached after 40–45 min in untreated cells but after only 7 or 8 min in cells pretreated with neuraminidase. Once asymptotic labeling had been reached, 25% of the ^{45}Ca was washed out in controls, but as much as 95% in cells exposed to neuraminidase; a similar treatment had no effect on washout of ^{42}K. In spheroidal aggregates of myocytes isolated from embryonic chick ventricle, uptake of ^{45}Ca increased at a mean rate of 1.3 ± 0.6 pmole/mg protein·min ($n = 4$) after 33–105 min of exposure to neuraminidase (0.2 – 0.6 U/ml); by 2 hr, such aggregates had taken up $54.3 \pm 4.9\%$ more ^{45}Ca than untreated controls (Nathan *et al.*, 1980). In contrast, phospholipase C (0.04 U/ml for 2 hr) increased ^{45}Ca uptake by as much as 42%, but this amount was not significantly different from that in the control. On the other hand, Langer *et al.* (1981) did observe a significantly greater amount of exchangeable Ca^{2+} (the amount of ^{45}Ca uptake reached asymptotically) when their neonatal rat myocytes were exposed to phospholipase C (1–2 U/ml for 5 min). However, this concentration altered the sarcolemma to such an extent that La^{3+} was found within the cytoplasm, and 72% of the intracellular ^{42}K was lost within 5 min.

Although these results suggest that both sialic acids and phospholipids are somehow involved in calcium homeostasis, there is little information on how such control might come about. One possibility is that sialic acid residues might exhibit a greater affinity for Ca^{2+} than do phospholipids. Once the former are removed, there might be a greater likelihood that calcium ions will bind to phospholipids, thereby increasing the local concentration of Ca^{2+} for transport through voltage-gated channels, leakage channels, or Na–Ca exchange (during depolarization of the membrane potential). In support of this idea, Burt and Langer (1983) found that pretreating isolated sarcolemmal membranes with neuraminidase (0.5 U/ml) produced a 28% increase in the fraction of bound ^{45}Ca that could be displaced by 0.1 mM polymyxin B, a multivalent cation that can penetrate the hydrophobic domain of the membrane. Alternatively, sialic acid residues could serve as functionally important parts of channels or exchangers, because these are likely to be glycoproteins. For example, the saxitoxin-binding component of sodium channels isolated from rat skeletal muscle sarcolemma is a glycoprotein that contains terminal sialic acid residues (Cohen and Barchi, 1981).

Although they probably are not structural constituents of membrane transport processes, phospholipids can influence membrane-bound enzymes (Wojtczak and Nalecz, 1979) as well as the single-channel conductance of membrane channels (Bell and Miller, 1984). Moreover, both phospholipase C (Philipson *et al.*, 1983) and phospholipase D (Philipson and Nishimoto, 1984) have been shown to stimulate Na–Ca exchange in cardiac sarcolemmal vesicles by enhancing the apparent affinity of the exchanger for Ca^{2+}. To explain these results, Philipson and Nishimoto suggested that phosphatidylserine and phosphatidylinositol (negatively charged phospholipids that are unaffected by phospholipase C) or phosphatidic acid (the product of phospholipase D) might augment negative surface charge in the vicinity of the Na–Ca exchange protein, thereby increasing the concentration of Ca^{2+} for exchange. This mechanism could also explain the enhancement of other membrane transport processes by negatively charged phospholipids (see Introduction).

D. Evidence from Studies of Electrical and Mechanical Activity

In frog sartorius muscle, the threshold voltage for activating a twitch was shifted by as much as 8.5 mV to more positive potentials when the fibers were pretreated for 2 hr with neuraminidase (3.3 – 5.0 U/ml) (Dörrscheidt-Käfer, 1979). Because this shift could be correlated with the amount of sialic acid released and because a pK_a of 2.75 (approximating the pK_a of sialic acid, 2.6) was appropriate to fit the dependence of threshold on $[Ca^{2+}]_o$, $[Mg^{2+}]_o$, or $[H^+]_o$, such shifts were attributed to the reduction of the sarcolemma's negative external surface potential, caused by release of these anionic residues. Stimulated by these findings, we initiated a series of experiments to determine whether sialic acids play a role in regulating the electrical activity of cardiac muscle. Table V summarizes the results for aggregates of embryonic chick heart cells (Bhattacharyya et al., 1981) and adult canine cardiac tissues (Woods et al., 1982; Kimura et al., 1984) treated with neuraminidase (0.5 – 1.0 U/ml).

The significant effects were (a) an initial increase in the sinus rate, which was followed by cessation of spontaneous activity; (b) depolarization of the maximum diastolic potential in embryonic chick ventricular myocytes and canine sinus node; (c) a decline in the maximum upstroke velocity in canine sinus node, atrial muscle, and Purkinje fibers; (d) shortening of the action potential duration (APD) in embryonic chick ventricular myocytes and canine Purkinje fibers, but lengthening of the duration in the canine sinus node; and (e) a reduction of conduction velocity in the canine sinus node and atrium.

With lower concentrations of neuraminidase (0.03 – 0.33 U/ml), the embryonic myocytes exhibited a significant slowing of spontaneous activity ($-12.8 \pm 4.0\%$, $n = 7$) and a slight hyperpolarization (3.3 ± 1.3 mV, $n = 7$; Nathan et al., 1980). As a control for possible contamination of our neuraminidase preparation, phospholipase C (0.012 U/ml) was also tested; it displayed no significant effect on the action potential but did slow beating significantly (-30.3%). Neither Woods et al. (1982) nor Kimura et al. (1984) observed a significant effect of neuraminidase on canine Purkinje fibers in the presence of either 1.3 or 2.7 mM Ca^{2+}; however, both $\dot{V}_{max}$ and APD were reduced significantly when the enzyme was added in the presence of 8.1 mM Ca^{2+} (Table V). In contrast, we have recorded a dose-dependent decline in the plateau, duration, maximum diastolic potential, and upstroke velocity of the action potential when canine Purkinje fibers were exposed to neuraminidase in the presence of 2.7 mM

TABLE V

Electrophysiological Effects of Neuraminidase (Neur) on Cardiac Preparations in Vitro[a]

Preparation	BR (beats/min)	MDP (mV)	APA (mV)	$\dot{V}_{max}$ (V/sec)	APD (msec)	v_{cond} (m/sec)
Embryonic chick ventricular aggregates, 1.8 mM [Ca^{2+}]$_o$ (Bhattacharyya et al., 1981)						
Control ($n=6$)	50 ± 6	−94 ± 2	123 ± 3	141 ± 5	136 ± 7[b]	
Neur (0.5 U/ml)	40 ± 7	[−85 ± 5][e]	111 ± 6	126 ± 9	[118 ± 8][f]	
Canine sinus node, 1.3 mM [Ca^{2+}]$_o$ (Woods et al., 1982)						
Control ($n=7$)	118 ± 24	−55 ± 4	54 ± 6	3 ± 2	91 ± 13[c]	0.015 ± 0.005
Neur (1.0 U/ml)	[150 ± 31][e]	[−37 ± 14][e]	44 ± 20	[1 ± 1][e]	[154 ± 46][e]	[0.001 ± 0.002][e]
Canine atrial muscle, 1.3 mM [Ca^{2+}]$_o$ (Woods et al. 1982)						
Control ($n=8$)		−75 ± 1	94 ± 8	50 ± 16	110 ± 30[c]	0.59 ± 0.14
Neur (1.0 U/ml)		−65 ± 14	81 ± 21	[37 ± 52][e]	86 ± 35	[0.29 ± 0.20][e]
Canine Purkinje fibers, 1.3 mM [Ca^{2+}]$_o$ (Woods et al., 1982)						
Control ($n=12$)		−85 ± 4	110 ± 7	231 ± 26	445 ± 78[c]	0.92 ± 0.20
Neur (1.0 U/ml)		−82 ± 8	109 ± 16	247 ± 74	361 ± 129	0.67 ± 0.34
Canine Purkinje fibers, 2.7 mM [Ca^{2+}]$_o$ (Kimura et al., 1984)						
Control ($n=9$)	8 ± 4	−88 ± 1	118 ± 2	412 ± 23	242 ± 15[d]	
Neur (1.0 U/ml)	13 ± 6	−89 ± 1	124 ± 1	396 ± 24	232 ± 18	
Canine Purkinje fibers, 8.1 mM [Ca^{2+}]$_o$ (Kimura et al., 1984)						
Control ($n=9$)	0.2 ± 0.2	−87 ± 1	118 ± 2	400 ± 19	235 ± 18[d]	
Neur (1.0 U/ml)	0.1 ± 0.1	−89 ± 1	122 ± 2	[328 ± 14][g]	[215 ± 17][e]	

[a] Abbreviations: BR = beat rate; MDP = maximum diastolic potential; APA = action potential amplitude; $\dot{V}_{max}$ = maximum upstroke velocity; APD = action potential duration; v_{cond} = conduction velocity. Values are mean ± S.E.M. at "steady state"; bracketed values are significantly different from the control.

[b] Measured at −40 mV.
[c] Measured at 50% of APA.
[d] Measured at −60 mV.
[e] $P < 0.05$
[f] $P < 0.01$
[g] $P < 0.001$.

$[Ca^{2+}]_o$ (Nathan and Bhattacharyya, 1981). These changes were potentiated by bubbling the Tyrode solution with 95% O_2, 5% CO_2 (as opposed to 95% air, 5% CO_2). Additional experiments are necessary to resolve these differences.

In addition to its effects on the action potential, neuraminidase has been shown to alter the stability of the resting potential and the rhythmicity of spontaneous activity. Figure 7 illustrates the influence of neuraminidase (0.5 U/ml) on the stability of the membrane potential in a dog Purkinje fiber after a period of rapid drive (cycle length = 0.3 sec) (R. D. Nathan and M. L. Bhattacharyya, unpublished results). Before exposure to the enzyme, the fiber depolarized smoothly (Fig. 7A), whereas after a 51-min exposure, the fiber depolarized more rapidly and exhibited 1- to 2-mV spontaneous fluctuations in the membrane potential (Fig. 7B). In canine Purkinje fibers exposed to neuraminidase (1.0 U/ml) for 2 hr, Kimura et al. (1984) also have observed a more rapid depolarization after stimulation. More importantly, when the fibers were treated with enzyme in the presence of 8.1 mM Ca^{2+} (cycle length = 0.2 sec), they exhibited depolarizing afterpotentials that were not seen in the controls.

Even in low $[Ca^{2+}]_o$ (1.8 mM), spontaneous voltage fluctuations and arrhythmic firing were recorded in aggregates of embryonic chick ventricular cells when more than 25% of the sarcolemma-bound sialic acid had been released by 0.5–1.0 U/ml of neuraminidase (Bhattacharyya et al., 1981). In aggregates whose spontaneous activity had been terminated by TTX, neuraminidase induced spontaneous voltage fluctuations and spontaneous firing. Quiescent canine Purkinje fibers also became spontaneously active after exposure to the enzyme (Woods et al., 1982). It is unlikely that such voltage fluctuations are caused by reentry of excitation from neighboring cells, because arrhythmic beating was seen also when *single* isolated myocytes were exposed to the enzyme (0.05 – 0.15 U/ml) (Nakamoto and Nathan, 1981), and similar voltage fluctuations

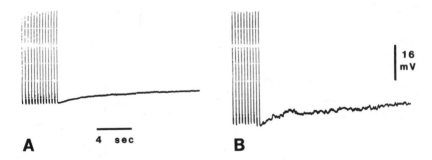

Fig. 7. Effect of neuraminidase (and release of sialic acid residues) on a canine Purkinje fiber. (A) Control stimulated (cycle length = 0.3 sec) for approximately 1 min before the slow diastolic depolarization; maximum diastolic potential = −60 mV. (B) Same fiber 51 min after exposure to neuraminidase (0.5 U/ml); maximum diastolic potential = −68 mV.

(induced by low $[Na^+]_o$) were recorded simultaneously from two cells well separated in an aggregate (Nathan and Bhattacharyya, 1984). Finally, voltage fluctuations were never seen in aggregates treated with phospholipase C (0.012–0.025 U/ml), even at concentrations up to 10 times the impurity level measured in neuraminidase (Bhattacharyya et al., 1981). Although the exact mechanisms for the voltage fluctuations are unknown, their similarity to perturbations induced by low $[Na^+]_o$ (Nathan and Bhattacharyya, 1984) and the ability of neuraminidase to increase ^{45}Ca uptake in similar cell aggregates (Nathan et al., 1980) suggest that elevated levels of intracellular Ca^{2+} are responsible. How sialic acid residues participate in the maintenance of calcium homeostasis is an important question that needs to be addressed in future work.

IV. SUMMARY

At present, our knowledge of the surface-charge properties of cardiac myocytes is surprisingly rudimentary. Tables I and II illustrate qualitative information such as Ca^{2+}- or H^+-induced shifts of activation– or inactivation–voltage relationships for most voltage-gated channels; however, few *quantitative* data are available. Thus, future work should be concerned with obtaining a catalog of surface-charge densities, surface potentials, and cation binding constants for fixed negative charges that lie in close proximity to each type of voltage-gated channel, in each type of cardiac cell. Because these values cannot be determined rigorously when cations *bind* to the fixed charges (for example, shifts could be caused by either a small ψ_o and large K_{Ca} or a large ψ_o and small K_{Ca}), investigators should determine the suitability of using screening cations such as dimethonium for these experiments. Once ψ_o and σ are known, the intrinsic binding constant can be determined for the cation of interest. When these parameters can be obtained with confidence, it will be important to know whether different channels or different gating structures (activation and inactivation) are influenced by the same surface potential. This information should be extremely helpful in understanding the electrophysiological consequences of alterations in serum pH, $[Mg^{2+}]$, or $[Ca^{2+}]$ that occur under pathological circumstances.

Although the available evidence suggests that calcium ions can bind to sarcolemmal phospholipids, sialic acids, and proteins and that sialic acid residues play some role in the maintenance of calcium homeostasis, there are no data to suggest that any one of these anionic moieties exerts a direct influence on the gating or permeation of ion channels or on the function of ion transport processes such as Na–Ca exchange or the Na–K pump. The best way to obtain this information would be first to collect a catalog of values for ψ_o, σ, and K_{Ca}, as described above, and then attempt to correlate changes in these parameters with *documented* alterations in sialic acid content, phospholipid content, and phospholipid or protein composition of the sarcolemma. Such experiments will be difficult because the enzymes used to alter each moiety might not have access to all the sites of interest. Nevertheless, these or similar experiments are essential for acquiring a comprehensive knowledge of sarcolemmal structure–function relationships in cardiac muscle.

ACKNOWLEDGMENTS

The author would like to thank Dr. Mohit L. Bhattacharyya for his collaboration in obtaining some of the unpublished results. This work was supported by Grant HL 20708 from the National Institutes of Health.

REFERENCES

Attwell, D., and Eisner, D. (1978). Discrete membrane surface charge distributions: Effect of fluctuations near individual channels. *Biophys. J.* **24,** 869–875.

Barron, E. A., Markwald, R. R., and Nathan, R. D. (1982). Localization of sialic acid at the surface of embryonic myocardial cells. *J. Mol. Cell. Cardiol.* **14,** 381–395.

Beeler, G. W., Jr., and Reuter, H. (1970). Voltage clamp experiments on ventricular myocardial fibres. *J. Physiol.* **207,** 165–190.

Bell, J. E., and Miller, C. (1984). Effects of phospholipid surface charge on ion conduction in the K^+ channel of sarcoplasmic reticulum. *Biophys. J.* **45,** 279–287.

Bhattacharyya, M. L., Nathan, R. D., and Shelton, V. L. (1981). Release of sialic acid alters the stability of the membrane potential in cardiac muscle. *Life Sci.* **29,** 1071–1078.

Brown, A. M., Lee, K. S., and Powell, T. (1981). Sodium current in single rat heart muscle cells. *J. Physiol.* **318,** 479–500.

Brown, R. H., Jr. (1974). Membrane surface charge: Discrete and uniform modelling. *Prog. Biophys. Mol. Biol.* **28,** 343–370.

Brown, R. H., Jr., and Noble, D. (1978). Displacement of activation thresholds in cardiac muscle by protons and calcium ions. *J. Physiol.* **282,** 333–343.

Brown, R. H., Jr., Cohen, I., and Noble, D. (1978). The interactions of protons, calcium, and potassium ions on cardiac Purkinje fibres. *J. Physiol.* **282,** 345–352.

Burt, J. M., and Langer, G. A. (1983). Ca^{2+} displacement by polymyxin B from sarcolemma isolated by 'gas dissection' from cultured neonatal rat myocardial cells. *Biochim. Biophys. Acta* **729,** 44–52.

Chandler, W. K., Hodgkin, A. L., and Meves, H. (1965). The effect of changing the internal solution on sodium inactivation and related phenomena in giant axons. *J. Physiol.* **180,** 821–836.

Chien, K. R., Reeves, J. P., Buja, L. M., Bonte, F., Parkey, R. W., and Willerson, J. T. (1981). Phospholipid alterations in canine ischemic myocardium: Temporal and topographical correlations with Tc-99-PPi accumulation and an in vitro sarcolemmal Ca^{++} permeability defect. *Circ. Res.* **48,** 711–719.

Cohen, I., and Van der Kloot, W. (1978). Effects of $[Ca^{2+}]$ and $[Mg^{2+}]$ on the decay of miniature endplate currents. *Nature* **271**, 77–79.

Cohen, I., Noble, D., Ohba, M., and Ojeda, C. (1979). Action of salicylate ions on the electrical properties of sheep cardiac Purkinje fibres. *J. Physiol.* **297**, 163–185.

Cohen, I., Attwell, D., and Strichartz, G. (1981). The dependence of the maximum rate of rise of the action potential upstroke on membrane properties. *Proc. R. Soc. Lond. B.* **214**, 85–98.

Cohen, S. A., and Barchi, R. L. (1981). Glycoprotein characteristics of the sodium channel saxitoxin-binding component from mammalian sarcolemma. *Biochem. Biophys. Acta* **645**, 253–261.

Cole, K. S. (1969). Zeta potential and discrete vs. uniform surface charges. *Biophys. J.* **9**, 465–469.

Delahay, P. (1965). "Double Layer and Electrode Kinetics." Wiley (Interscience), New York.

Desilets, M., and Horackova, M. (1982). Na^+-dependence of $^{45}Ca^{2+}$ uptake in adult rat isolated cardiac cells. *Biochim. Biophys. Acta* **721**, 144–157.

DiFrancesco, D. (1981). A new interpretation of the pace-maker current in calf Purkinje fibres. *J. Physiol.* **314**, 359–376.

DiFrancesco, D., and McNaughton, P. A. (1979). The effects of calcium on outward membrane currents in the cardiac Purkinje fibre. *J. Physiol.* **289**, 347–373.

Dörrscheidt-Käfer, M. (1979). Excitation–contraction coupling in frog sartorius and the role of the surface charge due to the carboxyl group of sialic acid. *Pflüg. Arch.* **380**, 171–179.

Drzeniek, R. (1973). Substrate specificity of neuraminidase. *Histochem. J.* **5**, 271–290.

Frank, J. S., Langer, G. A., Nudd, L. M., and Seraydarian, K. (1977). The myocardial cell surface, its histochemistry, and the effect of sialic acid and calcium removal on its structure and cellular ionic exchange. *Circ. Res.* **41**, 702–714.

Frank, J. S., Philipson, K. D., and Beydler, S. (1984). Ultrastructure of isolated sarcolemma from dog and rabbit myocardium: Comparison to intact tissue. *Circ. Res.* **54**, 414–423.

Frankenhaeuser, B. (1960). Sodium permeability in toad nerve and in squid nerve. *J. Physiol.* **152**, 159–166.

Frankenhaeuser, B., and Hodgkin, A. L. (1957). The action of calcium on the electrical properties of squid axons. *J. Physiol.* **137**, 218–244.

Gilbert, D. L. (1971). Fixed surface charges. *In* "Biophysics and Physiology of Excitable Membranes" (W. J. Adelman, Jr., ed.), pp. 359–378. Van Nostrand-Reinhold Co., New York.

Gilbert, D. L., and Ehrenstein, G. (1969). Effect of divalent cations on potassium conductance of squid axons: Determination of surface charge. *Biophys. J.* **9**, 447–463.

Goldman, D. E. (1943). Potential, impedance, and rectification in membranes. *J. Gen. Physiol.* **27**, 37–60.

Grahame, D. C. (1947). The electrical double layer and the theory of electrocapillarity. *Chem. Rev.* **41**, 441–501.

Gros, D., and Challice, C. E. (1975). The coating of mouse myocardial cells: A cytochemical electron microscopical study. *J. Histochem. Cytochem.* **23**, 727–744.

Hammond, K. S., and Papermaster, D. S. (1976). Fluorometric assay of sialic acid in the picomole range: A modification of the thiobarbituric acid assay. *Anal. Biochem.* **74**, 292–297.

Harding, S. E., and Halliday, J. (1980). Removal of sialic acid from cardiac sarcolemma does not affect contractile function in electrically stimulated guinea pig left atria. *Nature* **286**, 819–821.

Hauswirth, O., Noble, D., and Tsien, R. W. (1968). Adrenaline: Mechanism of action on the pacemaker potential in cardiac Purkinje fibers. *Science* **162**, 916–917.

Hescheler, J., Pelzer, D., Trube, G., and Trautwein, W. (1982). Does the organic calcium channel blocker D600 act from inside or outside on the cardiac cell membrane? *Pflüg. Arch.* **393**, 287–291.

Hille, B., Woodhull, A. M., and Shapiro, B. I. (1975). Negative surface charge near sodium channels of nerve: Divalent ions, monovalent ions, and pH. *Phil. Trans. R. Soc. Lond. Biol. Sci.* **270**, 301–318.

Hodgkin, A. L., and Huxley, A. F. (1952). The dual effect of membrane potential on sodium conductance in the giant axon of *Loligo. J. Physiol.* **116,** 497–506.

Hodgkin, A. L., and Katz, B. (1949). The effect of sodium ions on the electrical activity of the giant axon of the squid. *J. Physiol.* **108,** 37–77.

Irisawa, H., and Yanagihara, K. (1980). The slow inward current of the rabbit sino-atrial nodal cells. *In* "The Slow Inward Current and Cardiac Arrhythmias" (D. P. Zipes, J. C. Bailey, and V. Elharrar, eds.), pp. 265–284. Martinus Nijhoff Publishers, The Hague.

Isenberg, G., and Klöckner, U. (1980). Glycocalyx is not required for slow inward calcium current in isolated rat heart myocytes. *Nature* **284,** 358–360.

Jaques, L. W., Brown, E. B., Barrett, J. M., Brey, W. S., Jr., and Weltner, W., Jr. (1977). Sialic acid: A calcium-binding carbohydrate. *J. Biol. Chem.* **252,** 4533–4538.

Kass, R. S., and Tsien, R. W. (1975). Multiple effects of calcium antagonists on plateau currents in cardiac Purkinje fibers. *J. Gen. Physiol.* **66,** 169–192.

Kass, R. S., and Tsien, R. W. (1976). Control of action potential duration by calcium ions in cardiac Purkinje fibers. *J. Gen. Physiol.* **67,** 599–617.

Kimura, S., Hazama, S., Fujii, S., Nakaya, H., and Kanno, M. (1984). Delayed afterdepolarisations and triggered activity in canine Purkinje fibres treated with neuraminidase. *Cardiovasc. Res.* **18,** 294–301.

Kostyuk, P. G., Mironov, S. L., Doroshenko, P. A., and Ponomarev, V. N. (1982). Surface charges on the outer side of mollusc neuron membrane. *J. Membr. Biol.* **70,** 171–179.

Langer, G. A., and Nudd, L. M. (1983). Effects of cations, phospholipases, and neuraminidase on calcium binding to "gas-dissected" membranes from cultured cardiac cells. *Circ. Res.* **53,** 482–490.

Langer, G. A., Frank, J. S., and Philipson, K. D. (1981). Correlation of alterations in cation exchange and sarcolemmal ultrastructure produced by neuraminidase and phospholipases in cardiac cell tissue culture. *Circ. Res.* **49,** 1289–1299.

Lesseps, R. J. (1967). The removal by phospholipase C of a layer of lanthanun-staining material external to the cell membrane in embryonic chick cells. *J. Cell Biol.* **34,** 173–183.

Limas, C. J. (1977). Calcium-binding sites in rat myocardial sarcolemma. *Arch. Biochem. Biophys.* **179,** 302–309.

McLaughlin, A., Eng, W-K., Vaio, G., Wilson, T., and McLaughlin, S. (1983). Dimethonium, a divalent cation that exerts only a screening effect on the electrostatic potential adjacent to negatively charged phospholipid bilayer membranes. *J. Membr. Biol.* **76,** 183–193.

McLaughlin, S., Mulrine, N., Gresalfi, T., Vaio, G., and McLaughlin, A. (1981). Adsorption of divalent cations to bilayer membranes containing phosphatidylserine. *J. Gen. Physiol.* **77,** 445–473.

McLaughlin, S. G. A., Szabo, G., and Eisenman, G. (1971). Divalent ions and the surface potential of charged phospholipid membranes. *J. Gen. Physiol.* **58,** 667–687.

McNaughton, P. A., and Noble, D. (1973). The role of intracellular calcium ion concentration in mediating the adrenaline-induced acceleration of the cardiac pacemaker potential. *J. Physiol.* **234,** 53–54P.

Matsukubo, M. P., Singal, P. K., and Dhalla, N. S. (1981). Negatively charged sites and calcium binding in the isolated rat heart sarcolemma. *Basic Res. Cardiol.* **76,** 16–28.

Moffat, M. P., Singal, P. K., and Dhalla, N. S. (1983). Differences in sarcolemmal preparations: Cell surface material and membrane sidedness. *Basic Res. Cardiol.* **78,** 451–461.

Nakamoto, R. K., and Nathan, R. D. (1981). Arrhythmias induced in isolated heart cells by release of membrane sialic acid. *Fed. Proc.* **40,** 617.

Nathan, R. D. (1986). Two electrophysiologically distinct types of cultured pacemaker cells from rabbit sinoatrial node. *Am. J. Physiol.* **250,** H325–H329.

Nathan, R. D., and Bhattacharyya, M. L. (1981). Membrane sialic acid and electrophysiology of cardiac Purkinje fibers. *Biophys. J.* **33**, 34a.

Nathan, R. D., and Bhattacharyya, M. L. (1984). Perturbations in the membrane potential of cultured heart cells: Role of calcium. *Am. J. Physiol.* **247**, H273–H282.

Nathan, R. D., Fung, S. J., Stocco, D. M., Barron, E. A., and Markwald, R. R. (1980). Sialic acid: Regulation of electrogenesis in cultured heart cells. *Am. J. Physiol.* **239**, C197–C207.

Nathan, R. D., Kanai, K., Clark, R. B., and Giles, W. (1986). Selective block of calcium current by lanthanum in single bullfrog atrial cells. Submitted.

Noble, D., and Tsien, R. W. (1968). The kinetics and rectifier properties of the slow potassium current in cardiac Purkinje fibres. *J. Physiol.* **195**, 185–214.

Noma, A., and Irisawa, H. (1976). Effects of calcium ion on the rising phase of the action potential in rabbit sinoatrial node cells. *Jap. J. Physiol.* **26**, 93–99, 1976.

Ohmori, H., and Yoshii, M. (1977). Surface potential reflected in both gating and permeation mechanisms of sodium and calcium channels of the tunicate egg cell membrane. *J. Physiol.* **267**, 429–463.

Osterrieder, W., Yang, Q.-F., and Trautwein, W. (1982). Effects of barium on the membrane currents in the rabbit S-A node. *Pflüg. Arch.* **394**, 78–84.

Pang, D. C. (1980). Effect of inotropic agents on the calcium binding to isolated cardiac sarcolemma. *Biochim. Biophys. Acta* **598**, 528–542.

Philipson, K. D., and Nishimoto, A. Y. (1984). Stimulation of Na^+–Ca^{2+} exchange in cardiac sarcolemmal vesicles by phospholipase D. *J. Biol. Chem.* **259**, 16–19.

Philipson, K. D., Bers, D. M., and Nishimoto, A. Y. (1980). The role of phospholipids in the calcium binding of isolated cardiac sarcolemma. *J. Mol. Cell. Cardiol.* **12**, 1159–1173.

Philipson, K. D., Frank, J. S., and Nishimoto, A. Y. (1983). Effects of phospholipase C on the Na^+–Ca^{2+} exchange and Ca^{2+} permeability of cardiac sarcolemmal vesicles. *J. Biol. Chem.* **258**, 5905–5910.

Pierce, G. N., Kutryk, M. J. B., and Dhalla, N. S. (1983). Alterations in Ca^{2+} binding by and composition of the cardiac sarcolemmal membrane in chronic diabetes. *Proc. Natl. Acad. Sci. USA* **80**, 5412–5416.

Piper, H. M., Probst, I., Schwartz, P., Hütter, J. F., and Spieckermann, P. G. (1982). Culturing of calcium stable adult cardiac myocytes. *J. Mol. Cell. Cardiol.* **14**, 397–412.

Pressler, M. L., Elharrar, V., and Bailey, J. C. (1982). Effects of extracellular calcium ions, verapamil, and lanthanum on active and passive properties of canine cardiac Purkinje fibers. *Circ. Res.* **51**, 637–651.

Reuter, H. (1984). Ion channels in cardiac cell membranes. *Ann. Rev. Physiol.* **46**, 473–484.

Reuter, H., and Scholz, H. (1977). A study of the ion selectivity and the kinetic properties of the calcium dependent slow inward current in mammalian cardiac muscle. *J. Physiol.* **264**, 17–47.

Sauvé, R., and Ohki, S. (1979). Interactions of divalent cations with negatively charged membrane surfaces. I. Discrete charge potential. *J. Theor. Biol.* **81**, 157–179.

Schauf, C. L. (1975). The interactions of calcium with *Myxicola* giant axons and a description in terms of a simple surface charge model. *J. Physiol.* **248**, 613–624.

Takahashi, K., and Kako, K. J. (1984). Ischemia-induced changes in sarcolemmal (Na^+, K^+)-ATPase, K^+-pNPPase, sialic acid, and phospholipid in the dog and effects of the nisoldipine and chlorpromazine treatment. *Biochem. Med.* **31**, 271–286.

Tsien, R. W. (1974a). Effects of epinephrine on the pacemaker potassium current of cardiac Purkinje fibers. *J. Gen. Physiol.* **64**, 293–319.

Tsien, R. W. (1974b). Mode of action of chronotropic agents in cardiac Purkinje fibers: Does epinephrine act by directly modifying the external surface charge? *J. Gen. Physiol.* **64**, 320–342.

van Bogaert, P. P. (1985). Pace-maker current changes during intracellular pH transients in sheep cardiac Purkinje fibres. *Pflüg. Arch.* **404,** 29–40.

van Bogaert, P.-P., Vereecke, J. S., and Carmeliet, E. E. (1978). The effect of raised pH on pacemaker activity and ionic currents in cardiac Purkinje fibers. *Pflüg. Arch.* **375,** 45–52.

Van der Kloot, W. G., and Cohen, I. (1979). Membrane surface potential changes may alter drug interactions: An example, acetylcholine and curare. *Science* **203,** 1351–1353.

Warren, L. (1959). The thiobarbituric acid assay of sialic acids. *J. Biol. Chem.* **234,** 1971–1975.

Weidmann, S. (1955). Effects of calcium ions and local anaesthetics on electrical properties of Purkinje fibres. *J. Physiol.* **129,** 568–582.

Wilson, D. L., Morimoto, K., Tsuda, Y., and Brown, A. M. (1983). Interaction between calcium ions and surface charge as it relates to calcium currents. *J. Membr. Biol.* **72,** 117–130.

Wojtczak, L., and Nalecz, M. J. (1979). Surface charge of biological membranes as a possible regulator of membrane-bound enzymes. *Eur. J. Biochem.* **94,** 99–107.

Woods, W. T., Imamura, K., and James, T. N. (1982). Electrophysiological and electron microscopic correlations concerning the effects of neuraminidase on canine heart cells. *Circ. Res.* **50,** 228–239.

Yatani, A., Brown, A. M., and Akaike, N. (1984). Effect of extracellular pH on sodium current in isolated, single rat ventricular cells. *J. Membr. Biol.* **78,** 163–168.

4

Mechanisms of β-Adrenergic and Cholinergic Control of Ca and K Currents in the Heart

W. Trautwein and W. Osterrieder

I. INTRODUCTION

The afferent impulse traffic from the stellate ganglion and the ganglion nodosum is the essential control mechanism of the performance of the heart. The sympathetic fibers terminate in all parts of the heart and, via the transmitters epinephrine and norepinephrine, mediate the positive chronotropic effects on the sinus node, the shortening of atrioventricular (AV) conduction time, and the increase in the contractility of the myocardium. These effects are primarily the consequence of binding of the transmitters to β-adrenergic receptors that results in the stimulation of adenyl cyclase and, via cAMP, the activation of several intracellular enzymes. One pathway in the chain of events seems to be phosphorylation of a membrane protein related to the Ca channel, which thereby increases the Ca permeability of the cell.

The vagal fibers synapse on parasympathetic ganglia located in high density around the sinus and AV nodes and, to a lesser extent, in the atria and ventricles. The short postsynaptic fibers release acetylcholine (ACh), which slows the sinus rate and AV conduction and weakens the contraction of the atria and, under certain conditions, the ventricular myocardium as well. These effects of ACh are muscarinic (blocked by atropine) and consist of an increase in the K permeability and a decrease in the Ca permeability, the *latter* being antagonistic to that of β-adrenergic stimulation. This chapter focuses on the mechanism by which neurotransmitters control the membrane permeability of heart cells. For recent reviews

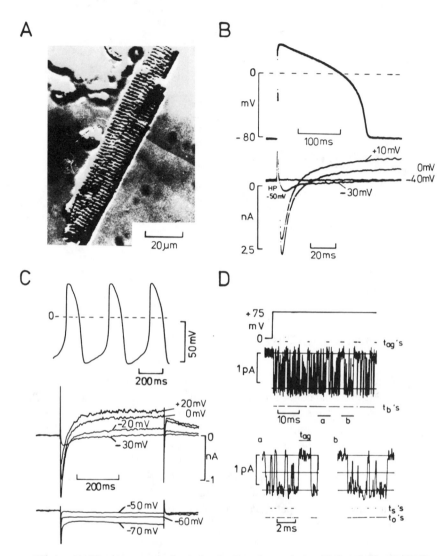

Fig. 1. (A) Photomicrograph of an isolated guinea pig ventricular cell (length 90 μm). (B) Top: action potential of a guinea pig ventricular cell. Bottom: membrane currents in response to depolarizing voltage-clamp steps from a holding potential of −50 mV to various test potentials indicated in the figure (from Cavalié *et al.*, 1983). (C) Action potentials and membrane currents of an isolated SA nodal cell from rabbit heart. The currents were recorded in response to voltage steps from a holding potential of −40 mV to various test potentials indicated in the figure (unpublished records from A. Noma, B. Sakmann, and W. Trautwein). (D) Top: single-Ca-channel activity recorded from an isolated guinea pig ventricular cell with the patch-clamp method. The elementary Ca currents were in response to a 300-msec depolarizing pulse by 75 mV from zero potential across the patch (=resting potential of approximately −65 mV). Channel activity occurred in bursts (duration t_b) of briefly

on this topic, see Reuter (1980, 1983), Trautwein (1982), Trautwein *et al.* (1981), and Tsien (1977, 1983).

II. ACTION POTENTIAL AND MEMBRANE CURRENT

Before turning to the action of neurotransmitters, we will summarize briefly the information on the pertinent conductances in the heart. Such information comes from studies of (1) the action potential, (2) membrane currents recorded from multicellular and unicellular preparations, and (3) currents through single ion channels in a small membrane patch of an isolated cell.

A. The Action Potential (AP)

After the rapid upstroke caused by a large, fast transient of inward sodium current, depolarization is maintained (during the plateau) as a result of a delicate balance between inward (depolarizing) and outward (repolarizing) currents. The inward current is carried predominantly by Ca ions (I_{Ca}), and the outward current predominantly by the inwardly rectifying K current (I_{K1}) and the delayed rectifier (I_K). Provided outward currents are affected only slightly by transmitter, a shift of the plateau in a positive or negative direction indicates a change in I_{Ca} (see Fig. 2A). Most of the information presented in this chapter has been obtained from single cells isolated from adult hearts by enzymatic digestion with collagenase (Powell and Twist, 1976; Powell *et al.*, 1980; Isenberg and Klöckner, 1980). Figure 1A shows a micrograph of a guinea pig ventricular cell isolated by a method modified from Taniguchi *et al.* (1981) and Isenberg and Klöckner (1982a). For details, see Cavalié *et al.* (1983). The cell bathed in Tyrode's solution containing 3.6 m*M* Ca is relaxed, quiescent, and rod shaped with a morphology similar to that of undissociated cells (Dow *et al.*, 1981). Most of these cells respond to electrical stimulation with action potentials whose configurations are typical of those in the multicellular host tissue (Fig. 1B).

In the sinus node, spontaneous diastolic depolarization in the potential range

---

spaced openings (t_o) interrupted by short closures (t_s). The bursts were separated by apparent gaps (t_{ag}). Bottom: two sections (a and b) of the current trace on top are plotted on an expanded time scale for better clarification of t_o, t_s, and t_{ag}. The closed state and the open state are indicated by horizontal lines obtained from amplitude histograms. See legend of Fig. 7 for explanation of the half-maximal amplitude and analyses of t_o, t_s, and t_{ag} (from Trautwein and Pelzer, 1985). The patch electrode was filled with a solution containing 2 m*M* NaCl, 4 m*M* KCl, 5 m*M* HEPES, 0.02 m*M* TTX, and 90 m*M* BaCl₂. Ba serves to increase the amplitude of the currents and to suppress the current through K channels for better resolution of currents through Ca channels.

of -60 to -40 mV, as well as the AP upstroke, is caused by the influx of Ca (Noma *et al.*, 1980). Thus if other conductances remain constant, changes in Ca current should alter the rate of beating. Action potentials have also been recorded from isolated cells of the sinoatrial (SA) and AV nodes, and an example is shown in Fig. 1C.

B. Membrane Current

1. The Ca Current (I_{Ca})

The ionic current that flows across the membrane in response to a depolarizing clamp step is the sum of several specific current components. On a step positive to the threshold of I_{Ca}, the current is directed first inward (I_{Na}, I_{Ca}) and later outward (I_{K1}, I_K). The problem is to dissect these specific components from the net current. When I_{Na} is eliminated (by removal of Na, application of TTX, or maintenance of the potential positive to -55 mV), the Ca current can be separated from the outward current (for details, see McDonald and Trautwein, 1978b).

Ca currents have been measured by a two-microelectrode voltage-clamp technique in short Purkinje fibers (Reuter, 1967) and small preparations of the rabbit SA node (Noma and Irisawa, 1976a) or by the sucrose-gap technique in frog atrial strips (Rougier *et al.*, 1969) and mammalian ventricular trabeculae of various species (Beeler and Reuter, 1970; New and Trautwein, 1972a; for reviews see Reuter, 1979, 1984; McDonald, 1982). Isolated cells are especially suitable for such studies, because technical difficulties such as cable complications and series resistance are largely reduced, especially when a low-resistance suction electrode is used (see below). Figure 1B is an example of a recording from a myocardial cell in which a barely suprathreshold depolarization to -30 mV elicited a small inward current (downward deflection). The maximum current increases in steps to approximately 0 mV, and the current amplitude decreases at more positive potentials, suggesting a bell-shaped current–voltage (I–V) relation. Such bell-shaped I–V relations with reversal potentials of approximately $+60$ mV have been found in multicellular preparations (Beeler and Reuter, 1970; Ochi, 1970; New and Trautwein, 1972a,b) as well as in isolated ventricular cells (Isenberg and Klöckner, 1980, 1982b; Lee and Tsien, 1982). The rise in I_{Ca} (activation) to its peak is fast compared to its decay (inactivation), which in multicellular preparations has been reported to follow a monoexponential time course but in isolated cells is better described by two exponentials (for reviews on I_{Ca}, see Reuter, 1979; McDonald, 1982).

Ca currents have been recorded also in single SA and AV nodal cells (see Fig. 1C). In these structures, I_{Ca} is activated at potentials as negative as -55 mV and can hence depolarize the membrane during the second half of diastole. Similar to that in ventricular cells, inactivation of I_{Ca} in nodal cells occurs with voltage-dependent time constants on the order of 30 msec (Nakayama et al., 1984). Unitary Ca currents through single ionic channels can now be recorded by the patch-clamp technique (Hamill et al., 1981). In brief, a fine-tipped fire-polished pipette is pressed against the cell, and, by application of gentle suction, a gigaohm seal is formed between the glass wall and the membrane surface. Under this condition, the current flow across the membrane patch can be recorded with high resolution and fast clamp control. Upon depolarization of the membrane patch by voltage-clamp pulses to the vicinity of maximal I_{Ca}, single-channel activity (about 1.2 pA at −10 mV, solid lines in Fig. 1D, bottom) appears as closely spaced bursts of brief channel openings and closings separated by longer periods of inactivity (t_o, t_s, and t_{ag}, respectively, in Fig. 1D). Statistical analyses of a large number of current records in response to step depolarizations of a given amplitude yield the approximate time constants for opening and closing. This allows interpretation of the kinetics of Ca-channel activation on the basis of a model that consists of three states in series: C_1 (a closed state with a lifetime of 1–2 msec); C_2 (a closed state with a lifetime of a fraction of 1 msec); and O, an open state with a lifetime of approximately 1 msec (cf. Colquhoun and Hawkes, 1981; see also below, Section IV). Comparison with the current recorded from the whole cell is possible by averaging an ensemble of many elementary current records (see Fig. 7).

2. Potassium Currents

Potassium currents appear in Figs. 1B and C as outward currents toward the end of the voltage-clamp pulse. From such traces, two components can be dissected (cf. McDonald and Tautwein, 1978a,b), the inward rectifier I_{K1} and the time-dependent outward current I_K. I_{K1} or background current is zero close to the resting potential and increases at more negative and positive voltages, but decreases again at potentials positive to −55 mV (Trautwein and McDonald, 1978a; Isenberg and Klöckner, 1982b). The unitary current through single I_{K1} channels has recently been studied in ventricular cells by Sakmann and Trube (1984a,b), and an example is shown in Fig. 12A. I_{K1} sets the resting potential close to the potassium equilibrium potential. In the SA node, I_{K1} is not so well developed; the current is zero at a much more positive voltage than E_K, and the current–voltage relation does not show a negative slope resistance (Nakayama et al., 1984). Hence when the cell becomes quiescent, the resting potential is approximately −40 mV. It is shown below that I_{K1} channels are rare in the SA and AV nodes; however, another potassium channel has been observed. It has a very low probability of opening that can be increased greatly by acetylcholine (see Section V,D).

Important in the context of β-adrenergic stimulation is the time-dependent potassium current (delayed rectifier I_K) observed in all cardiac tissues. In Purkinje fibers (Noble and Tsien, 1968), ventricular fibers (McDonald and Trautwein, 1978a), and small SA nodal preparations (Noma and Irisawa, 1976b), I_K is activated approximately between −45 and +10 mV with voltage-dependent time constants between 100 and 300 msec. The reversal potential depends on the external concentration of potassium in a way that suggests the current is carried primarily by potassium ions.

3.   Hyperpolarization-Activated Inward Current (i_f)

This very slow inward current is activated at membrane potentials between −50 (beginning of activation) and −100 mV (current fully saturated). In Fig. 1C, i_f appears as an increasing inward current upon hyperpolarization to −70 mV. The current is carried by sodium and potassium ions (DiFrancesco, 1981b) and has a reversal potential positive to −50 mV. Activation and deactivation follow a monoexponential time course with time constants of 2–4 sec. Investigators have observed i_f in rabbit SA and AV nodes (Noma and Irisawa, 1976a; Yanagihara and Irisawa, 1980), in the frog's sinus venosus (Brown et al., 1977; for review see Brown, 1982), in Purkinje fibers (DiFrancesco, 1981a), and in isolated Purkinje cells (Callewaert et al., 1984), but, apparently, i_f does not exist in working myocardial cells. In Purkinje fibers, i_f is activated in the voltage range of diastolic depolarization and is the main mechanism of spontaneous impulse formation (DiFrancesco, 1981a; Callewaert et al., 1984). In SA and AV node cells with maximum diastolic potentials of −50 to −60 mV, i_f seems to play only a minor role in spontaneous depolarization (Noma et al., 1980; but see Brown and DiFrancesco, 1980).

III.   β-ADRENERGIC STIMULATION

A.   Adrenaline: Action Potential and Membrane Current

A typical effect of catecholamines is to shift the plateau of the action potential to a more positive level. For example, this has been shown in mammalian ventricular tissue by Gargouil et al. (1958) and Beresewicz and Reuter (1977), and in Purkinje fibers by Otsuka (1958), Carmeliet (1967), and Reuter (1967). The adrenaline effect is especially pronounced when the plateau has been depressed by a high concentration of potassium in Tyrode's solution (Engstfeld et al., 1961). Figure 2A shows the effects of adrenaline on an isolated ventricular

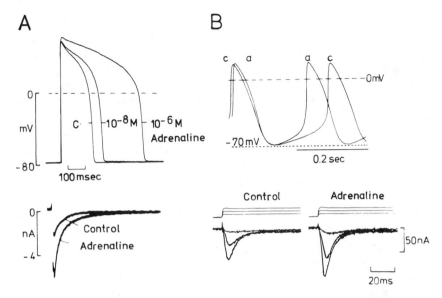

Fig. 2. (A) Effect of adrenaline on action potential and membrane current of an isolated guinea pig ventricular cell. Top: the superimposed action potentials were recorded in control and during superfusion with 10^{-8} and 10^{-6} M adrenaline (steady state). Bottom: the superimposed currents were in response to a step depolarization from -50 to 0 mV and were recorded before and during superfusion with 10^{-6} M adrenaline. Note the increase in maximum I_{Ca}. (B) Top: effect of adrenaline (5.5×10^{-6} M) on the pacemaker depolarization in a cluster of SA nodal cells. Action potentials recorded in presence of adrenaline (a) and control (c) superimposed at the initial phase of diastolic depolarization. Bottom: effect of adrenaline (5.5×10^{-7} M) of I_{Ca} measured as the difference between control currents and those in presence of D600. Currents in response to three voltage steps to -30, -20, and -10 mV from -40 mV are superimposed. (Part B from Noma *et al.* (1980).)

cell: both the plateau and the Ca current are enhanced greatly. Evidence of an increase in Ca current was first reported by Reuter (1967) in Purkinje fibers and by Vassort *et al.* (1969) in frog atrial strips and has since been confirmed in various other cardiac preparations (for review, see Reuter, 1980). The increase in Ca current should elevate the plateau and prolong the action potential. In fact, the same concentration–response relationships of catecholamines were reported for the plateau height and the amplitude of I_{Ca} (Reuter, 1974). The increase in amplitude of I_{Ca} by catecholamines occurs without any change in the kinetics. Neither the steady-state activation or inactivation nor the current reversal or ion selectivity of the channel is altered (Reuter and Scholz, 1977). These authors concluded that adrenaline increases the amplitude of the current by increasing the *number* of functional channels. In the SA node the increased rate of spontaneous firing induced by adrenaline or sympathetic stimulation is caused by a more rapid diastolic depolarization and upstroke of the action potential (Hutter and Traut-wein, 1956; Otsuka, 1958). An example of diastolic depolarization in a small SA nodal preparation is shown in Fig. 2B together with the Ca current in response to three voltage steps before and during application of adrenaline. The current traces were measured as the differences between control currents and currents recorded in the presence of D600 (a Ca entry blocker) and are hence pure Ca currents, which are increased in amplitude by adrenaline (Fig. 2B). This increase may be the most important factor in the positive chronotropic action of adrenaline (Noma et al., 1980). These authors attributed little importance to the increase in i_f because the latter occurred only at potentials too negative to affect pacemaker activity in the SA node (but see Brown et al., 1979a; Brown, 1982). In Purkinje fibers, where i_f contributes to pacemaker activity, adrenaline shifts the activation curve in the depolarizing direction, resulting in a larger i_f current in the voltage range of diastolic depolarization; this is the likely explanation of the positive chronotropic action of adrenaline in this tissue (cf. Tsien, 1974).

Adrenaline increases the magnitude of the potassium current I_K, also. Depending on the relative effects on I_{Ca} and I_K, either a longer or a shorter duration of the action potential will prevail, in contrast to the consistent elevation of the plateau height. The effect on the duration of the action potential depends on the concentration (Quadbeck and Reiter, 1975). In Purkinje fibers, small concentrations prolong and larger concentrations shorten the action potential because of the larger responsiveness of I_K as compared to I_{Ca} at saturating doses of noradrenaline (Kass and Wiegers, 1982). Using a computer reconstruction, Kass and Wiegers (1982) have shown that the changes in current produced by noradrenaline account quantitatively for changes in the configuration of the action potential. The effect on duration of the action potential depends also on the rate of stimulation. At very low rates, or after a long rest, catecholamines prolong the action potential, whereas at a higher rate of stimulation, the duration is not changed (Beresewicz and Reuter, 1979). An increase in the magnitude of I_K by adrenaline with little change in current kinetics has also been observed in the SA node (Brown et al., 1979a,b; Noma et al., 1980). In quiescent atrial and coronary sinus preparations from dogs, hyperpolarization by adrenaline has been reported by Dudel and Trautwein (1956) and by Boyden et al. (1983). The most likely mechanism is an increase in K permeability (Boyden et al., 1983).

B.   cAMP and cAMP-Dependent Protein Kinase

It is now generally accepted that binding of β-agonists to the β-receptor activates the membrane-bound adenyl cyclase, leading thereby to an increase in the intracellular concentration of cyclic AMP, which acts as an intracellular messenger for β-adrenergic stimulation (Robison et al., 1971; Watanabe and Besch, 1974). Indirect evidence for this hypothesis was provided by experiments with inhibitors of phosphodiesterase and with membrane-permeable derivatives

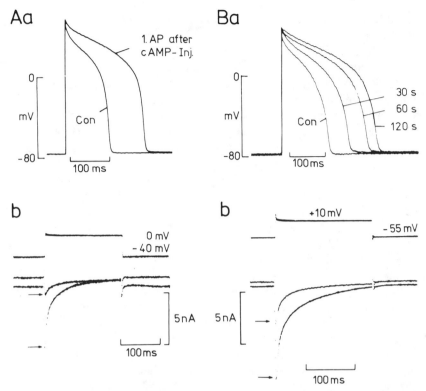

Fig. 3. Pressure injection of cAMP and of catalytic subunit of cAMP-dependent protein kinase into isolated guinea pig ventricular cells. (Aa) Injection of cAMP (50 sec, 500 kPa) prolonged the action potential and increased its amplitude (height of the plateau). Control was recorded shortly before the injection. The cell was stimulated at 0.33 Hz. Estimated increase in cellular cAMP: 5 × 10^{-6} M/liter. (Ab) Increase of Ca current after injection of cAMP. The membrane potential (top) was held at −40 mV, and 200-msec pulses were applied at a rate of 0.33 Hz. Below: current shortly before and a few seconds after injection of cAMP. The arrows indicate the amplitude of I_{Ca}. (Ba) Injection of catalytic subunit increased the duration and amplitude of the action potential. The pressure was increased from 0 to 500 kPa within 1 min and then maintained for 1 min. Estimated elevation of intracellular concentration of catalytic subunit was 10 μM. The cell was stimulated at 0.33 Hz. The control action potential and those recorded 30, 60, and 120 sec after the beginning of the injection are shown. (Bb) Increase in the amplitude of the Ca current on injection of catalytic subunit. Superimposed voltage traces (top) and current traces (bottom) are shown. The upper current trace was recorded before, and the lower current 2 min after injection of the catalytic subunit (500 kPa). Arrows indicate the amplitude of the Ca current before and after injection. [From Brum *et al.* (1983).]

of cAMP (Carmeliet and Vereecke, 1969; Tsien *et al.*, 1972). Such agents produced adrenaline-like effects in Purkinje fibers. These effects were not blocked by propranolol; however, the finding that the effects of adrenaline and theophylline were mutually occlusive suggested a final common mechanism (Tsien, 1974). Furthermore, in guinea pig hearts rendered inexcitable by elevated potassium, methylxanthines restored excitability and promoted Ca-mediated action potentials with pronounced plateaus (Schneider and Sperelakis, 1975). In ventricular myocytes, theophylline changes the configuration of the action potential in the same way as adrenaline (W. Osterrieder, G. Brum, and W. Trautwein, unpublished observations).

A more direct approach was to inject cAMP iontophoretically into Purkinje fibers, inducing initially an elevation of the plateau height and prolongation of the action potential and thereafter a shortening of the action potential. The spontaneous firing rate was enhanced also (Tsien, 1973). These changes in the configuration of the action potential suggested that at least two conductances are increased: I_{Ca}, which elevates the plateau, and I_K, which shortens the action potential. In addition, the magnitude of i_f, which depolarized Purkinje fiber membrane during diastole, was presumably increased. Pressure injection of cAMP into isolated ventricular cells elevated the plateau and prolonged the action potential consistently. Intracellular injection within a small cluster of AV nodal cells enhanced the diastolic depolarization (Trautwein *et al.*, 1981). Prolongation of an action potential recorded in a ventricular myocyte and a large increase in Ca current are shown in Fig. 3A (a and b, see arrows). As with adrenaline, the I_{Ca}-voltage relation was unchanged except in amplitude. The effects of a short (1–10 sec) injection vanished within 1–3 min, presumably because of the activity of the cAMP-phosphodiesterase. Several authors have suggested that the increase in Ca conductance depends on activation of a cAMP-dependent protein kinase (Greengard, 1976; Schneider and Sperelakis, 1975; Niedergerke and Page, 1977; Reuter and Scholz, 1977). It was thought that the kinase phosphorylates membrane proteins associated with the Ca channel, thus enabling the channel to open during depolarization. Such a mechanism predicts the opening of more Ca channels during β-adrenergic stimulation than during control conditions and hence a larger amplitude of the macroscopic current without a change in its kinetics (Reuter and Scholz, 1977).

The protein kinase that depends on cAMP has been isolated in high purity from bovine heart (Rubin *et al.*, 1972; Hofmann *et al.*, 1975). The inactive holoenzyme is a tetramer consisting of two catalytic (C) and two regulatory (R) subunits. cAMP activates the enzyme by binding to the regulatory subunit and dissociating the tetramer: $R_2C_2 + 4cAMP \rightleftharpoons R_2(cAMP)_4 + 2C$. The reaction yields a free catalytic subunit, which is then able to phosphorylate substrate proteins (Flockhart and Corbin, 1982; Rinaldi *et al.*, 1982) and, when injected into a myocyte, should produce adrenaline- and cAMP-like alterations of the action potential and I_{Ca}.

Injection of the catalytic subunit of the cAMP-dependent protein kinase elevated the plateau and prolonged the action potential as expected. Simultaneously, the Ca current was much increased (see Figs. 3B and 4). These effects were detectable approximately 3 sec after the onset of injection, reached a steady state after 2 min, and persisted for the time of observation (30 min) (Osterrieder *et al.*, 1982; Brum *et al.*, 1983). The I_{Ca}–voltage relation after each of two injections was not changed except in amplitude (Fig. 4). In multiple-injection experiments, the first or second injection produced considerable effects on the action potential; however, subsequent injections had little effect, suggesting that

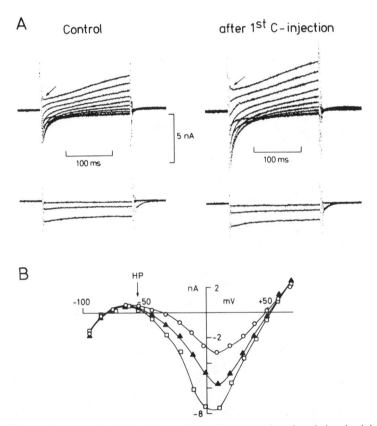

Fig. 4. Current–voltage relations during control and after injection of catalytic subunit into an isolated guinea pig ventricular cell. (A) Currents in response to 200-msec clamp pulses from −55 mV (holding potential) in 10-mV steps up to +65 mV (top) and to −75, −85, and −95 mV (bottom). Left: control; right: same clamp protocol 1 min after injection. Arrows indicate reversal potential. (B) Current–voltage relations of the peak current (same experiment as in A). Current amplitudes were measured 6 msec after onset of the clamp pulses. Open circles, before injection; solid triangles, after initial injection; open squares, after a second enzyme injection. Holding potential marked by arrow.

the Ca conductance of the cell membrane is saturable. Furthermore, the effects of catalytic subunit and adrenaline were mutually occlusive; even high concentrations of adrenaline did not alter the ventricular action potential when the Ca conductance was maximal (Brum *et al.*, 1983). This would not have been the case had adrenaline and the catalytic subunit influenced different populations of sarcolemmal Ca channels. The results suggest strongly that adrenaline, cAMP, and cAMP-dependent protein kinase increase I_{Ca} by the same basic mechanism.

The action of cAMP or catalytic subunit was not confined to I_{Ca}; the outward current was enhanced as well (see Fig. 4A). Although these effects have not yet been studied in detail, the current traces in Fig. 4A suggest that the amplitude of the time-dependent outward current is increased (see also Brum *et al.*, 1983). How these effects on potassium current relate to those on I_{Ca} is not clear. They could be secondary to Ca entry (Ca-induced potassium conductance); it is more likely, however, that K channels are tied to metabolism via phosphorylation induced by the catalytic subunit.

C. Regulatory Subunit of cAMP-Dependent Protein Kinase (R)

The regulatory subunit (R) binds the catalytic subunit (Krebs and Beavo, 1979); hence, when injected into the cell, it should decrease the latter's ability to phosphorylate Ca channels. Thus, injection of R should have effects opposite to those of the catalytic subunit, provided that in the absence of β-stimulation, a basal phosphorylation keeps channels functional. In Tyrode's solution with normal or elevated potassium (Ca-mediated action potentials), injection of regulatory subunit depressed the plateau and shortened the action potential (Fig. 5A). This result is in line with a decrease in Ca conductance (Osterrieder *et al.*, 1982), which has been substantiated in voltage-clamp experiments (Fig. 5B and M. Kameyama and W. Trautwein, unpublished observations). Effects opposite to those of cAMP and catalytic subunit are seen also in recordings of the potassium current, which is depressed by injection of regulatory subunit (see Fig. 5B). In those myocytes that possess, under control conditions, a large outward current, injection of regulatory subunit does not alter or even shorten the action potential, presumably because of a relatively larger depression of I_K than I_{Ca}. The plateau height of the action potential is, however, lowered in all cells. The results in this section do indeed suggest that protein phosphorylation of the Ca channel plays a role not only during β-stimulation but also in its absence; furthermore, both the Ca conductance and the potassium conductance (I_K) are likely to be under metabolic control.

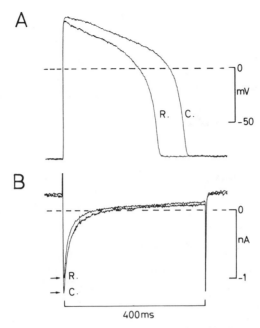

Fig. 5. Effect of intracellular application of regulatory subunit (R) on action potential and membrane current in an isolated guinea pig ventricular myocyte. (A) Superimposed action potentials: control (C) and after 5 min of perfusion of the electrode tip with a solution containing 15 μM R in 50 mM KCl, 100 mM K-Aspartate, and 1 mM MgCl$_2$; whole-cell recording (patch electrode with disrupted sarcolemma in the patch). (B) Superimposed membrane currents: control (peak, arrow C) and after perfusion with 40 μM R for 5 min (peak, arrow R); step depolarizations from -40 to 0 mV. Same experimental conditions as in A. [Unpublished experiment from M. Kameyama and W. Trautwein.]

IV. SINGLE-Ca-CHANNEL ACTIVITY, ADRENALINE, AND cAMP

   This section discusses the mechanism, at the level of the single Ca channel, by which β-adrenergic stimulation brings about an increase in Ca current recorded from the whole cell. Generally, the amplitude of a current (I) is given by the product $I = N \cdot i \cdot p$, where N is the number of conducting channels, i is the single-channel current, and p is the (time-dependent) probability that the channel will be in the open (conducting) state. An increase in I_{Ca} could result from a larger N, i, or p, or any combination is possible. The factors involved can be clarified by recording single-Ca-channel currents in a small membrane patch (see Fig. 1D)

A Control   B Adrenaline (1μM)

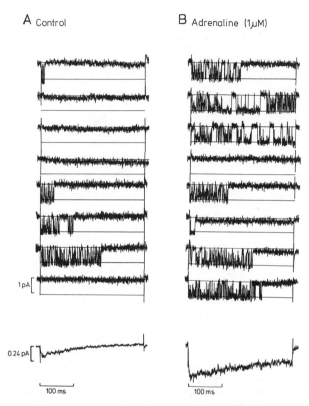

Fig. 6. Ca-channel activity in response to step depolarizations from −65 (holding potential) to +5 mV at a rate of 0.5 Hz. Single myocyte from guinea pig ventricle. (A) Before and (B) during bath perfusion with 1 μM adrenaline. The amplitude of the single-channel current (distance between horizontal lines) was obtained from amplitude histograms. Note the smaller number of blanks and the increase in activity in the presence of adrenaline. The average currents, each of 180 traces, under control and during adrenaline perfusion are shown at the bottom of A and B. [From Trautwein and Kameyama (1985).]

before and during perfusion of adrenaline or pressure injection of cAMP. Such an experiment is shown in Fig. 6. The current traces were recorded during a series of 180 consecutive depolarizations; each series was obtained under control conditions (Fig. 6A) or during bath application of adrenaline (Fig. 6B). The records show that the activity of a single channel is burst-like, i.e., brief openings are separated by shorter or longer times in the closed state (see also Fig. 1D). However, some traces (blanks) do not show activity, i.e., the channel was apparently unavailable at that time to open in response to the depolarizing step. Adrenaline did not increase the amplitude of the unitary current (*i*). In the experiment of Fig. 6, the patch contained only one channel. This was inferred from the observation that, in response to all 360 depolarizations in this experiment, superposition of unitary currents never occurred, i.e., the number of channels (N) in the patch did not increase. This conclusion is supported by the observation that, in patches from which activity could not be recorded and that apparently did not contain a channel (approximately 90% of all patches), adrenaline never produced a channel (i.e., channel activity). The only effect of adrenaline and cAMP is to increase greatly the probability that the channel will be in the open state (p_o). Most obviously, p_o is increased by decreasing the proportion of blanks in the ensemble of current traces. In this experiment, for example, there were no blanks during 50% of the current traces recorded under control conditions; this number was reduced to 11% by adrenaline (see dots in Figs. 7Aa and 7Ba).

The p_o was increased also in those traces that displayed activity. For the 180 traces recorded in the experiment illustrated in Fig. 6, the overall open probability, measured as the fraction of time the channel was open during the depolarizing pulse (integrated activity), is shown as vertical bars in Fig. 7Aa before and in Fig. 7Ba during β-stimulation. The increase in p_o was studied by computing distribution histograms of open and shut times. Open-time distributions were monoexponential (Figs. 7Ab and 7Bb), whereas the closed-time distributions consisted of the sum of two exponentials. The short closed times (<1msec) correspond with the brief closures within bursts (t_s in Fig. 1D) and the longer closed times (1–2 msec; t_{ag} in Fig. 1D) with separate bursts. Adrenaline or injection of cAMP alters these fast gating properties in several ways. The mean channel lifetime (t_o) is prolonged by a factor of 1.5–2, and the frequency of openings is increased. The duration of the long closures between bursts is decreased by approximately one-half. Adrenaline must have little effect on the duration of short closures, because the shortening in Fig. 7Bc is not a regular finding.

The existence of two closed-time distributions suggests that there are at least two closed states. If C_1 and C_2 denote these states and O the open state, a possible model for Ca-channel activation is

$$C_1 \underset{K_2}{\overset{K_1}{\rightleftharpoons}} C_2 \underset{K_4}{\overset{K_3}{\rightleftharpoons}} O \qquad (1)$$

(Fenwick et al., 1982). The rate constants in the model can be computed from the time histograms (cf. Cavalié et al., 1983). It was found that β-adrenergic stimulation altered the constants in such a way that for both partial reactions in the model, the chemical equilibrium was shifted to the right, thus favoring opening of the channel (Brum et al., 1984; Cachelin et al., 1983).

An even more important effect of adrenaline was to reduce the number of blanks. The dots beneath the base lines in Figs. 7Aa and 7Ba indicate the failure

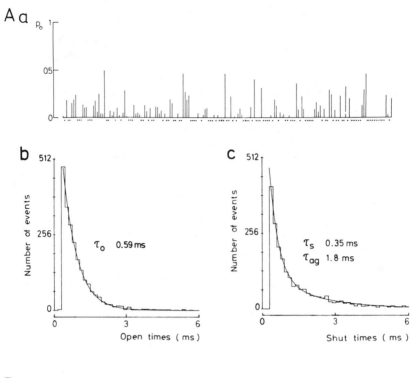

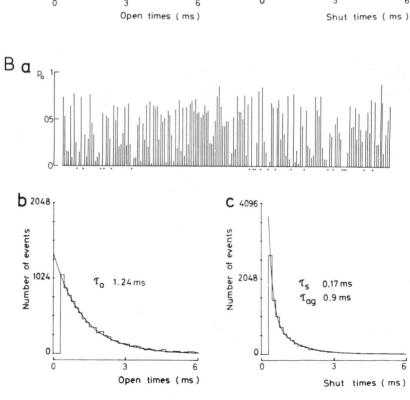

of channel activity. In the control, the blanks were more frequent and tended to occur in clusters. This pattern suggests there is a very slow (on the order of 10 sec) transition between available and nonavailable states of the channel, which we believe results from the state of phosphorylation of a protein. Recently Rinaldi *et al.* (1982) have shown that β-adrenergic stimulation phosphorylates a protein that they called calciductin. The relation of this protein to the Ca channel is, however, not yet clear. The three-state model for Ca-channel activation (see above) does not include such a state in which the Ca channel is unable to respond to depolarization. A more complete model of the Ca-channel behavior would be

$$C_1, C_2 \underset{\displaystyle U}{\overset{\displaystyle O}{\lessgtr}} \qquad (2)$$

where U, the state of unavailability (having a duration on the order of 100 msec), can be reached from both the open and closed states (which are combined for simplicity). Thus, when the channel is in the U state it is nonfunctional (perhaps dephosphorylated), and this time is reduced greatly by adrenaline. Another state of nonresponsiveness of the channel, voltage-dependent inactivation, is not included in the model. It was found recently that, similar to the voltage relation of steady-state inactivation, the less negative the conditioning potential, the greater the number of blanks observed after a depolarizing pulse to a given potential (Trautwein and Pelzer, 1984).

The whole-cell I_{Ca} is the average response, to one depolarization, of the activity and failures of 2,000–10,000 channels. Averaging the single-channel traces in response to many consecutive depolarizations yields $\bar{I}$, the average current. $\bar{I}$ is increased in amplitude by adrenaline (see Figs. 6A and B, bottom) as a result of the large open probability, which both reduces the number of blanks and increases the open time during activity. For voltage-dependent inactivation, a close relationship was recently found between conditioning voltage and both the number of blanks and the amplitude of $\bar{I}$. We assume, therefore, that in the

Fig. 7. Analysis of data from the experiment of Fig. 6. (A) Control and (B) during perfusion with adrenaline. (Aa) and (Ba), open probability given as vertical bars (integrated activity of each trace) for 180 consecutive depolarizations. Dots mark blanks. Note the larger probability of opening and the smaller number of blanks during perfusion with adrenaline. (Ab) and (Bb), monoexponential distributions of open times. Note the longer open time in the presence of adrenaline. (Ac) and (Bc), biexponential distributions of closed times τ_s within bursts and τ_{ag} between bursts. Note the shortening of the closed times in the presence of adrenaline. For analysis of open- and closed-time distributions, a horizontal line halfway between the base line and the average elementary current amplitude was drawn (see Fig. 1D at expanded time scale). The computer program detected transitions between the conducting (lower level in Fig. 1D) and nonconducting (upper level) states as crossings of this line. Mono- and double-exponential curves were fitted to the displayed histograms by a nonlinear, unweighted, least-squares method. The respective time constants are given in the figure. Temperature during the experiment was 35°C. [From Trautwein and Kameyama (1985).]

A   Control   B 10⁻⁵M/l Adrenaline

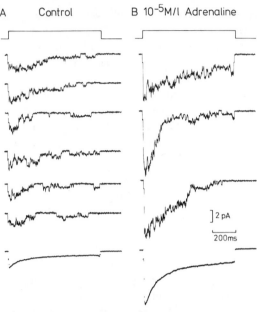

Fig. 8.   Effect of adrenaline on a multichannel patch current (bovine myocyte). (A) Six original records and the average of 180 current traces (bottom). (B) Three current records from the same patch during bath application of 10^{-5} M adrenaline, and the average current from 150 records (bottom). The currents (corrected for leakage and capacitive currents) were in response to depolarizing pulses of 80 mV applied from the resting potential at a rate of 0.33 Hz; the pulse duration was 1 sec (indicated schematically on top). [From Brum *et al.* (1984).]

case of β-adrenergic stimulation, the smaller number of blanks is primarily responsible for the increase in $\bar{I}$ and I_{Ca} recorded from the whole cell.

The analysis of the effects of β-adrenergic stimulation has been confined so far to single-channel patches. In cat and bovine myocytes, however, patches that contained one to three (as seen by the superpositions of unitary currents) or even more active channels were observed. The current activity of such a cluster of channels was increased dramatically by adrenaline (Fig. 8) or injection of cAMP (Brum *et al.*, 1984), resulting in an increase in the average current by a factor of 4 (bottom traces in Fig. 8). Activity of such multichannel patches has been analyzed by nonstationary fluctuation analysis, which gives information on the single-channel conductance, the open probability, and the number of functional channels in the patch.

Every individual patch current deviates from the average current, the deviations being expressed adequately by the variance (σ^2). Only if the channels are identical and independent from each other and have only one conducting state (as seen in the patch-clamp records) can the variance be expressed as $\sigma^2 = N \cdot p(t) \cdot (1-p(t)) \cdot i^2$ (Sigworth, 1980). When $I = N \cdot i \cdot p(t)$ is solved for $p(t)$ and substituted in the equation above, the variance can be written $\sigma^2 = i \cdot I - (I^2/N)$.

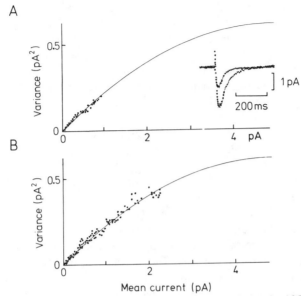

Fig. 9. Relation between variance and mean current to determine the number of Ca channels in a multichannel patch, and the maximum probability of opening of individual channels in a cat myocyte. Injection of cAMP (pressure 500 kPa) increased the mean current as compared to control (inset of A). The original data (stored on FM tape) were transferred to the computer (NICOLET MED 80) and digitized (sampling interval, 1 msec). Each of n patch currents (I_j) was corrected for leakage and capacitive currents, and all currents were averaged to obtain $\bar{I}$, the mean current. For each of the 1024 digitized values, the variance (σ^2) was calculated according to the equation

$$\sigma^2 = \sum_{j=1}^{n} (\bar{I}_j - I)^2/(n-1)$$

The parabolas in A (control) and B (during cAMP injection) were both computed according to the equation $\sigma^2 = i \cdot I - I^2/N$ (see text). [From Brum *et al.* (1984).]

Thus, the relation between variance and mean current is parabolic, and by fitting the parabola to the data one obtains the number of channels (N) and the single-channel current (i).

With only one channel in the patch, the variance–current relation before and during β-adrenergic stimulation could readily be fitted by a single parabola. The data extended over a wider range of the parabola (Brum *et al.*, 1984), indicating that at the peak of the average current the probability of opening was increased (Sigworth, 1980). An example of a multichannel patch in which intracellular injection of cAMP had increased the average current from 1.2 to 2.5 pA is shown in Fig. 9. The plots of variance against average current (Figs. 9A and B) show a large increase of variance during injection of cAMP. The data for both control and injection of cAMP could be fitted using the same parameters, namely, $i = 1.2$ pA (also measured in the original traces) and $N = 8$. The analysis suggested that the number of channels was unaffected by cAMP and that the increase in peak I_{Ca} was caused by an increase in the maximum probability of opening. In many multichannel patches, the data deviated largely from a parabola (Brum *et al.*, 1984), suggesting the existence of inhomogeneity or independence, either of which could preclude this type of analysis (Sigworth, 1980). In favor of the first alternative was the observation of two inactivation time constants in the average currents. Under this condition, plots of variance vs. mean current resulted in complex curves from which the number and probability of opening of the channels could not be determined (Brum *et al.*, 1984).

It should be mentioned that this result contrasts with a report on fluctuation analysis of the whole-cell current in frog myocytes; it suggests that isoprenaline increases the *number* of functional channels (Bean *et al.*, 1984). In these experiments, the parabola extended over a wider range, and the increase in Ca current was much larger (factor up to 15). The reason for this discrepancy seems not to be intrinsic but rather to result from different analytical approaches.

In summary, there is good evidence that in cardiac myocytes β-adrenergic stimulation increases the Ca current by increasing the probability of opening of the Ca channel both during activity and by removing some kind of inactivation.

V. MECHANISM OF ACTION
OF ACETYLCHOLINE

The effects of vagal stimulation, or of ACh, are shortening of the SA, AV, and atrial action potential, slowing of the sinus rate and AV conduction, and hyperpolarization. The effects on rate, conduction, and AP configuration could be explained by either inhibition of the Ca current or an increase in the permeability of the cell membrane to K. Because inward Ca current contributes progressively to the slow depolarization during the second half of diastole (Brown *et al.*, 1977; Noma *et al.*, 1980), inhibition of Ca influx by ACh would be expected to slow the rate in much the same way as the Ca-channel blockers manganese and D600. Depression of the plateau and shortening of the action potential would also result from such inhibition. Alternatively, an increase in K current could bring about similar effects and could, in addition, explain hyperpolarization of the membrane, i.e., the classical muscarinic response. The following sections show that ACh can in fact alter *both* conductances (g_{Ca} and g_K).

A. ACh and K Current

There is abundant literature reporting an increase of the K conductance in heart by ACh (for review see Trautwein, 1982). Such an ACh-induced increase has

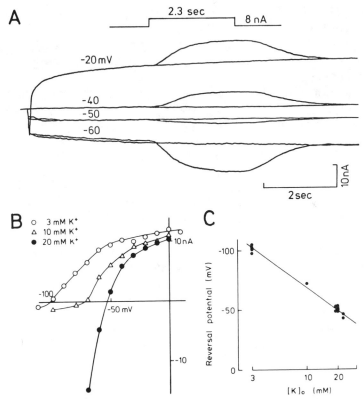

Fig. 10. Properties of ACh-activated K current in the rabbit SA node. (A) Reversal of currents activated by ACh. Iontophoretic application of ACh (8 nA, 2.3-sec duration) during voltage steps to levels indicated in the figure. Current traces with and without ACh application were superimposed. Note current reversal was approximately -50 mV in 20 mM K_o. (B) Steady-state current–voltage relations of the ACh-induced current for three concentrations of K_o. ACh was applied iontophoretically (10 nA, 2.3 sec, essentially the same experiment as in A). In the presence of low K_o, the bending of curves toward the abscissa at potentials negative to reversal is caused probably by depletion of extracellular K in the vicinity of plasma membrane. (C) Semilogarithmic plot of reversal potential of ACh-induced current. Reversal potentials were determined by intercept of K current with voltage axis as in B. [From Noma and Trautwein (1978).]

been shown directly in radiotracer studies, in which the rate of uptake of ^{42}K was found to be increased in frog sinus venosus and to a lesser extent in the atrium (Hutter, 1961; Rayner and Weatherall, 1959; Nawrath, 1977). In electrophysiological experiments, we have obtained evidence of an increase in g_K, such as shortening of the length constant (Trautwein *et al.*, 1956), and have demonstrated that the reversal potential of the ACh response depends on K_o (Trautwein and Dudel, 1958). Figure 10A shows such an experiment, in which the extracellular K was 20 mM and ACh was released iontophoretically. Positive to -50

mV (the value of E_K), release of ACh resulted in an outward current, whereas at more negative potentials it resulted in an inward current.

The voltage relations of the ACh-activated current shown in Fig. 10B display anomalous rectification, i.e., at more positive potentials, the curves are bent strongly toward the abscissa. The curves bear strong similarities to the voltage relation of the inward rectifier I_{K1}. In Fig. 10B, for example, the ACh-activated current at approximately 0 mV is nearly equal at different K_o despite the strong reduction in driving force. Such behavior has been described also for I_{K1} in Purkinje fibers (Dudel et al., 1967; Noble and Tsien, 1968) and in ventricular trabeculae (McDonald and Trautwein, 1978b). In addition, cesium ions block the inward rectifier channel I_{K1} (Isenberg, 1976; Trautwein and McDonald, 1978) and the ACh-activated K current (Ojeda et al., 1981). Because of these similarities, it has been suggested that ACh increases the conductance of the inward rectifying channel I_{K1} (Garnier et al., 1978). The validity of this conclusion has been questioned by Noma and Trautwein (1978) and Noma et al. (1979a), primarily because the ACh-activated current exhibits a time dependence in contrast to I_{K1}, which was thought to depend only on voltage.

The increase in the K conductance produced by ACh is very specific. This is suggested by Fig. 10C, which plots the reversal potentials against the logarithm of different extracellular K concentrations. The line is a least squares fitted to the experimental data and has a slope of 61 mV for a 10-fold change in K_o. This is in accord with the observation that anion fluxes are unaffected by ACh (Hutter, 1961).

B. Kinetics

The time course of hyperpolarization in quiescent atria during stimulation of postganglionic parasympathetic nerve endings (Glitsch and Pott, 1978; Pott, 1979) or after iontophoretic application of ACh to the atrial septum of the frog (Hill-Smith and Purves, 1978; Hartzell, 1979) is characterized by (1) a relatively long delay (100 msec at 36°C) between release of ACh and onset of response and (2) a slow rise to the peak response (Taniguchi et al., 1981). Recently, the time course of the muscarinic response to iontophoretic application of ACh has been studied in isolated AV nodal cells. Even when the tip of the ACh-releasing electrode was attached to the clean cell surface, the apparent delay of the response was never shorter than 20 msec (Taniguchi et al., 1981). There are two basic hypotheses that attempt to explain this delay. Pott (1979) has postulated a model in which three rate-limiting reactions lead to channel opening after the ACh molecule has bound to its receptor. Such a scheme seems to be supported by the strong temperature dependence ($Q_{10} = 11$) of the early rise time (Hartzell et al., 1977). The prolongation of the rise time of the response by caffeine, a phosphodiesterase inhibitor, indicates that cyclic nucleotides might be involved in the reactions (Pott, 1979). The alternative hypothesis attributes the delay and slow response to the kinetics of opening and closing of the K channel activated by ACh. This model, which has been applied to the muscarinic receptor in the heart, had been applied previously to the nicotinic receptor in the motor endplate (Katz and Miledi, 1972):

$$A + R \underset{k_2}{\overset{k_1}{\rightleftharpoons}} AR \underset{\alpha}{\overset{\beta}{\rightleftharpoons}} AR^+ \tag{3}$$

where A is the agonist, R the receptor, AR the closed conformation, and AR^+ the open conformation of the ACh–receptor complex. The rate constants for each reaction step are k_1, k_2, α, and β. Dose–response relations (current or hyperpolarizations) revealed Hill coefficients of 1 (Glitsch and Pott, 1978; Osterrieder et al., 1980, 1981) and K_D ($=k_2/k_1$) of approximately 1.5×10^{-6} M. The second step, which was considered to be rate-limiting, implies that the receptor–agonist complex exists in two states, closed (C) with conductance zero and open (O) with conductance γ:

$$C \underset{\alpha}{\overset{\beta'(A)}{\longleftrightarrow}} O \tag{4}$$

The apparent rate constant for channel opening, $\beta'(A)$, is related to β, the agonist concentration (A), and the dissociation constant (K_D) by the equation $\beta'(A) = \beta/(1 + K_D/A)$. The rate constant can be obtained from the time dependence (relaxation) of the ACh-activated K current (Noma and Trautwein, 1978). In Fig. 11, the current in response to a given depolarization in the absence of ACh is subtracted from the current in response to the same depolarization in the presence of ACh. The result is an outward current, which increases upon depolarization and then decays exponentially to a steady value. The voltage-dependent time constant (larger at negative potentials) was approximately 100 msec (rabbit SA node). It was interpreted as the average open time of the channel activated by ACh and is $\tau = [\alpha + \beta'(A)]^{-1}$. Relaxation of ACh-induced current has been observed also in isolated AV nodal cells of the rabbit heart. The time constants were significantly smaller, approximately 20 msec (Sakmann et al., 1983). Although the rate constants α and β cannot be measured directly, it is possible to measure the dependence of the apparent rate constant $\beta'(A)$ on ACh concentration. Then, β can be extracted using the equation $\beta'(A) = \beta/(1 + K_D/A)$, which describes the concentration dependence of the binding step (for details, see Osterrieder et al., 1980). Values for α and β' of 10 sec^{-1} and 12 sec^{-1}, respectively, were obtained. With these values and allowances for diffusion, we have computed the time course of the muscarinic response with an apparent delay of 30 msec (Osterrieder et al., 1981). These results suggest that in the rabbit

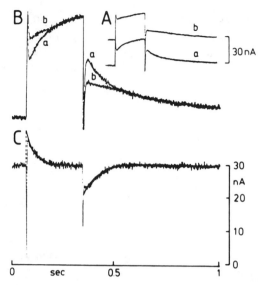

Fig. 11. Relaxation of ACh-activated current recorded from an SA node preparation (200 μm × 100 μm). (A) Two current traces at low gain: (a) control and (b) 2×10^{-6} M ACh. The Tyrode solution contained 5×10^{-7} gm/ml D600. Note the shift in holding current in the presence of ACh. (B) The current recorded in the presence of 2×10^{-6} M ACh (b) is superimposed upon the control (a) with both normalized to the same holding current (vertical shift). (C) Difference a-b (relaxation current). The lines drawn are single exponentials obtained by a least-squares fit of the experimental curves. The time constants were 40 and 65 msec at −40 and −60 mV, respectively. Clamp pulses were from −40 to −10 mV. The steady-state ACh-induced current was 30 nA. The dashed line connects the onset of the pulse with extrapolation of the relaxation to t=0. [From DiFrancesco *et al.* (1980).]

sinus node, the slow response to ACh results from slow channel kinetics and diffusion of the agonist in the tissue. The hypothesis assumes further that ACh opens a special K channel—not I_{K1} channels—when the agonist binds to a receptor that is coupled closely to the channel gate.

C.   ACh-Induced Noise

Further information on the cholinergic activation of K channels has come from studies on ACh-induced fluctuations (noise) in currents recorded from small preparations of the rabbit sinus node. The ACh-activated current recorded from the whole preparation was generated by a large number of channels that open and close independently. This resulted in statistical fluctuations of the current, which could be analyzed by either their variance or the frequency distribution of the power density (see Armstrong, 1975; Neher and Stevens, 1977). The analysis yields information on the single-channel conductance and the kinetics of the channel. The noise increased with increasing agonist concentration, and the relationship between the ACh-induced variance and mean current could be fitted by a parabola (Noma et al., 1979a). From such relationships the single-channel conductance was inferred to be approximately 4 pS (at 3 mM extracellular K), which corresponds to a single-channel current of 0.25 pA at -40 mV.

Current fluctuations from ACh channels were analyzed also by computation of the frequency distribution of power density. Such an analysis yielded Lorentzian curves (in a low frequency range) from which a value of approximately 4 pS for the single-channel conductance and a time constant of relaxation of 100–200 msec were obtained (Noma et al., 1979a).

Technical limitations that might have affected these measurements were caused by the multicellular preparation and the recording system. The latter had a relatively high background noise and a frequency response of approximately no more than 50 Hz (cf. Noma et al., 1979a). In the relaxation measurements, other problems such as accumulation or depletion of potassium in the vicinity of the cells might have affected the time constant. Relaxation of the ACh-induced current can be separated from currents caused by accumulation of K ions (DiFrancesco et al., 1980); however, the problem can never be ignored completely in any given experiment.

D.   Single-K-Channel Activity and ACh

1.   Two Classes of K Channels

With the advent of the patch-clamp technique, direct answers regarding the nature of the ACh-activated K channel could be expected. Recording of single-channel currents in SA and AV nodal cells (Sakmann et al., 1983) and atrial cells (Soejima and Noma, 1984) revealed two classes of K channels that differ primarily in their mean open time. Figure 12A shows elementary currents with a mean open time of 50 msec and a single-channel conductance of 34 ± 6 pS. The voltage and ion dependence of this channel suggests that it is the classical inward rectifier I_{K1} (Sakmann and Trube, 1984a,b). The channel has been observed in almost every patch in ventricular (Sakmann and Trube, 1984a) and atrial (Soejima and Noma, 1984) cells but rarely in SA and AV nodal cells (Sakmann et al., 1983). Effects of ACh on the conductance and kinetics of the channel were not observed. The second type of K channel (Fig. 12B) has a similar single-channel conductance but a much shorter mean open time (approximately 1 msec) and has been observed in atrial as well as SA and AV nodal cells (which are known to respond to ACh with an increase in K conductance) but apparently not in ventricular cells. It should be pointed out that channel openings occurred at a low frequency in the absence of ACh and that the frequency was then greatly increased in the presence of the agonist. The low frequency of short openings and

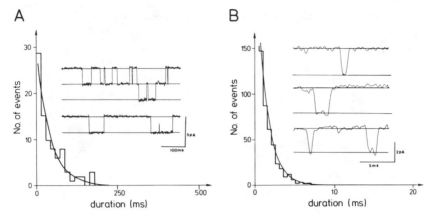

Fig. 12. Two classes of K channels observed in isolated, quiescent AV nodal cells from the rabbit heart. Recordings in the absence of ACh in the bath or pipette solution. Bath solution was normal Tyrode. The pipette contained 70 mM K. (A) The resting K currents of the ventricular inward rectifier type shown in the inset had a mean amplitude of 2.5 pA at the resting potential (-20 mV). The histogram of open channel durations was fitted by a single exponential with a time constant of 48 msec. (B) The resting K currents of the nodal type shown in the inset occurred as short pulses 2.4 pA in amplitude at the resting potential (-20 mV). The histogram represents the distribution of current pulse durations and was fitted by a single exponential with a time constant of 1.4 msec. [From Sakmann *et al.* (1983).]

hence a small mean current accompanied by an apparently low density of I_{K1} channels in SA and AV nodal cells were in accord with the current–voltage relation of the whole-cell current, which displayed little inward rectification and a zero current potential at approximately -60 mV (Nakayama *et al.*, 1984). In contrast, in ventricular and atrial cells, the mean current of I_{K1} was much larger, setting the resting potential close to E_K.

2.   Conductance Properties
of the ACh-Activated K Channel

Figure 13A shows current through an ACh-regulated K channel recorded with a pipette that contained 2×10^{-7} M ACh and 20 mM KCl. At the resting membrane potential (trace marked 0 mV), current steps were inward and increased in amplitude with increasing hyperpolarization. The direction of single-channel current reversed on depolarization of the membrane potential by more than $+20$ mV (3 mM K in the perfusate). The distribution of outward and inward current step amplitudes for approximately the same absolute driving force shows a step amplitude that is approximately five times larger when the current is inward (Fig. 13B). The strong rectification of the current was observed also for ACh-activated K current from the whole cell. With 20 mM K in the pipette, the

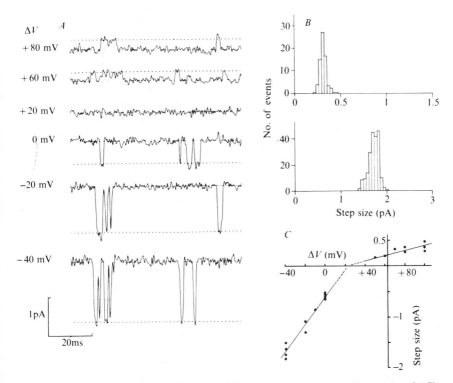

Fig. 13. Conductance properties of single ACh-activated K channels. (A) Examples of ACh-activated inward and outward unitary currents recorded from a rabbit AV nodal cell at various patch membrane potentials. The current recording pipette contained (in mM): NaCl, 120; KCl, 20; CaCl$_2$, 4; and Na-HEPES, 5; as well as 2×10^{-7} M ACh. The numbers on the left of each trace indicate the shift in patch potential, ΔV, with respect to the cell's resting potential (V_r); e.g., -20 mV indicates a patch potential 20 mV more negative than V_r. Current steps reverse in polarity when the patch potential is approximately 20 mV more positive than the resting potential. Inward current steps are downward; the extrapolated reversal potential is approximately 20 mV more positive than V_r. The continuous line indicates the fitted zero current base line; the dotted line, the average step size (i) at each potential. (B) Distribution of outward current step-amplitudes when the membrane patch potential was 80 mV more positive than V_r (upper graph) and of inward current steps when the patch potential was 40 mV more negative than V_r (lower graph). The net driving force in both cases is approximately 60 mV. The mean step sizes in the distributions are 0.32 and 1.68 pA, respectively. (C) Current–voltage relation of ACh-activated single-channel currents obtained with 20 mM K in the pipette. The mean amplitude obtained from step size distributions as in B was plotted as a function of the patch potential. $\Delta V = 0$ represents the cell's resting potential. The chord conductance of the K channel was 25 pS for inward current and 5 pS for outward current. The lines represent linear regression fits of the data points. Zero current intercept is extrapolated to 22 mV more positive than V_r. [From Sakmann *et al.* (1983).]

single-channel chord conductance was 25 pS for inward and 5 pS for outward current steps (Fig. 13C), in fair agreement with previous values obtained from the variance and power spectrum of whole-cell current recorded in multicellular preparations. At -40 mV, the single-channel conductance was 3.5 and 6 pS at 3 and 12 mM K_o, respectively (Noma *et al.*, 1979b). Also, in regard to the ACh concentration–response curve, very similar results were obtained in patch-clamp experiments and multicellular preparations. The mean patch current increased with increasing ACh concentrations from 0.48 $\pm$ 2 pA at 10^{-7} M ACh to 3.1 $\pm$ 0.8 pA at 10^{-6} M, with an apparent equilibrium constant of approximately 1.6 $\times$ 10^{-6} M (Sakmann *et al.*, 1983).

E.   Kinetics: Gating of ACh-Modulated K Channels

There is only one available study of the gating behavior of the ACh-activated K channel in the heart (Sakmann *et al.*, 1983). With 2 $\times$ 10^{-7} M ACh in the pipette, elementary currents were well separated at a low overall frequency (see Fig. 14A, inset). The openings of channels did not occur at random intervals because a large proportion were grouped into bursts of current pulses (Fig. 14B, inset). The distribution of intervals between the pulses shown in Fig. 14A can be fitted by the sum of two clearly separated exponential components representing the short closed times within a burst (τ = 1.3 msec) and long closed times between the bursts (τ = 80 msec, Fig. 14A). The distribution of burst durations can also be fitted by the sum of two exponentials with time constants of 11 and 1 msec.

These results were interpreted on the basis of the two-step model (Reaction (3)). The rate constants obtained were k_1 = 17 sec^{-1}, k_2 = 150 sec^{-1}, α = 510 sec^{-1}, and β = 460 sec^{-1}. In this analysis, the rate constants for opening and closing were one order of magnitude larger than those derived from the relaxation experiments and noise analysis in multicellular SA nodal preparations. From the kinetics, a time constant of relaxation of approximately 1 msec (20 times shorter than that actually observed in SA nodal cells) had to be expected (Sakmann *et al.*, 1983). Even a burst is much too short an event to account for relaxation of the slow muscarinic response on iontophoretic application of ACh. Single-channel activity in response to voltage steps has not yet been measured. It remains to be seen whether activity is enhanced after a hyperpolarizing step and reduced in response to a depolarizing step. Such activity, occurring perhaps in a cluster of bursts, would result in an apparent open time of larger duration as if it were recorded with low-frequency resolution. Relaxation of the ACh-activated current recorded from the whole cell is in fact an average of the responses of many channels, and the time course of relaxation may no longer be determined by the open-closed times within bursts. The same consideration holds for the time course of the ACh-induced hyperpolarization. Thus, there is not necessarily

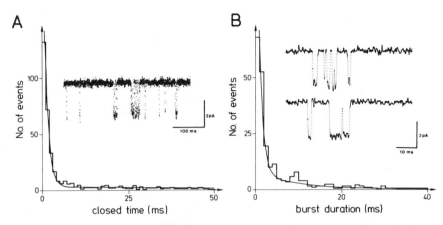

Fig. 14. Bursts of single-channel currents with low concentrations of ACh in the patch pipette (70 mM K and 2 × 10^{-7} M ACh). Isolated rabbit AV nodal cell. The bath was Tyrode solution. The membrane patch was hyperpolarized by 20 mV. (A) The histogram shows the distribution of intervals between 1021 single-current pulses (closed-time durations). Currents occur as single pulses or as bursts. The inset shows a digitized sample recorded with poor time resolution. The distribution was fitted by the sum of a slow and a fast exponential component (continuous line). The time constants were 80 and 1.3 msec, respectively. (B) The histogram shows the distribution of current bursts (defined as any sequence of current pulses separated by intervals no longer than 6 msec). The inset shows digitized records (with greater time resolution) of current bursts. The distribution was fitted by the sum of two exponentials (continuous line) with time constants of 11 and 1.3 msec. [From Sakmann *et al.* (1983).]

a discrepancy between the results obtained from the single-channel analysis and kinetic analysis of current relaxation and fluctuations. The latter results do not reflect, however, the kinetics of the single channel, but yield averages and apparent open times obtained by recording (with low-frequency resolution) the activity of many channels.

F. Intracellular Messenger Unlikely

In regard to the delay of the muscarinic response, the hypothesis of an intracellular messenger like cGMP has been discussed widely (for references, see Goldberg *et al.*, 1975). George *et al.* (1973) applied ACh to the perfused rat heart and found that the decrease in heart rate was correlated strongly with an increase in cGMP. If an intracellular messenger were involved in the increase in K conductance by ACh, one would expect that ACh applied outside the membrane patch would activate K channels in the patch isolated from the rest of the cell. In an elegant experiment, Soejima and Noma (1984) have shown that ACh applied to the bath does not increase the occurrence of elementary currents in the patch. When the pipette interior was perfused, however, the number of current

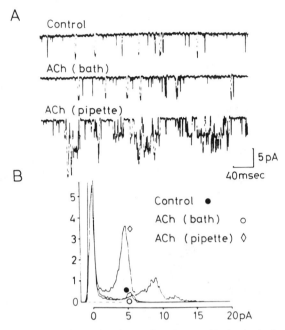

Fig. 15. Effects of ACh on the patch and the cell surface outside the patch of an isolated rabbit atrial cell. The recordings were made 20 mV negative to the resting membrane potential of −20 mV. The pipette contained 70 mM K. (A) The top trace, control, was recorded before the application of ACh (basal activity); the middle trace, during the application of ACh in the bath; and the bottom trace, during perfusion of the patch electrode with 0.1 μM ACh. The channel activity increased markedly, with up to three unitary currents overlapping. (B) Probability–density histograms of the current level. The solid circle indicates the basal activity; the open circle, activity during application of ACh in the bath; and the diamond, ACh in the patch electrode. [From Soejima and Noma (1984).]

events increased dramatically; at times, as many as three channels were open simultaneously (see Fig. 15A). Soejima and Noma's analysis, in the form of a probability density histogram, showed that the probability of an opening was great when the pipette was perfused with ACh but not significantly greater than control on bath application of ACh (Fig. 15B). These results suggest strongly that intracellular mechanisms are not involved in the activation of K channels by ACh. This conclusion is supported by the observation that when the patch is disrupted from the cell and an outside-out configuration is achieved (the outside of the membrane patch sees the bath), ACh continues to increase the number of elementary K currents. It should be added that all attempts to show that either cGMP or its membrane-permeable derivative, 8-bromo-cGMP, plays a role in the context of the ACh-induced increase in K fluxes have failed (Fleming *et al.*, 1981; Nawrath, 1977). Furthermore, injection of cGMP into aggregates of 2–5 cells of AV node did not produce hyperpolarization, nor did it affect the amplitude or time course of the hyperpolarization on iontophoretic application of ACh (Trautwein *et al.*, 1982). It is, therefore, altogether unlikely that the increase in K conductance by ACh is mediated by an intracellular messenger.

VI.   THE SECOND MUSCARINIC RESPONSE

A.   Inhibition of Ca Current by ACh

This section describes a second mechanism of action of ACh that may also lead to slowing of the spontaneous sinus rate and atrioventricular conduction as well as to shortening of the action potential.

That ACh might depress a slow inward current was suspected by Paes de Carvalho *et al.* (1969) because of the agonist's suppression of the slower final portion of the upstroke of AV and SA nodal action potentials. The same suggestion was raised by Prokopczuk *et al.* (1973), who reported effects of ACh similar to those of manganese on the action potential and tension of mammalian atrial preparations. This notion was substantiated in voltage-clamp experiments in which ACh was found to depress the slow inward Ca current in bullfrog atrial strips (Ikemoto and Goto, 1975; Giles and Noble, 1976) and mammalian atrial trabeculae (Ten Eick *et al.*, 1976). Figure 16A shows an example of depression of slow inward current by ACh. In response to a voltage step from -80 to 0 mV, the Ca current was reduced significantly in the presence of $3 \times 10^{-8} M$ and nearly suppressed in the presence of $1.2 \times 10^{-7} M$ ACh. The strong depression of the Ca current is seen also in the current–voltage relation (Fig. 16B). It is noteworthy that in this preparation, the bullfrog atrial strip, the K current was not increased at these two ACh concentrations. Ikemoto and Goto (1975) reported that the agonist had little effect on the kinetics of the Ca current. The steady-state activation and inactivation curves were unchanged, as were the time constants of activation, inactivation, and recovery from inactivation. The only effect was a decrease in the maximum conductance $\bar{g}_{Ca}$. Thus the effect of ACh on the Ca current seems to be opposite to that of adrenaline.

For a long time, the ventricular myocardium has been considered insensitive even to high concentrations of ACh (cf. Hoffman and Suckling, 1953). In recent experiments with mammalian papillary muscles, however, Hino and Ochi (1980) found an ACh-induced depression of the plateau and slight shortening of the action potential as well as a depression of the slow inward Ca current in voltage-clamp experiments. As in the experiments on frog atrial strips by Ikemoto and Goto (1975), Giles and Noble (1976), and Garnier *et al.* (1978), the concentration dependence of the Ca-current depression correlated strongly with the negative inotropic effect. In isolated ventricular cells, an effect of ACh on the action

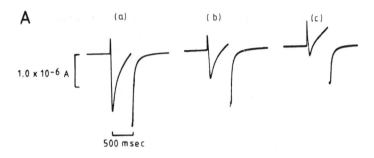

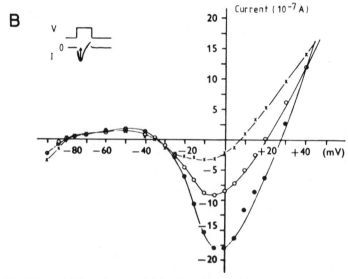

Fig. 16. Effect of ACh on I_{Ca} recorded from a bullfrog atrial strip superfused continually with Ringer's solution containing TTX (2×10^{-6} gm/liter). (A) Pen recorder tracings of slow inward current in response to 500-msec, 80-mV depolarizations from the resting potential (-80 mV): (a) control; (b) and (c) were recorded after application of 3×10^{-8} and 1.2×10^{-7} M ACh, respectively. (B) Peak inward or minimum outward current in response to each rectangular voltage-clamp pulse was measured as shown in inset, and current–voltage relations were then constructed. Solid circles, control; open circles, values obtained during application of 3×10^{-8} M ACh; asterisks, values obtained in 1.2×10^{-7} l ACh. [From Giles and Noble (1976).]

potential and membrane currents cannot be reproduced reliably. Most cells do not respond, but some exhibit shortening of the action potential and depression of the Ca current (Pelzer and Trautwein, 1981). Responsiveness seems to depend somehow on the state of the preparation. In this context, it is interesting that ACh depressed the Ca current in ventricular cells only when the level of intracellular cAMP was high, an effect that was blocked by atropine (Josephson and Sperelakis, 1978; cf. Bailey *et al.*, 1979; Inui and Imamura, 1977).

B. Possible Mechanisms of the Depression of Ca Current by ACh

Both the depression of I_{Ca} without alteration of the kinetics (Ikemoto and Goto, 1975) and the inhibitory action of ACh predominantly in isoproterenol-treated ventricular fibers (Josephson and Sperelakis, 1978) suggest that ACh does interfere with a step in the β-adrenergic stimulation. In mammalian myocardium, muscarinic inhibition of catecholamine-stimulated adenylate cyclase has been described (Jakobs *et al.*, 1979). The receptors mediating the inhibition are distinct from those coupled to the activation of adenylate cyclase. Inhibition of basal or stimulated adenylate cyclase is never complete; 40 to 60% of the control activity is retained in the presence of the inhibitor. The presence of GTP is required for the inhibition, which is not detected in the presence of GTPase-resistant analogues of GTP (e.g., Gpp(NH)p). Further information substantiating the concept that muscarinic agonists interfere with activation of cardiac adenylate cyclase can be found in Murad *et al.* (1962), Lee *et al.* (1971), and Watanabe *et al.* (1978), and in electrophysiological experiments by Biegon and Pappano (1980).

Another alternative could be that the ACh-induced depression is caused by another cyclic nucleotide, namely, 3, 5-cyclic guanosine monophosphate (cGMP). It has been shown that muscarinic agonists stimulate guanylate cyclase and increase intracellular levels of cGMP in cardiac muscle (George *et al.*, 1973; reviewed in Goldberg *et al.*, 1975). In accord with such a hypothesis, Nawrath (1977) found a reduction of ^{45}Ca uptake in rabbit atria by both ACh and cGMP. In addition, Kohlhardt and Haap (1978) have shown that both 8-bromo-cGMP and ACh inhibit the Ca-dependent, slow-response action potential in guinea pig atria. Similarly, Ikemoto and Goto (1978) have described depression of the overshoot and plateau of the frog's atrial action potential upon iontophoretic injection of cGMP. A depression of the plateau and shortening of the action potential have been observed on injection of cGMP or 8-bromo-cGMP into isolated ventricular cells (Fig. 17A). In the case of the former, the effect was biphasic: after an initial shortening, the action potential became prolonged beyond control, presumably an effect of the metabolite GMP, which, when injected, prolonged the action potential without a preliminary shortening. Injection of the more slowly degraded dB-cGMP did not produce the secondary prolongation (Fig. 17B). Changes in cGMP would affect the regulatory protein G, activating the adenylate cyclase. Because GTP is a substrate for cGMP, an increase in cGMP by ACh might deplete GTP and

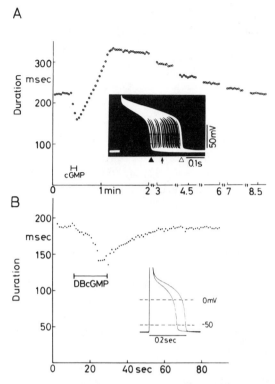

Fig. 17.   Effects of pressure injection (100 kPa) of cGMP or dB-cGMP on configuration of the action potential of an isolated guinea pig ventricular cell. (A) Time course of the biphasic change in action potential duration induced by injection of cGMP. Period of injection indicated above the scale. During recovery phase the scale is interrupted for 60 sec every 80 sec. Inset: same experiment; arrow indicates the control action potential. Solid triangle marks the shortest action potential; open triangle, the longest one. Stimulus interval 2.5 sec. (B) During injection of dB-cGMP, the duration of the action potential was shortened. The effect was reversible. Inset: action potentials recorded before the application (rightmost) and during maximum shortening. Stimulus rate, 1 sec^{-1}. [From Trautwein *et al.* (1982).]

thereby inhibit the activation of adenylate cyclase (Watanabe *et al.*, 1978). Finally, Flitney and Singh (1980) reported that 8-bromoguanosine-cGMP depressed the concentration of cAMP and that this effect was attenuated by theophylline. They supposed that the depression was caused by stimulation of phosphodiesterase rather than by the suppression of adenylate cyclase. Whether the depression of the Ca current by ACh is related to cGMP in the sense of an intracellular mediator remains to be seen.

VII. SUMMARY AND PERSPECTIVES FOR FUTURE RESEARCH

This chapter has dealt with mechanisms involved in the control of Ca and K currents by β-adrenergic and cholinergic stimulation. Beta-adrenergic stimulation results in a cascade of steps. Recent progress in the isolation of cardiac cells from the adult heart and development of the patch-clamp technique have made it possible to track these steps in an intact myocyte and to study the mechanisms at the level of a single Ca channel. When the agonist was applied to the outer side of the cell and when cAMP or the catalytic subunit of the cAMP-dependent protein kinase was applied intracellularly, the effect was to increase both Ca and K (I_K) currents. The mechanisms for the increase in Ca current were an alteration in gating of the channel, which resulted in longer open and shorter closed times during activity, and removal of a chemical inactivation that made more channels available to open upon depolarization. We have assumed that the relatively long periods of unavailability and of responsiveness of the channel are related to a phosphorylation–dephosphorylation cycle that is altered by β-adrenergic stimulation.

A related problem is to find further, perhaps metabolic, requirements for Ca-channel availability. In channels separated from the cell (inside-out patches), activity ceases. This observation and the result with the regulatory subunit suggest that in the absence of a β-stimulation, cAMP-dependent protein kinase is involved only slightly in the control of Ca-channel activity. It will be interesting to discover possible metabolic factors, or perhaps a protein, that keep Ca channels available in a membrane patch separated from the cell.

Another promising direction of research will be the reconstruction of cardiac Ca and other ionic channels in lipid membranes. Such simpler models would allow one to study the requirements for the channel's normal activity and its modulation by neurotransmitters. Perhaps in not too long a time biochemists and biophysicists will acquire sufficient knowledge of the chemical structure of the Ca channel and other ionic channels to explain their biophysical behavior. It may then be clear what protein is phosphorylated by β-adrenergic stimulation and why such phosphorylation alters the channel's gating properties and its state of chemical inactivation.

The classical muscarinic response, hyperpolarization of the membrane potential, results from an increase in potassium conductance. The gating behavior of the respective channel is much faster than that of the inward rectifier (I_{K1}). Acetylcholine increases the probability that the channel will open, which is very low in the absence of the agonist. Thus by binding to its receptor, acetylcholine modulates the behavior of the channel, but does not produce a channel. The kinetics of the ACh-modulated K channel, as studied by relaxation experiments and current fluctuation analyses in a multicellular preparation, could explain the long delay in the onset of hyperpolarization as well as its slow time course. In contrast, single channels displayed very short open times (two orders faster) and bursting behavior. Obviously the macroscopic response (hyperpolarization or increased outward current) does not reflect the gating behavior of the single channel. The former is a continuous average of the activity of several thousand K channels in each of the 200 to 500 cells of the preparation. Further experiments are required to clarify the events within the 20 msec that elapse between the application of agonist and the onset of an increase in conductance.

REFERENCES

Armstrong, C. M. (1975). Ionic pores, gates, and gating currents. *Quart. Rev. Biophys.* **7**, 179–210.

Bailey, I. C., Watanabe, A. M., Besch, H. R., Jr., and Lathrop, D. R. (1979). Acetylcholine antagonism of the electrophysiological effects of isoproterenol on canine cardiac Purkinje fibers. *Circ. Res.* **44**, 378–383.

Bean, B. P., Nowycky, M. C., and Tsien, R. W. (1984). β-Adrenergic modulation of calcium channels in frog ventricular heart cells. *Nature* **307**, 371–375.

Beeler, G. W., and Reuter, H. (1970). Membrane calcium current in ventricular myocardium fibres. *J. Physiol. (Lond.)* **207**, 191–209.

Beresewicz, A., and Reuter, H. (1977). The effects of adrenaline and theophylline on action potential and contraction of mammalian ventricular muscle under 'rested-state' and 'steady-state' stimulation. *Naunyn-Schmiedebergs Arch. Exp. Path. Pharmakol.* **301**, 99–107.

Biegon, R. L., and Pappano, A. (1980). Dual mechanism for inhibition of calcium-dependent action potentials by acetylcholine in avian ventricular muscle. *Circ. Res.* **46**, 353–362.

Boyden, P. A., Cranefield, P. F., and Gadsby, D. C. (1983). Noradrenaline hyperpolarizes cells of the canine coronary sinus by increasing their permeability to potassium ions. *J. Physiol. (Lond.)* **339**, 185–206.

Brown, H. F. (1982). Electrophysiology of the sinoatrial node. *Physiol. Rev.* **62**, 505–530.

Brown, H. F., and DiFrancesco, D. (1980). Voltage-clamp investigations of membrane currents underlying pacemaker activity in rabbit sino-atrial node. *J. Physiol.* **308**, 331–351.

Brown H. F., Giles W., and Noble S. J. (1977). Membrane currents underlying activity in frog sinus venosus. *J. Physiol.* **271**, 783–816.

Brown, H. F., DiFrancesco, D., and Noble, S. J. (1979a). How does adrenaline accelerate the heart? *Nature* **280**, 235–236.

Brown, H. F., DiFrancesco, D., and Noble, S. J. (1979b). Cardiac pacemaker oscillation and its modulation by autonomic transmitters. *J. Exp. Biol.* **81**, 175–204.

Brum, G., Flockerzi, V., Hofmann, F., Osterrieder, W., and Trautwein, W. (1983). Injection of catalytic subunit of cAMP-dependent protein kinase into isolated cardiac myocytes. *Pflügers Arch.* **398**, 147–157.

Brum, G., Osterrieder, W., and Trautwein, W. (1984). β-Adrenergic increase in the calcium conductance of cardiac myocytes studied with the patch clamp method. *Pflügers Arch.* **401**, 111–118.

Cachelin, A. B., De Peyer, J. E., Kokubun, S., and Reuter, H. (1983). Ca^{2+} channel modulation by 8-bromocyclic AMP in cultured heart cells. *Nature* **304**, 462–466.

Callewaert, G., Carmeliet, E., and Vereecke, J. (1984). Single cardiac Purkinje cells: General electrophysiology and voltage-clamp analysis of the pacemaker current. *J. Physiol.* **349**, 643–661.

Carmeliet, E. (1967). Adrenaline effects on the plateau of the cardiac action potential. *Arch. Intern. Phsyiol. Biochem.* **75**, 542–543.

Carmeliet, E., and Vereecke, J. (1969). Adrenaline and the plateau phase of the cardiac action potential. Importance of Ca^{++}, Na^+ and K^+ conductance. *Pflügers Arch. Ges. Physiol.* **315**, 300–315.

Cavalié, A., Ochi, R., Pelzer, D., and Trautwein, W. (1983). Elementary currents through Ca^{2+} channels in guinea pig myoctyes. *Pflügers Arch.* **398**, 284–297.

Colquhoun, D., and Hawkes, A. G. (1981). On the stochastic properties of single ion channels. *Proc. R. Soc. Lond. B.* **211**, 205–235.

DiFrancesco, D. (1981a). A new interpretation of the pacemaker current in calf Purkinje fibres. *J. Physiol.* **314**, 359–376.

DiFrancesco, D. (1981b). A study of the ionic nature of the pacemaker current in calf Purkinje fibres. *J. Physiol.* **314**, 377–393.

DiFrancesco, D., Noma, A., and Trautwein, W. (1980). Separation of current induced by potassium accumulation from acetylcholine-induced relaxation current in the rabbit S-A node. *Pflügers Arch.* **387**, 83–90.

Dow, J. W., Harding, N. G. L., and Powell, T. (1981). Isolated cardiac myocytes. I. Preparation of adult myocytes and their homology with the intact tissue. *Cardiovasc. Res.* **15**, 483–514.

Dudel, J., and Trautwein, W. (1956). Die Wirkung von Adrenalin auf das Ruhepotential von Myokardfasern des Vorhofs. *Experientia (Basel)* **12**, 396–398.

Dudel, J., Peper, K., Rüdel, R., and Trautwein, W. (1967). The potassium component of membrane current in Purkinje fibres. *Pflügers Arch.* **296**, 308–327.

Engstfeld, G., Antoni, H., and Fleckenstein, A. (1961). Die Restitution der Erregungsfortleitung und Kontraktionskraft des K^+-gelähmten Frosch- und Säugetiermyokards durch Adrenalin. *Pflügers Arch. Ges. Physiol.* **273**, 145–163.

Fenwick, E. M., Marty, A., and Neher, E. (1982). Sodium and calcium channels in bovine chromaffin cells. *J. Physiol.* **331**, 599–635.

Fleming, B. P., Giles, W., and Lederer, J. (1981). Are acetylcholine-induced increases in ^{42}K efflux mediated by intracellular cyclic GMP in turtle cardiac pacemaker tissue? *J. Physiol.* **314**, 47–64.

Flitney, F. W., and Singh, J. (1980). Depressant effect of 8-bromo guanosin 3′,5′-cyclic monophosphate on endogenous adenosine 3′,5′-cyclic monophosphate levels in frog ventricle. *J. Physiol (Lond.)* **302**, 29P.

Flockhart, D. A., and Corbin, J. D. (1982). Regulatory mechanisms in the control of protein kinases. *CRC Critical Rev. Biochem.* **12**, 133–186.

Gargouil, Y. M., Tricoche, R., Fromenty, D., and Coraboeuf, E. (1958). Effects de l'adrénaline sur l'activité électrique du coeur de mammifères. *C.R. Acad. Sci. (Paris)* **246**, 334–336.

Garnier, D., Nargeot, J., Ojeda, C., and Rougier, O. (1978). The action of acetylcholine on background conductance in frog atrial trabeculae. *J. Physiol. (Lond.)* **274**, 381–396.

George, W. J., Wilkerson, R. D., and Kadowitz, P. J. (1973). Influence of actylcholine on contractile force and cyclic nucleotide levels in the isolated perfused rat heart. *J. Pharmacol. Exp. Ther.* **184**, 228–235.

Giles, W. R., and Noble, S. J. (1976). Changes in membrane currents in bull-frog atrium produced by acetylcholine. *J. Physiol. (Lond.)* **261**, 103–123

Glitsch, G. H., and Pott, L. (1978). Effects of acetylcholine in parasympathetic nerve stimulation on membrane potential in quiescent guinea-pig atria. *J. Physiol. (Lond.)* **279**, 655–668.

Goldberg, N. D., Haddox, M. K., Nicol, S. E., Glass, D. B., Sanford, C. H., Kuehl, F. A., Jr., and Estensen, R. (1975). Biological regulation through opposing influences of cyclic GMP and cyclic AMP: The yin yang hypothesis. *In* "Advances in Cyclic Nucleotide Research" (G. I. Drummond, P. Greengard, G. A. Robinson, eds.), Vol. 5, pp. 307–330. Raven Press, New York.

Greengard, P. (1976). Possible role for cyclic nucleotides and phosphorylated membrane proteins in postsynaptic actions of neurotransmitters. *Nature* **269**, 101–108.

Hamill, O. P., Marty, A., Neher, E., Sakmann, B., and Sigworth, F. J. (1981). Improved patch-clamp techniques for high resolution current recording from cells and cell-free membrane patches. *Pflügers Arch.* **391**, 85–100.

Hartzell, H. C. (1979). Distribution of muscarinic acetylcholine receptors in amphibian cardiac muscle. *Nature (Lond.)* **278**, 569–571.

Hartzell, H. C., Kuffler, S. W., Stickgold, R. S., and Yoshikami, D. (1977). Synaptic excitation and inhibition resulting from direct action of acetylcholine on two types of chemoreceptors on individual amphibian parasympathetic neurones. *J. Physiol.* **271**, 817–846.

Hill-Smith, I., and Purves, R. D. (1978). Synaptic delay in the heart: An iontophoretic study. *J. Physiol. (Lond.)* **279**, 31–54.

Hino, N., and Ochi, R. (1980). Effect of acetylcholine on membrane currents in guinea-pig papillary muscle. *J. Physiol. (Lond.)* **307**, 183–197.

Hoffman, B. F., and Suckling, E. E. (1953). Cardiac cellular potentials: Effect of vagal stimulation and acetylcholine. *Am. J. Physiol.* **173**, 312–320.

Hofmann, F., Beavo, J. A., Bechtel, P. J., and Krebs, E. G. (1975). Comparison of adenosine 3',5'-monophosphate-dependent protein kinases from rabbit skeletal and bovine heart muscle. *J. Biol. Chem.* **250**, 7795–7780.

Hutter, O. F. (1961). Ion movements during vagus inhibition of the heart. *In* "Nervous Inhibition" (E. Florey, ed.), pp. 114–123. Pergamon Press, Oxford.

Hutter, O. F., and Trautwein, W. (1956). Vagal and sympathetic effects on the pacemaker fibers in the sinus venosus of the heart. *J. Gen. Physiol.* **39**, 715–733.

Ikemoto, Y., and Goto, M. (1975). Nature of the negative inotropic effect of acetylcholine on the myocardium. An elucidation of the bullfrog atrium. *Proc. Japan Acad.* **51**, 501–505.

Ikemoto, Y., and Goto, M. (1978). Effects of acetylcholine and cyclic nucleotides on the bullfrog atrial muscle. *In* "Recent Advances in Studies on Cardiac Structure and Metabolism" (T. Kobayashi, T. Sano, and N. S. Dhalla, eds.), Vol. II, pp. 57–61. University Park Press, Baltimore.

Inui, J., and Imamura, H. (1977). Effects of acetylcholine on calcium-dependent electrical and mechanical responses in the guinea-pig papillary muscle partially depolarized by potassium. *Naunyn-Schmiedebergs Arch. Exp. Pharmakol.* **299**, 1–7.

Isenberg, G. (1976). Cardiac Purkinje fibers: Cs as a tool to block inward rectifying potassium currents. *Pflügers Arch.* **365**, 99–106.

Isenberg, G., and Klöckner, U. (1980). Glycocalyx is not required for slow inward calcium current in isolated rat heart myocytes. *Nature* **284**, 358–360.

Isenberg, G., and Klöckner, U. (1982a). Calcium tolerant ventricular myocytes prepared by prein-cubation in "KB medium." *Pflügers Arch* **395**, 6–18.

Isenberg, G., and Klöckner, U. (1982b). Calcium currents of isolated bovine ventricular myocytes are fast and of large amplitude. *Pflügers Arch.* **395**, 30–41.

Jakobs, K. H., Aktories, K., and Schultz, G. (1979). GTP-dependent inhibition of cardiac adenylate cyclase by muscarinic cholinergic agonists. *Naunyn-Schmiedebergs Arch. Pharmakol.* **310**, 113–119.

Josephson, I., and Sperelakis, N. (1978). 5'-Guanylimidodiphosphate stimulation of slow Ca^{2+} current in myocardial cells. *J. Mol. Cell. Cardiol.* **10**, 1157–1166.

Kass, R. S., and Wiegers, S. E. (1982). The ionic basis of concentration-related effects of nor-adrenaline on the action potential of calf cardiac Purkinje fibers. *J. Physiol.* **322**, 541–558.

Katz, B., and Miledi, R. (1972). The statistical nature of the acetylcholine potential and its molecular components. *J. Physiol (Lond.)* **224**, 665–699.

Kohlhardt, M., and Haap, K. (1978). 8-Bromo-guanosine-3′,5′-monophosphate mimics the effect of acetylcholine on slow response action potential and contractile force in mammalian atrial myocardium. *J. Mol. Cell. Cardiol.* **10**, 573–586.

Krebs, E. G., and Beavo, J. A. (1979). Phosphorylation-dephosphorylation of enzymes. *Ann. Rev. Biochem.* **48**, 923–959.

Lee, K. S., and Tsien, R. W. (1982). Reversal of current through calcium channels in dialysed single heart cells. *Nature* **297**, 498–501.

Lee, T. P., Kuo, J. F., and Greengard, P. (1971). Regulation of myocardial cyclic AMP by isoproterenol, glucagon and acetylcholine. *Biochem. Biophys. Res. Comm.* **45**, 991–997.

McDonald, T. F. (1982). The slow inward calcium current in the heart. *Ann. Rev. Physiol.* **44**, 425–434.

McDonald, T. F., and Trautwein, W. (1978a). The potassium current underlying delayed rectification in cat ventricular muscle. *J. Physiol.* **274**, 217–246.

McDonald, T. F., and Trautwein, W. (1978b). Membrane currents in cat myocardium: Separation of inward and outward components. *J. Physiol. (Lond.)* **274**, 193–216.

Murad, F., Chi, Y. M., Rall, W. T., and Sutherland, E. W. (1962). Adenyl cyclase. III. The effect of catecholamines and choline esters on the formation of adenosine 3′,5′-phosphate by preparations from cardiac muscle and liver. *J. Biol. Chem.* **237**, 1233–1238.

Nakayama, T., Kurachi, Y., Noma, A., and Irisawa, H. (1984). Action potential and membrane currents of single pacemaker cells of the rabbit heart. *Pflügers Arch.* **402**, 248–257.

Nawrath, H. (1977). Does cyclic GMP mediate the negative inotropic effect of acetylcholine in the heart? *Nature* **267**, 72–74.

Neher, E., and Stevens, C. F. (1977). Conductance fluctuations and ionic pores in membranes. *Ann. Rev. Biophys. Bioeng.* **6**, 345–381.

New, W., and Trautwein, W. (1972a). Inward membrane currents in mammalian myocardium. *Pflügers Arch.* **334**, 1–23.

New, W., and Trautwein, W. (1972b). The ionic nature of slow inward current and its relation to contraction. *Pflügers Arch.* **334**, 24–38.

Niedergerke, R., and Page, S. (1977). Analysis of catecholamine effects in single atrial trabeculae of the frog heart. *Proc. R. Soc. Lond. B* **197**, 333–362.

Noble, D., and Tsien, W. (1968). The kinetics and rectifier properties of the slow potassium current in cardiac Purkinje fibres. *J. Physiol.* **195**, 185–214.

Noma, A., and Irisawa, H. (1976a). Membrane currents in the rabbit sinoatrial node cell as studied by the double microelectrode method. *Pflügers Arch.* **364**, 45–52.

Noma, A., and Irisawa, H. (1976b). A time- and voltage-dependent potassium current in the rabbit sinoatrial node cell. *Pflügers Arch.* **366**, 251–258.

Noma, A., and Trautwein, W. (1978). Relaxation of the ACh-induced potassium current in the rabbit sinoatrial node cell. *Pflügers Arch.* **377**, 193–200.

Noma, A., Peper, K., and Trautwein, W. (1979a). Acetylcholine-induced potassium current fluctuations in the rabbit sino-atrial node. *Pflügers Arch.* **381**, 255–263.

Noma, A., Osterrieder, W., and Trautwein, W. (1979b). The effect of external potassium on the elementary conductance of the ACh-induced potassium channel in the sinoatrial node. *Pflügers Arch.* **381**, 263–269.

Noma, A., Kotake, H., and Irisawa, H. (1980). Slow inward current and its role mediating the chronotropic effect of epinephrine in the rabbit sinoatrial node. *Pflügers Arch.* **388**, 1–9.

Ochi, R. (1970). The slow inward current and the action of manganese ions in guinea pig's myocardium. *Pflügers Arch.* **316**, 81–94.

Ojeda, C., Rougier, O., and Tourneur, Y. (1981). Effects of Cs on acetylcholine-induced current; is i_{K1} increased by ACh in frog atrium? *Pflügers Arch.* **391,** 57–59.

Osterrieder, W., Noma, A., and Trautwein, W. (1980). On the kinetics of the potassium channel activated by acetylcholine in the S-A node of the rabbit heart. *Pflügers Arch.* **386,** 101–109.

Osterrieder, W., Yang, Q-F., and Trautwein, W. (1981). The time course of the muscarinic response to ionophoretic acetylcholine application to the S-A node of the rabbit heart. *Pflügers Arch.* **389,** 283–291.

Osterrieder, W., Brum, G., Hescheler, J., Trautwein, W., Flockerzi, V., and Hofmann, F. (1982). Injection of subunits of cyclic AMP-dependent protein kinase into cardiac myocytes modulates Ca^{2+} current. *Nature* **298,** 576–578.

Otsuka, M. (1958). Die Wirkung von Adrenalin auf Purkinje-Fasern von Saügetierherzen. *Pflügers Arch. Ges. Physiol.* **266,** 512–517.

Paes de Carvalho, A. P., Hoffman, B. F., and de Carvalho, M. P. (1969). Two components of the cardiac action potential. I. Voltage–time course and the effect of acetylcholine on atrial and nodal cells of the rabbit heart. *J. Gen. Physiol.* **54,** 607–635.

Pelzer, D., and Trautwein, W. (1981). Zum Mechanismus der negativ inotropen Acetylcholin (ACh)-Wirkung auf das Ventrikelmyokard. *German J. Cardiol.* **70,** 308, R202.

Pott, L. (1979). On the time course of the acetylcholine-induced hyperpolarization in quiescent guinea pig atria. *Pflügers Arch.* **380,** 71–77.

Powell, T., and Twist, V. W. (1976). A rapid technique for the isolation and purification of adult cardiac muscle cells having respiratory control and a tolerance to calcium. *Biochem. Biophys. Res. Comm.* **72,** 327–333.

Powell, T., Terrar, D. A., and Twist, V. W. (1980). Electrical properties of individual cells isolated from adult rat ventricular myocardium. *J. Physiol. (Lond.)* **302,** 131–153.

Prokopczuk, A., Lewartowski, B., and Czarnecka, M. (1973). On the cellular mechanism of the inotropic action of acetylcholine on isolated rabbit and dog atria. *Pflügers Arch. Ges. Physiol.* **339,** 305–316.

Quadbeck, J., and Reiter, M. (1975). Cardiac action potential and inotropic effect of noradrenaline and calcium. *Naunyn-Schmiedebergs Arch. Exp. Path. Pharmakol.* **286,** 337–351.

Rayner, B., and Weatherall, N. (1959). Acetylcholine and potassium movements in rabbit auricles. *J. Physiol. (Lond.)* **146,** 392–409.

Reuter, H. (1967). The dependence of slow inward current in Purkinje fibers on the extracellular calcium-concentration. *J. Physiol. (Lond.)* **192,** 479–492.

Reuter, H. (1974). Localization of beta adrenergic receptors and effects of noradrenaline and cyclic nucleotides on action potentials, ionic currents and tension in mammalian cardiac muscle. *J. Physiol. (Lond.)* **242,** 429–451.

Reuter, H. (1979). Properties of two inward membrane currents in the heart. *Ann. Rev. Physiol.* **41,** 413–424.

Reuter, H. (1980). Effects of neurotransmitters on the slow inward current. *In* "The Slow Inward Current and Cardiac Arrhythmias" (D. P. Zipes, J. C. Bailey, and V. Elharrar, eds.), pp. 205–219. Martinus Nijhoff Publishers, The Hague, Boston, London.

Reuter, H. (1983). Calcium channel modulation by neurotransmitters, enzymes and drugs. *Nature* **301,** 569–574.

Reuter, H. (1984). Ion channels in cardiac cell membranes. *Ann. Rev. Physiol.* **46,** 473–484.

Reuter, H., and Scholz, H. (1977). The regulation of the Ca conductance of cardiac muscle by adrenaline. *J. Physiol. (Lond.)* **264,** 49–62.

Rinaldi, M. L., Capony, J. P., and Demaille, J. G. (1982). The cyclic AMP-dependent modulation of cardiac sarcolemma slow calcium channels. *J. Mol. Cell. Cardiol.* **14,** 279–289.

Robison, G. A., Butcher, R. W., and Sutherland, E. W. (1971). "Cyclic AMP," pp. 22–29. Academic Press, New York and London.

Rougier, O., Vassort, G., Garnier, D., Gargouil, Y. M., and Coraboeuf, E. (1969). Existence and role of a slow inward current during the frog atrial action potential. *Pflügers Arch.* **308**, 91–110.

Rubin, C. S., Ehrlichman, J., and Rosen, O. M. (1972). Molecular forms of a cyclic adenosine 3',5'-monophosphate-dependent protein kinase purified from bovine heart muscle. *J. Biol. Chem.* **247**, 36–44.

Sakmann, B., and Trube, G. (1984a). Conductance properties of single inwardly rectifying potassium channels in ventricular cells from guinea pig-heart. *J. Physiol. (Lond.)* **347**, 641–657.

Sakmann, B., and Trube, G. (1984b). Voltage-dependent inactivation of inward-rectifying single channel currents in the guinea-pig heart cell membrane. *J. Physiol. (Lond.)* **347**, 659–683.

Sakmann, B., Noma, A., and Trautwein, W. (1983). Acetylcholine activation of single muscarinic K+ channels in isolated pacemaker cells of the mammalian heart. *Nature* **303**, 250–253.

Schneider, J. A., and Sperelakis, N. (1975). Slow Ca^{2+} and Na^+ responses induced by isoproterenol and methylxanthines in isolated perfused guinea-pig hearts exposed to elevated K^+. *J. Mol. Cell. Cardiol.* **7**, 249–273.

Sigworth, F. J. (1980). The variance of sodium current fluctuations at the node of Ranvier. *J. Physiol.* **307**, 97–129.

Soejima, M., and Noma, A. (1984). Mode of regulation of the ACh-sensitive K-channel by the muscarinic receptor in rabbit atrial cells. *Pflügers Arch.* **400**, 424–431.

Taniguchi, J., Kokubun, S., Noma, A., and Irisawa, H. (1981). Spontaneously active cells isolated from the sino-atrial and atrio-ventricular nodes from the rabbit heart. *Japan. J. Physiol.* **31**, 547–558.

Ten Eick, R., Nawrath, H., McDonald, T. F., and Trautwein, W. (1976). On the mechanism of the negative inotropic effect of acetylcholine. *Pflügers Arch.* **316**, 207–213.

Trautwein, W. (1982). Effect of acetylcholine on the S-A node of the heart. *In* "Cellular Pacemakers" (D. O. Carpenter, ed.), Vol. 1, pp. 127–160. John Wiley & Sons, Baltimore.

Trautwein, W., and Dudel, J. (1958). Zum Mechanismus der Membranwirkung des Acetylcholin an der Herzmuskelfaser. *Pflügers Arch. Ges. Physiol.* **266**, 324–334.

Trautwein, W., and Kameyama, M. (1985). The mechanism of β-adrenergic regulation of calcium channels: Intracellular injections and patch-clamp studies. *In* "Electrophysiology of Single Cardiac Cells" (D. Noble and T. Powell, eds.), Academic Press, London. In press.

Trautwein, W., and McDonald, T. F. (1978). Current–voltage relations in ventricular muscle preparations from different species. *Pflügers Arch.* **374**, 79–89.

Trautwein, W., and Pelzer, D. (1984). Gating of single calcium channels in the membrane of enzymatically isolated ventricular myocytes from adult mammalian hearts. *In* "Cardiac Electrophysiology and Arrhythmias" (D. P. Zipes, and J. Jalife, eds.). Grune and Stratton, New York. In press.

Trautwein, W., and Pelzer, D. (1985). Voltage-dependent gating of single calcium channels in cardiac cell membranes and its modulation by drugs. *In* "Calcium and Cell Physiology" (D. Marmé, ed.), pp. 55–93. Springer-Verlag Berlin and New York.

Trautwein, W., Kuffler, S. W., and Edwards, C. (1956). Changes in membrane characteristics of heart muscle during inhibition. *J. Gen. Physiol.* **40**, 135–145.

Trautwein, W., Osterrieder, W., and Noma, A. (1981). Potassium channels and the muscarinic receptor in the sino-atrial node of the heart. *In* "Drug Receptors and Their Effectors" (N. Birdsall, ed.), pp. 5–22, Macmillan, London.

Trautwein, W., Taniguchi, J., and Noma, A. (1982). The effects of intracellular cyclic nucleotides on the action potential and the acetylcholine response of isolated cardiac cells. *Pflügers Arch.* **392**, 307–314.

Tsien, R. E., Giles, W., and Greengard, P. (1972). Cyclic AMP mediates the effects of adrenaline on cardiac Purkinje-fibers. *Nature New Biol.* **240**, 181–183.

Tsien, R. W. (1973). Adrenaline-like effects of intracellular iontophoresis of cyclic AMP in cardiac Purkinje fibers. *Nature New Biol.* **245**, 120–122.

Tsien, R. W. (1974). Mode of action of chronotropic agents in cardiac Purkinje fibers. *J. Gen. Physiol.* **64**, 320–345.

Tsien, R. W. (1977). Cyclic AMP and contractile activity in the heart. *Adv. Cyclic Nucleotide Res.* **8**, 363–420.

Tsien, R. W. (1983). Calcium channels in excitable cell membranes. *Ann. Rev. Physiol.* **45**, 341–358.

Vassort, G., Rougier, O., Garnier, D., Sauviat, P., Coraboeuf, E., and Gargouil, Y. M. (1969). Effects of adrenaline on membrane inward currents during the cardiac action potential. *Pflügers Arch.* **309**, 70–81.

Watanabe, A. M., and Besch, H. R. (1974). Cyclic adenosine monophosphate modulation of slow calcium influx channels in guinea pig heart. *Circ. Res.* **35**, 316–324.

Watanabe, A. M., McConnaughey, M. M., Strawbridge, R. A., Fleming, J. W., Jones, L. R., and Besch, H. R. (1978). Muscarinic cholinergic receptor modulation of β-adrenergic receptor affinity for catecholamines. *J. Biol. Chem.* **253**, 4833–4836.

Yanagihara, K., and Irisawa, H. (1980). Inward current activated during hyperpolarization in the rabbit sinoatrial node cell. *Pflügers Arch.* **385**, 11–19.

NOTE

Due to the lengthy process of publication, much new information, for example on the Ca channel phosphorylation hypothesis of the β-adrenergic stimulation, on the basal regulation of Ca conductance, on the existence of a second Ca channel, on the muscarinic regulation of both Ca and K channels, etc., is not included. Hence we must appologize to those colleagues whose relevant work is not quoted.

5

Modulation of Cell Electrical Properties by Peptide Hormones

Robert L. DeHaan

I. INTRODUCTION

Starling (1905) coined the term "hormone" and gave birth to the field of endocrinology shortly after he and Bayliss discovered the first gastrointestinal peptide, secretin (Bayliss and Starling, 1902). In the past 80 years, a wide variety of chemical coordinators of various bodily functions (Gardner and Jensen, 1983) have been included among the hormones. These are biologically active agents of varied molecular structure that are carried through the bloodstream from their site of synthesis to a target cell, where they exert their effects by binding to specific receptors. Peptide hormones include molecules in a wide range of sizes and amino acid sequences: the neurohypophyseal agonists, vasopressin and oxytocin; pituitary peptides, such as adrenocorticotropic hormone (ACTH), luteinizing hormone (LH), and growth hormone; a group of releasing hormones, such as corticotropin-releasing factor (CRF), thyrotropin-releasing hormone (TRH), gonadotropin-releasing hormone, and somatostatin; the peptide components of the gastrointestinal endocrine system (Walsh, 1981), including cholecystokinin (CCK), gastrin, bombesin, substance P, and vasoactive intestinal polypeptide (VIP); and a group of agents that encompasses insulin and the polypeptide growth factors (James and Bradshaw, 1984). Each of these polypeptides has metabolic or secretagogic effects that are amply documented; in addition, many produce changes in the bioelectric properties of target cells that are less often recognized. Our purpose here is to determine how widespread these effects may be and to consider what role they may have in regulation of cell function.

Peptide hormones can exhibit pleiotropic actions by binding to different recep-

129

tors or by activating more than one type of intracellular mediator. Although many hormones are known to utilize cyclic AMP as a second messenger, most of the peptide regulators exert some or all of their actions by postreceptor mechanisms that do not involve the adenyl cyclase system. Many work instead through a calcium messenger system (Rasmussen and Barrett, 1984) and have therefore come to be termed the calcium-releasing hormones. For example, vasopressin exerts its antidiuretic effects through a cAMP-dependent process, whereas its vasoactive and glycogenolytic actions are mediated by cAMP-independent Ca-regulating mechanisms (Michell et al., 1979; Jard, 1983). Similarly, insulin binds with low affinity to IGF-I receptors (Czech et al., 1983) to modulate a sequence of growth-promoting processes, including some that involve the adenyl cyclase system (Gospodarowicz, 1981). Occupancy of the high-affinity insulin-specific receptor is thought, however, to regulate membrane transport of ions and other components, as well as cell membrane potential, through a multiplicity of cAMP-independent processes (Avruch et al., 1982a; Resh et al., 1980; Moore, 1983; Jarett et al., 1985).

Many of the peptide regulators found originally in the gut, skin, or mesodermally derived tissues have been reported to be synthesized also in cells of the brain or peripheral nervous system (Krieger, 1983; Rehfeld et al., 1985). In addition to those associated with the neurosecretory system (for review, see Sladek and Sladek, 1985), such as vasopressin, oxytocin, ACTH, LH, and others, these brain peptides include CCK, bombesin, substance P, and VIP, as well as insulin, enkephalin, and glucagon. These substances are not distributed homogeneously, but are localized in cells in different parts of the brain. Insulin is present at high concentrations in the hypothalamus and limbic areas and in certain cell bodies in the neocortex. CCK and VIP are found primarily in cortical areas. Indeed, CCK appears to be present at higher concentrations in the mammalian neocortex than in the gastrointestinal tract (Krieger, 1983). Peptides can be found also in peripheral nerves, often localized with classical neurotransmitters. Hoekfelt et al. (1980) have found serotonin, substance P, and thyrotropin-releasing hormone together in individual neurons of the medulla oblongata; mesencephalic cells contain CCK and dopamine; and VIP and acetylcholine coexist in cells of certain autonomic ganglia. The brain peptide, neuropeptide Y (NPY) (Tatemoto et al., 1982) has been localized in high concentrations in nerve fibers supplying the human heart (Gu et al., 1983). NPY was especially rich in the innervation of the SA and AV nodes and the coronary vessels and was found intermingled with cholinergic and adrenergic neurons (Gu et al., 1984). This close association of neuropeptides and neurotransmitters suggests that substances that function as secretagogues or endocrine hormones in the gut or other organs may serve as modulators of neural or neurotransmitter function in the nervous system and heart (Bousfield, 1985).

Bayliss and Starling chose "hormone" from the Greek word meaning to set in motion. We have tried to assemble here a body of evidence showing that a

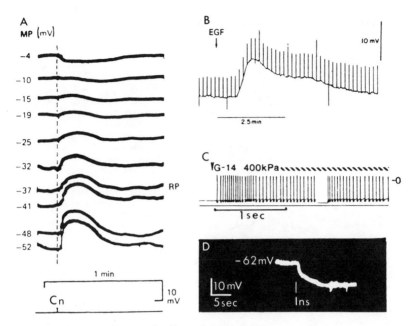

Fig. 1. Representative bioelectric effects of peptide hormones.

(a) Transient depolarization of a pancreatic acinar cell, recorded at different membrane potentials with a microelectrode, in response to repeated 100-msec iontophoretic pulses of caerulein. The resting membrane potential (RP) was −37 mV. The membrane potential of the cell was shifted by passing hyperpolarizing or depolarizing currents through a second microelectrode inserted into a neighboring cell. The ejection current applied to the caerulein micropipette was −100 nA. The null potential at which the peptide-evoked response reversed direction was approximately −10 mV. [Reproduced from Petersen and Philpott (1979) with permission.]

(b) Depolarization of a mitotically quiescent cultured BSC-1 cell in response to rapid superfusion with solution containing 12 ng/ml EGF. Resting membrane potential was −52 mV; cell input resistance was monitored by constant current pulses passed through the microelectrode at 10-sec intervals. Exchange of bath dead space took about 50 sec, indicating that the latency for onset of depolarization was 5–10 sec. [Reproduced from Rothenberg *et al.* (1982) with permission.]

(c) The excitatory action of G-14 on spontaneous firing of a CA1 pyramidal neuron in a rat, isolated hippocampal-slice preparation. The downward arrow indicates onset of pressure ejection of the peptide from a multibarreled pipette located near the cell body. The gastrin response shown was virtually identical to that of CCK-8. [Reproduced from Dodd and Kelly (1981) with permission.]

(d) Hyperpolarizing response of a rat caudofemoralis muscle fiber to abrupt superfusion with porcine insulin. The hormone was pressure ejected from a wide-bore pipette positioned near the surface of the muscle. The electrode was inserted in a surface fiber resting at −62 mV. [Reproduced from Zierler and Rogus (1981b) with permission.]

substantial number of the peptide hormones act on the electrical properties of target cells. In many cases, the resulting changes in transmembrane ion fluxes or cell membrane potential have been demonstrated to precede the metabolic or other effects of hormone binding. Most of the brain–gut peptides evoke depolarizing or excitatory responses, as exemplified in Figs. 1a–c. Insulin and the

TABLE I

Peptides That Alter Membrane Electrical Properties

Hormone	Amino acids	Bioelectric effects
		Brain–gut peptides
TRH	3	Stimulates Ca action potentials in pituitary cells [35,36,37].
Oxytocin	8	Depolarizes and stimulates action potentials in uterine smooth muscle [1,25] and in molluscan ganglion cells [24].
Vasopressin	9	Activates Na influx in toad urinary bladder [2] and in Swiss 3T3 cells [4]; depolarizes and stimulates firing of rat CNS neurons [3] and molluscan ganglion cells [24].
Caerulein	10	Depolarizes pancreatic acinar cells; decreases input resistance [7].
Substance P	11	Depolarizes parotid acinar cells [26] and spinal neurons [6].
Bombesin	14	Depolarizes pancreatic acinar cells [7,8]; depolarizes and stimulates hippocampal neurons [5].
Somatostatin	14	Depolarizes and increases firing rate of CNS neurons [5].
CCK-PZ	33	Depolarizes and decreases input resistance of acinar cells [9]; activates Ca-dependent cation channels [10]; depolarizes and stimulates firing of CNS neurons [5,27].
Gastrin	34	Depolarizes and decreases input resistance of pancreatic acinar cells [8]; depolarizes and stimulates firing of CNS neurons [5,27].
NPY	36	Stimulates contraction of arterial smooth muscle [14].
CRF	41	Stimulates firing and blocks afterhyperpolarization of CNS neurons [23].
		Polypeptide growth factors
Insulin	51	Hyperpolarizes skeletal muscle [20,28], heart [30,31], fat cells [18], and gastric mucosa [19]; hyperpolarizes [22] or depolarizes [15] liver; stimulates Na–K pump [17,20,34] and Na–K ATPase [29,34]; stimulates Na influx [20] and microsomal Ca uptake [21]; slows cardiac beat rate [30,32]; activates K current [33].
EGF	53	Depolarizes BSC-1 monkey kidney and A431 carcinoma cells [11,12]; increases cytosolic Ca [12,13].
IGF-II (MSA)	67	Slows beat rate of heart cell aggregates [32].
NGF	118	Stimulates Na–K pump; increases intracellular Na [16].
PDGF	165	Stimulates increase of cytosolic Ca [13].

Abbreviations: CCK-PZ, cholecystokinin-pancreozymin; CRF, corticotropin-releasing factor; EGF, epidermal growth factor; IFG-II, insulin-like growth factor (multiplication-stimulating activity); NGF, nerve growth factor; NPY, neuropeptide Y; PDGF, platelet-derived growth factor; TRH, thyrotropin-releasing hormone.

References: [1] Woodbury and McIntyre (1954); [2] Palmer and Edelman (1981); [3] Muhlethaler et al. (1982); [4] Mendoza et al. (1980); [5] Dodd and Kelly (1981); [6] Konishi and Otsuka (1974); [7] Petersen and Philpott (1979); [8] Iwatsuki and Petersen (1978); [9] Iwatsuki et al. (1977); [10] Maruyama and Petersen (1982); [11] Rothenberg et al. (1982); [12] Sawyer and Cohen (1981); [13] Moolenaar et al. (1984); [14] Edvinsson et al. (1983); [15] Wondergem (1983); [16] Yankner and Shooter (1982); [17] Flatman and Clausen (1979); [18] Beigelman and Hollander (1965); [19] Rehm et al. (1961); [20] Moore (1981); [21] McDonald et al. (1978); [22] Frol'kiss (1977); [23] Siggins et al. (1985); [24] Barker and Smith (1980); [25] Creed (1979); [26] Gallacher and Petersen (1980); [27] Phillis and Kirkpatrick (1979); [28] Zierler (1957); [29] McGeoch (1983); [30] LaManna and Ferrier (1981); [31] Lantz et al. (1980); [32] DeHaan et al. (1984); [33] Ayer et al. (1986); [34] Hougen et al. (1978); [35] Kidokoro (1975); [36] Ozawa and Kimura (1979); [37] Barker et al. (1983).

insulin-like growth factors tend to have hyperpolarizing effects on target cells (Fig. 1d). In Table I, a number of brain–gut peptides and peptide growth factors are listed in order of increasing molecular size, with documented examples of their effects on ion transport, cell membrane potential, excitability, or other membrane electrical properties.

II. THE BRAIN–GUT PEPTIDES

A. Thyrotropin-Releasing Hormone

TRH was isolated orginally from the hypothalamus as the tripeptide amide pyroGlu—His—Pro—NH_2 and was shown to cause release of thyrotropin and prolactin from the pituitary. It is widely distributed in neurons and nerve terminals in the central and peripheral nervous systems and has generally excitatory effects, including antagonism of sedative drugs, tachycardia, tachypnea, and increased blood pressure (Walsh, 1981). In pituitary tumor (GH_3) cells in culture, TRH causes a biphasic response consisting of an initial hyperpolarization (Barker et al., 1983; Dubinsky and Oxford, 1985) followed by a long-lasting depolarization that stimulates trains of Ca action potentials (Ozawa and Kimura, 1979).

B. Oxytocin and Vasopressin

The neurohypophyseal hormones of mammals are nonapeptides whose cyclic structure results from a disulfide bridge between cysteine residues 1 and 6 (for review, see Muhlethaler et al., 1984). In addition to being secreted into the circulation as neuroendocrine hormones, these peptides are found in the nervous system of most vertebrates (Crim and Vigna, 1983), where accumulating evidence suggests that they act as neurotransmitters or neuromodulators (Dreifuss et al., 1982; Muhlethaler et al., 1983). Similar peptides are also widespread in invertebrates, suggesting that these molecules are evolutionarily stable (Greenberg and Prince, 1983).

In mammals, vasopressin (VP) has multiple effects on a range of target cells. It is a potent stimulant of vascular smooth-muscle contraction and liver-glycogen breakdown, and it has well-known effects on the kidneys, from which it derives its alternate name of antidiuretic hormone. The antidiuretic and vasopressor effects of VP are mediated via different mechanisms involving occupancy of separate isoreceptors (Michell et al., 1979; Jard, 1983). VP reduces water permeability of the renal collecting ducts and solute transport of the ascending limb of Henle's loop through V_2 receptors, with an increase in cAMP production.

Conversely, stimulation of liver glycogenolysis and contraction of vascular smooth muscle, which are mediated by VP binding to V_1 receptors, are not accompanied by an increase in intracellular cAMP, but are associated with increased phosphatidylinositol breakdown (Michell et al., 1979; Nishizuka et al., 1984).

Four examples of VP effects on the bioelectric properties of cell membranes are available. (1) Recording membrane potential with intracellular micro-electrodes, Muhlethaler et al. (1982) reported that VP caused depolarization and a sustained increase in firing rate of pyramidal cells in the CA1 area of the rat hippocampus. Threshold concentration of the hormone was about 10 nM. (2) Palmer and Edelman (1981) measured current–voltage curves of toad, urinary-bladder epithelia in the presence and absence of sodium transport and were able to derive an I_{Na}–V relationship representing the amiloride-sensitive sodium permeability of the apical membrane (Lewis et al., 1984). Sodium transport increased rapidly, reaching a peak approximately 15 min after application of the hormone. This effect resulted from activation of quiescent sodium channels in the apical membrane, rather than from a change in single-channel properties (Li et al., 1982). Similar conclusions were reached by Helman et al. (1981) regarding VP-induced increases in sodium conductance in frog skin. (3) The addition of VP to Swiss 3T3 or MDCK cells caused a rapid increase in sodium ion influx across the membrane (Mendoza et al., 1980; Reznik et al., 1985). Elevation of Rb transport by the Na–K pump was detectable within 2 min after application of the hormone, as a result of an increased rate of Na entry. When the Na–K pump was inhibited by ouabain, VP increased intracellular Na concentration markedly, whereas cell K was unaltered. These results suggest that the primary effect of VP was increased Na entry, which resulted in stimulation of the Na–K pump. Thus VP action on Swiss 3T3 cells resembled that on bladder and skin epithelia. (4) Ganglion cell 11 of the mollusc Otala is either silent or displays a low frequency of rhythmic spiking. Vasopressin at nanomolar concentrations initiated dose-dependent bursting by increasing a voltage-sensitive sodium current (Barker and Smith, 1980). Oxytocin (OX) had a similar effect and was equally potent.

In mammalian uterine smooth muscle, OX has pronounced electrophysiological effects. The nonpregnant uterus shows slow bursts of action potential spikes. During pregnancy, the uterus becomes progesterone dominated, and bursting ceases as the smooth muscle is hyperpolarized. As parturition approaches, the sensitivity of the muscle to OX increases dramatically, and exposure to the hormone yields rapid, spontaneous spike bursts (Creed, 1979; Kuriyama and Suzuki, 1976). With intracellular microelectrodes, Woodbury and McIntyre (1954) recorded stable resting potentials averaging -44.7 mV from segments of pregnant rabbit uterus. After application of a supramaximal dose of OX, V_m shifted to $+22$ mV and remained at that level for several hours. The authors postulated that oxytocin reversal of V_m resulted from a sharp increase in membrane sodium permeability to a point greatly exceeding that for potassium.

C. Substance P

Substance P is an undecapeptide, isolated originally from equine gut and brain by von Euler and Gaddum (1931) and analyzed structurally by Chang *et al.* (1971). Lembeck (1953) found the peptide concentrated in the dorsal root of mammalian spinal nerves and suggested that it could act as an excitatory transmitter for spinal neurons. This hypothesis was confirmed by Konishi and Otsuka (1974) when their isolated spinal cord preparation from newborn rat was superfused with micromolar concentrations of substance P. These workers found that a depolarization accompanied by spike discharges could be recorded within seconds. The preparation's sensitivity to the depolarizing action of substance P was approximately 200 times greater than that to L-glutamate, which is regarded as an effective excitatory neurotransmitter in the spinal cord. Substance P has been reported also to cause excitation in the Betz cells of the cerebral cortex (Phillis and Limacher, 1974), but was not excitatory when applied to glutamate-sensitive pyramidal neurons of the mammalian hippocampus (Dodd and Kelly, 1981). In the chick dorsal root ganglion, all of the cell bodies that exhibited immunoreactivity to substance P were found to derive from the embryonic neural crest (Fontaine-Perus *et al.,* 1985). Interestingly, substance P inhibits nicotinic release from adrenal chromaffin cells (another neural crest derivative) and reduces their Ach-activated current (Clapham and Neher, 1985; Livett, 1984). In a nonneural tissue, Gallacher and Petersen (1980) found that substance P produced a 10- to 15-mV depolarization and decrease in input resistance of rat parotid gland acinar cells that resembled the response to acetylcholine. Minimal latency of the response was 1.7 msec. The null potential for the salivary gland response was approximately -60 mV, indicating that the induced ionic permeabilities included a substantial K component (Roberts *et al.,* 1978). In this tissue, the depolarization was followed within a few seconds by a transient 5- to 10-mV afterhyperpolarization (AHP). The AHP was ouabain sensitive and could be blocked by perfusion with Na-free or K-free solution, indicating that it was caused by an electrogenic Na–K pump. Haddas *et al.* (1979) found, however, that the pump stimulation was also Ca dependent and could be mimicked by exposure of cells to the Ca ionophore A23187. This suggests the possible involvement of a calcium-activated K current.

D.   Bombesin, Gastrin, Caerulein, and Cholecystokinin

Cholecystokinin (CCK) was isolated originally as a 33 amino-acid peptide (CCK-33) from hog intestine along with a 39 amino-acid variant (CCK-39). More recent studies have shown that the amidated C-terminal octapeptide (CCK-8) has all of the biological activity of the parent molecule, but is approximately 10 times more potent (for reviews, see Walsh, 1981; Gardner and

Jensen, 1983). As a gut peptide, a major role of CCK is to increase enzyme secretion from the pancreas. Two other peptide secretagogues that are structurally similar to CCK, and seem to interact with the same glycoprotein receptor (Rosenzweig *et al.*, 1984), are gastrin and caerulein. Like CCK, gastrin has been found in different molecular sizes, containing 34, 17, and 14 amino acids (G-34, G-17, and G-14), and it shares a common C-terminal pentapeptide amide sequence with CCK. Caerulein is a decapeptide, isolated originally from the skin of the frog *Hyla caerulea*, that shares seven of its eight C-terminal amino acids with CCK.

There are two other classes of cAMP-independent peptide secretagogues that can produce bioelectric effects in target cells. One includes a family of bombesin-like molecules, which were also isolated originally from the skins of various frogs, for which they were named (see Crim and Vigna, 1983). Bombesin, from *Bombina bombina*, has 14 residues. The 27 amino-acid, gastrin-releasing peptide (GRP), shares 9 of the 10 C-terminal amino acids with bombesin. The physalaemin-like dodecapeptides form the third group of compounds with secretagogic activity. This group includes substance P.

It appears that the CCK peptides serve as excitatory neurotransmitters or neuromodulators. They are widely distributed in the central and peripheral nervous systems (Hoekfelt *et al.*, 1980, 1985; Krieger, 1983). CCK-33, CCK-8, and the biologically active C-terminal tetrapeptide (CCK-4) are present in the neocortex, hippocampus, amygdala, hypothalamus, and spinal cord, whereas bombesin has been identified in vagal and enteric neurons. Snyder *et al.* (1981) suggested that CCK-4 may be the specific brain-type peptide. An excitatory action of iontophoretically applied CCK was first observed in hypothalamic neurons by Oomura *et al.* (1978), and the peptide was shown to cause tetrodotoxin-insensitive depolarization of both dorsal and ventral roots in the toad spinal-cord preparation (Phillis and Kirkpatrick, 1979). CCK-8 and CCK-4 are potent excitants of pyramidal cells in rat hippocampal-slice preparations (Dodd and Kelly, 1981), and of granule cells in the dentate gyrus (Brooks and Kelly, 1985). Within seconds after application, these peptides caused depolarization that initiated firing or produced a dramatic increase in rate of CA1 cells. Similar effects were produced by gastrin fragments G-13 and G-14 (Fig. 1c) and by bombesin. In some preparations, substance P also had CCK-like effects (Willetts *et al.*, 1985).

In pancreatic acinar cells impaled with intracellular microelectrodes, short iontophoretic pulses of bombesin or caerulein at micromolar levels caused a muscarinic-like depolarization of 7–10 mV (Fig. 2a) with latencies of 500–1400 msec (Petersen and Philpott, 1979). By applying depolarizing or hyperpolarizing current in a neighboring coupled cell, Petersen and Philpott (1979) found that the amplitude of the peptide-evoked response could be decreased or increased, and its polarity reversed (Fig. 1a). The reversal potential for both caerulein and

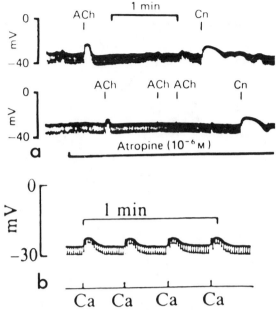

Fig. 2. Transient depolarizations in pancreatic acinar cells. (a) Similar effects of iontophoresis of acetylcholine (ACh) and caerulein (Cn) on cell membrane potential and input resistance. In the presence of atropine (1 μM), the response to ACh was blocked with no effect on the Cn-evoked depolarization, indicating that the two ligands acted through different receptors. Brief hyperpolarizing currents (2 nA, 100 msec) were passed through the intracellular electrode to monitor input resistance. [Reproduced from Petersen and Philpott (1979) with permission.] (b) Response of a similar cell to intracellular iontophoretic injection of $CaCl_2$. [From Iwatsuki and Petersen (1977). Reprinted with permission from *Nature* Vol. 268, pp. 147–149. Copyright © 1977 Macmillan Journals Limited.]

bombesin was −10 to −15 mV. A similar response with a reversal potential at −16 mV could be elicited by injections of calcium into the cells (Fig. 2b; Petersen and Iwatsuki, 1978). Gastrin had a similar depolarizing effect (Iwatsuki *et al.*, 1977). Because of the sequence homologies among gastrin, caerulein, and the terminal sequence of CCK, these substances are believed to share a common receptor on the acinar cell membrane. From CCK-binding studies, Jensen *et al.* (1980) estimated that there were approximately 10,000 receptors per acinar cell. Separate receptors exist for bombesin and substance P. But all three receptor types seem to share a common postreceptor mechanism with the muscarinic ACh receptor. This mechanism does not involve the adenyl cyclase system (Petersen, 1981), but depends on mobilization of intracellular calcium (Michell *et al.*, 1979; Gardner and Jensen, 1983). Using the patch-clamp technique of Sakmann and Neher (1983), Maruyama and Petersen (1982) identified a nonspecific cation channel in the acinar cell membrane that could account for the peptidergic

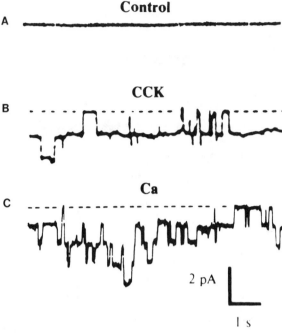

Fig. 3. Cholecystokinin activation of single-channel currents in pancreatic acinar cells. Patch-electrode recordings from a cell-attached membrane patch superfused with (a) control solution or (b) CCK-8 reveal the presence of a 35-pS peptide-activated channel. When a patch was excised from the cell in the presence of the CCK antagonist, dibutyryl cyclic GMP, similar channels could be activated (c) by exposing the cytoplasmic membrane surface to a Ca-containing solution. [Reproduced from Maruyama and Petersen (1982) with permission.]

depolarization. In cell-attached experiments, the channel was activated equally well by ACh or CCK-8 applied outside the patch pipette (Figs. 3a,b). With either agonist, a delay of 10–40 sec between exposure and channel activation allowed ample time for intracellular diffusion of second messenger molecules and a variety of possible metabolic events. In its conductance properties, this channel was shown to resemble the Ca-activated channel in the cardiac cell membrane (Colquhoun *et al.*, 1981): the channel did not discriminate strongly between monovalent cations; it had a conductance of approximately 35 pS; and it could be blocked by dibutyryl cGMP. In excised membrane patches, no channel activity was seen in calcium-free solution, but the CCK activation of the channel could be mimicked (Fig. 3c) by raising the calcium concentration on the cytoplasmic surface to 300 μM (Petersen and Maruyama, 1983). In more recent experiments, using the same techniques, Petersen and Maruyama (1984) have seen a Ca-activated potassium-selective channel, as well, in the acinar cell membrane.

Thus calcium must be considered an obvious candidate for the second messenger in peptide-evoked changes in membrane potential. (Willetts *et al.*, 1985).

E. Neuropeptide Y

Tatemoto *et al.* (1982) isolated a 36 amino-acid peptide amide from porcine brain (NPY), which resembles the pancreatic hormonal peptide PP and the gut peptide known as PYY. The nerve supply to the cerebral arteries, the coronary vessels of the heart, and the sinoatrial and atrioventricular nodes includes subpopulations of fibers that are immunoreactive for NPY (Gu *et al.*, 1984; Allen *et al.*, 1985). Isolated segments of cat middle-cerebral arteries contracted when exposed to NPY. The response had a rapid onset (seconds), it was concentration dependent in the range of 20–200 nM, and it could be blocked by removal of calcium from the bathing medium or by calcium antagonists (Edvinsson *et al.*, 1983; Edvinsson, 1985). Because of this prominent vasoconstrictor effect and the rich innervation of cardiac nodal tissue with NPY-containing fibers, Gu *et al.* (1983) proposed that NPY may serve as a major cardiac neuropeptide.

F. Corticotropin-Releasing Factor

CRF is a 41-residue neuropeptide with potent corticotropin-releasing activity, first isolated by Vale *et al.* (1981). Ehlers *et al.* (1983) suggested that the peptide may be a regulator of brain excitability. Valentino *et al.* (1983) demonstrated that CRF injections caused increases in spontaneous spike discharge of individual neurons in the rat locus coeruleus. In an *in vitro* hippocampal-slice preparation, superfusion with CRF concentrations greater than 250 nM depolarized both CA1 and CA3 pyramidal neurons and caused increases in spontaneous firing rate and input resistance. At lower concentrations (10–200 nM), CRF reduced the magnitude and duration of the afterhyperpolarizations that normally followed current-evoked bursts of action potentials (Siggins *et al.*, 1985). Because these AHPs were tetrodotoxin resistant and were prevented by calcium blockers, Siggins *et al.* (1985) concluded that CRF functions by reducing a calcium-activated K conductance in the neurons.

III. THE POLYPEPTIDE GROWTH FACTORS

Approximately 40 peptide growth factors (PGFs) have now been recognized; many of these have been isolated and purified. All have specific high-affinity receptors. These substances appear to be synthesized as part of larger precursor molecules and are released slowly from the site of synthesis into the bloodstream in a steady flow. The PGFs can be grouped structurally by amino-acid-sequence homology into three categories: (1) the insulin-like growth factors such as IGF-I and IGF-II, nerve growth factor (NGF), relaxin, and insulin (Bradshaw and Niall, 1978; Blundell *et al.*, 1983); (2) a group that includes epidermal growth factor (EGF) and several transforming growth factors (TGFs) (Marquardt *et al.*, 1983); and (3) a subset comprising platelet-derived growth factor (PDGF), fibroblast-derived growth factor (FDGF), and osteosarcoma-derived growth factor (ODGF) (Dicker *et al.*, 1981). All of these substances are known to regulate a wide variety of metabolic and transport processes in cells and to trigger a cascade of biochemical and physiological changes in many cells (for reviews, see Bradshaw and Rubin, 1980; James and Bradshaw, 1984).

A.   Insulin and the Insulin-Like Growth Factors

All vertebrates possess a family of polypeptide hormones that includes insulin and several insulin-like growth factors, or somatomedins. The latter include IGF-I (which is homologous to somatomedin C), IGF-II or multiplication-stimulating activity, relaxin, and the more distantly related nerve growth factor. All of these peptides share substantial sequence homology with insulin (Blundell *et al.*, 1983), and they exhibit an overlapping series of regulatory functions, some prominent only during embryonic development. These include modulation of membrane transport, stimulation of RNA, DNA, and protein synthesis, and mitogenesis. It has been reported recently that insulin initiates development of electrotonic coupling between sympathetic neurons (Kessler *et al.*, 1984). The role and mechanism of action of insulin and the IGFs have been reviewed by Bradshaw and Rubin (1980) and Czech (1984).

1.   Receptors for Insulin and the IGFs

Mammalian cells share three different receptors to which insulin-like peptides can bind (Czech *et al.*, 1983; Jacobs and Cuatracasas, 1983; Rechler and Nissley, 1985). These have been isolated and purified (Jacobs *et al.*, 1980; Yip *et al.*, 1980; Czech and Massague, 1982; Endo and Elsas, 1984), and the complete 1370 amino-acid sequence of the human insulin proreceptor has been deduced (Ullrich *et al.*, 1985). The insulin receptor and that for IGF-I are similar in structure. Both are integral-membrane heterotetrameric-glycoprotein complexes, with a native relative molecular weight (M_r) of approximately 350,000. The complex consists of two 125,000-Da alpha subunits and two 90,000-Da beta subunits, joined by disulfide linkages. After isolation with cross-linking agents, insulin is found associated with the alpha subunit. But the minimal insulin binding site is apparently the alpha–beta dimer (Fujita-Yamaguchi *et al.*, 1983; Czech, 1985). The two subunits are found together in the membrane even when they are not linked by disulfide bonds (Chvatchko *et al.*, 1984) and are apparently synthesized intracellularly as a single-chain proreceptor (Deutsch *et al.*, 1983). This macromolecule is later cleaved into mature disulfide-linked subunits and glycosylated before insertion into the plasma membrane (Ronnett *et al.*, 1984). It is now clear that the beta subunit has a tyrosine-selective protein kinase catalytic site at the inner surface of the cell membrane, which causes autophosphorylation of the subunit when insulin occupies the extracellular binding site on the alpha subunit (Avruch *et al.*, 1982b; Kasuga *et al.*, 1982; Blackshear *et al.*, 1984), but the role of this autophosphorylation is unknown (Simpson and Hedo, 1984; Czech, 1985).

The IGF-II receptor is a single polypeptide chain of M_r 220,000 (Massague and Czech, 1982). Jacobs and Cuatracasas (1983) have suggested that this may be a form of the alpha–beta proreceptor that has not been subjected to the same posttranslational cleavage and processing before insertion into the membrane.

As indicated, each PGF has its own specific receptor to which binding is strongest. However, insulin and the IGFs all cross-react to some extent with receptors for other members of the IGF family. For example, IGF-I and IGF-II bind to each other's receptors with affinities only slightly less than to their own (Massague and Czech, 1982). Both peptides bind to the insulin receptor, but with considerably lower affinities; in isolated adipocytes, the IGF-II binding coefficient is approximately 2.5%, and the IGF-I is less than 1% that of insulin (Blundell *et al.*, 1983). Insulin binds weakly to the IGF-I receptor and with even lower affinity to the IGF-II receptor. In both mammalian and avian cells, insulin binding gave curvilinear Scatchard plots, demonstrating more complex kinetics than expected from a single ligand–receptor interaction (Olefsky and Chang, 1978; Wheeler *et al.*, 1980; Serravezza *et al.*, 1981). Such binding behavior reflects negatively cooperative receptor events (DeMeyts and Roth, 1975), conformational changes within the receptor, or occupancy of two or more receptor classes with different affinities (for review, see Gammeltoft, 1984). When we analyzed insulin binding to embryonic chick heart cells according to a two-receptor model (Wheeler *et al.*, 1980; Serravezza *et al.*, 1981), two distinct functional responses to insulin could be identified and correlated with occupancy of either the high- or low-affinity receptor class. One response was an insulin-induced hyperpolarization (IIH), which occurred rapidly, with a half-maximal effective hormone concentration of 1.7 n*M* (Lantz *et al.*, 1980). This ouabain-insensitive response resulted from an increase in net outward current (Fischmeister *et al.*, 1983) and was sufficient to account for the prolongation of the interbeat interval of spontaneously beating heart cell aggregates (DeHaan *et al.*, 1984; see below). The second response was stimulation of A-amino-acid transport. This response was slower to develop and required approximately 25 n*M* hormone for half-maximal effect (Elsas *et al.*, 1975; Wheeler *et al.*, 1978). Moreover, the lower-affinity receptor effect could be mimicked by IGF-II, which demonstrated preferential binding (Wheeler *et al.*, 1980).

2. Postreceptor Events

After insulin binds to its surface receptor, there occur several rapid responses that are analogous to receptor activation in other systems. These include covalent modification of the receptor (Petruzelli *et al.*, 1982) and tyrosine-specific auto-phosphorylation of its beta subunit (Kasuga *et al.*, 1982; Blackshear *et al.*, 1984), stimulation of transmembrane transport of ions (Fehlmann and Freychet, 1981; Moore, 1983; Gelehrter *et al.*, 1984) and organic molecules (Wheeler *et al.*, 1978), generation of intracellular insulin mediators (Jarett *et al.*, 1985), stimulation of phospholipid methylation (Kelly *et al.*, 1984), increased incorporation of ^{32}P into phosphatidylinositol (Garcia-Sainz and Fain, 1980), uptake of Ca by endoplasmic reticulum (McDonald *et al.*, 1978), and a negative shift in membrane potential (Zierler, 1972).

3. Electrophysiological Effects of Insulin

In 1957, Zierler reported that insulin increased the potential difference and altered the distribution of Na and K across rat skeletal-muscle membrane. This observation has since been confirmed and extended (Zierler, 1972; Flatman and Clausen, 1979; Zierler and Rogus, 1981a,b). A similar hyperpolarizing effect of the hormone has been described in other tissues (reviewed in Zierler and Rogus, 1981a; Moore, 1983; Zierler, 1985; see Table I). These include frog skeletal muscle (Moore, 1973; Moore and Rabovsky, 1979); rat, dog, kitten (LaManna and Ferrier, 1981), and embryonic chick (Lantz *et al.*, 1980) cardiac tissue; and rat skeletal muscle *in vivo* (Frol'kis, 1977). In frog heart, Voorhees *et al.* (1978) found that insulin blocked the cardioacceleratory action of epinephrine. The hormone caused a similar negative voltage shift in rat adipocytes (Beigelman and Hollander, 1965), in frog gastric mucosa (Rehm *et al.*, 1961), and in rat liver *in situ* (Frol'kis, 1977). In contrast, Wondergem (1983) found that insulin (1.3–130 n*M*) caused a slowly developing depolarization in rat hepatocytes in culture, accompanied by an increase in cell input resistance. Most of the IIH effects were on the order of 3–10 mV. However, Beigelman and Hollander (1965) reported a mean hyperpolarization of 22 mV. With 14-day chick embryo ventricle cells, Lantz *et al.* (1980) obtained negative voltage shifts of up to 19 mV, and occasionally more than 50 mV, in low-K (1.3 m*M*) medium. In frog skeletal muscle and mammalian heart, these responses were blocked by cardiac glycosides, suggesting that the effect depended on stimulation of the electrogenic Na–K pump (Moore, 1983); however, in chick embryo heart (Lantz *et al.*, 1980) and in rat skeletal muscle (Zierler and Rogus, 1981c), the effect was ouabain resistant. In both of these cases, the response was evoked by physiological (nanomolar) concentrations of hormone and began within seconds after exposure (Zierler and Rogus, 1981b).

In a spontaneously beating cardiac preparation, a hyperpolarizing response would slow the beat rate. This is the mechanism of the negative chronotropic effects of muscarinic agonists and adenosine on the heart (Galper et al., 1982; Creazzo et al., 1985; Halvorsen et al., 1983; Belardinelli and Isenberg, 1983). In this laboratory, insulin-induced slowing of the beat rate was observed first in preliminary experiments with spherical aggregates prepared from 7-day embryonic chick ventricle cells, exposed to high concentrations of the hormone (Shipley and DeHaan, 1981), and a similar response has been reported in canine false tendons (LaManna and Ferrier, 1981). Recently, we have determined the dose response for insulin slowing by measuring the spontaneous beat rate of groups of superfused aggregates (DeHaan et al., 1984). During steady superfusion with insulin-free bovine serum albumin (BSA) buffer, the mean beat rate of aggregates fluctuated generally by less than 10% over several hours. Switching to a solution that contained insulin resulted consistently in a prolongation of the interbeat interval (Fig. 4, inset). The response began with a latency of less than 1 min and was maximal after approximately 20 min (23°C). The degree of slowing was dose dependent, with a half-maximal effect at 1.7 nM (Fig. 4, main curve). IGF-II at similar concentrations was equally effective. At supramaximal concentrations above 100 nM, the response was attenuated, and at very low concentrations, into the femtomolar range, there was a consistent, statistically significant response that was 10–20% of the maximum.

The physiological effect can be related to receptor occupancy by superimposing the dose–response curve of Fig. 4 on binding curves obtained with ^{125}I-labeled insulin on 7-day heart cells under identical culture conditions (Fig. 5; R. L. DeHaan, E. Strumlauf, and L. J. Elsas, unpublished). Here, binding was analyzed, according to a two-receptor model (Wheeler et al., 1980), to yield a population of approximately 600 high-affinity receptors ($K_A = 6 \times 10^8\ M^{-1}$) and 9000 low-affinity receptors ($K_A = 1.5 \times 10^7\ M^{-1}$) per cell. Although the exact correspondence of the concentration (1.7 nM) that produces half-maximal slowing and 50% occupancy of the high-affinity receptor is probably fortuitous, the similarity of the two curves suggests that the slowing response may be mediated by hormone binding to the high-affinity receptor. By similar logic, we might speculate that occupancy of the low-affinity (IGF?) receptor counters insulin's hyperpolarizing action to produce the observed supramaximal reversal of the slowing response. This idea is given some credence by observations of the interaction between insulin and the jack bean lectin concanavalin A (Con A). Con A is known to bind to the free mannosyl end groups of the insulin receptor (Katzen et al., 1981; Hedo et al., 1981), and the lectin displays many insulin-

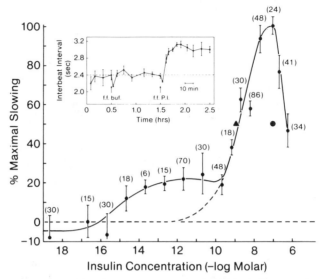

Fig. 4. Effect of insulin superfusion on interbeat interval (IBI) of spontaneously beating 7-day embryonic ventricle cell aggregates. Inset: mean IBI ($\pm$S.D.) of a group of six aggregates superfused with bovine serum albumin (BSA) buffer. At "ff buf" the chamber was rapidly flushed with BSA buffer, resulting in a transient decrease in IBI. At "ff PI" the chamber was reflushed with BSA buffer containing 17 nM porcine insulin. Main curve: dose response of insulin-evoked slowing of the beat rate. IBIs were measured before and 20 min after superfusion with control buffer and again before and 20 min after reflushing with PI at concentrations ranging from 1.7×10^{-19} to $8.5 \times 10^{-7} M$. At each concentration, net change in IBI was calculated as the increment in IBI caused by hormone minus the increment produced by the buffer flush, taken as a percentage of the maximal effect (100 nM). Each point represents the mean ($\pm$S.E.) of N aggregates (N shown in parentheses). Dissociation constants for high-affinity ($\blacktriangle$) and low-affinity ($\bullet$) insulin receptor populations from 7-day aggregates are shown for comparison. [Reproduced from DeHaan et al. (1984) with permission.]

like properties (Williams et al., 1980). Moreover, at low concentrations, Con A converts the Scatchard curve for insulin binding to erythrocytes from a curvilinear to linear form (Herzberg et al., 1980), that is, the lectin either blocks all of the high-affinity sites or converts all receptors into a low-affinity configuration. Thus it was of some interest to find that this lectin caused depolarization and shortening of the interbeat interval in heart cell aggregates and blocked insulin's slowing action (Myrdal and DeHaan, 1983). These results are consistent with the hypothesis that the slowing response requires an interaction between insulin and the high-affinity receptor, whereas occupancy of the low-affinity binding site has an opposite effect.

Despite such consistencies, these ideas must be entertained with caution. An alternative interpretation may be worth considering. According to the calculations of the two-receptor model shown in Fig. 4, half of the high-affinity sites

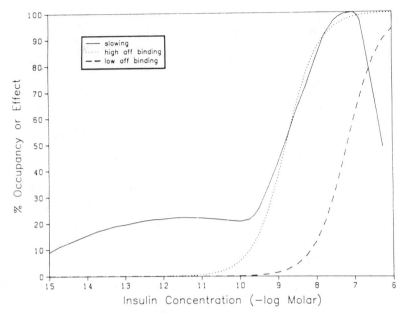

Fig. 5. Comparison of the dose dependence of receptor occupancy with the insulin-evoked reduction in beat rate. The percentage of insulin-evoked slowing (solid line) from Fig. 4 is superimposed on insulin binding curves. These were determined from measurements of ^{125}I-labeled insulin binding to 7-day ventricular aggregates, under conditions identical to those used during the beat rate studies (R. L. DeHaan, E. Strumlauf, and L. J. Elsas, unpublished), and calculated as percentage ligand binding to high-affinity (dotted line) and low-affinity (dashed line) receptors according to a two-receptor model (Wheeler *et al.*, 1980).

(i.e., 300) carry insulin when the concentration is at 1.7 n*M*. At that hormone concentration, only approximately 2% of the low-affinity receptors are occupied, but because there are 9000 of these in all, that represents 200 receptors, almost as many as those binding to the high-affinity population. At 4 n*M* insulin, when the high-affinity population is 70% saturated (440 occupied receptors), there are actually more low-affinity receptors (approximately 500) that carry insulin. If the slowing response depends not on binding to a particular receptor class but merely on the amount of insulin bound to the cell surface, the low-affinity receptors would have a more significant role at hormone concentrations of 4 n*M* and greater. It should be remembered that there is a precedent for misinterpreting such a correspondence between an insulin-evoked effect and a high-affinity binding curve. Cuatracasas (1972) compared the binding kinetics of insulin receptors in rat adipose tissue with the dose response for insulin-evoked lipogenesis. From the similarity of the binding K_d and the concentration that elicited half-maximal response, he concluded that insulin action was directly proportional to the fractional occupancy of that receptor and that binding and action were coupled linearly (Cuatracasas, 1971). In an extended analysis of this work, Gammeltoft (1984) discusses the possible errors in this interpretation.

Not all workers have found similar bioelectric effects of insulin. Malinow (1958) obtained only small variable decreases in action potential duration and no change in maximum diastolic potential upon application of 1.3 μM insulin to driven rat ventricle strips. But he allowed only 20 min for equilibration of the muscle with the superfusing Tyrode solution. This was probably not long enough for the endogenous insulin to be released from receptors, considering the slow off-rate of the hormone (Kahn and Baird, 1978; Serravezza et al., 1983). Moreover, such a high dose would have been in the supramaximal range in which insulin responsiveness is suppressed. More recently, Stark and O'Doherty (1982) found no change in intracellular concentrations of Na or K, nor in rest potential, in rat soleus muscle exposed to 650 nM porcine insulin. This concentration stimulated glucose uptake by the preparation approximately fourfold; however, these workers superfused the muscle with Ringer's solution containing 5 mM K. In this solution, the Na–K pump would be fully activated (Gadsby, 1982), and resting membrane potential would lie close to the potassium equilibrium potential (E_K). Insulin is known to cause a significant enhancement of Na–K pump activity only if K and/or Na is present at suboptimal concentrations (Gavryck et al., 1975), and it could cause an increase in outward current only if the cell were to rest sufficiently far from E_K to generate an appreciable driving force.

B.   Epidermal Growth Factor

EGF is a single-chain polypeptide that stimulates DNA replication and cell division in a wide variety of both epidermal and nonepidermal cells (see Das, 1983, for review). It was isolated first from mouse submaxillary glands by Cohen (1962), but is present in mammalian urine as urogastrone and is found in normal human serum at concentrations of 0.1–0.2 nM.

Binding of EGF to its receptor causes phosphorylation of both membrane-associated and nonmembrane proteins. Carpenter et al. (1978) showed that tyrosine-specific protein kinase activity was associated with the receptor. The EGF receptor bears substantial sequence homology with the insulin receptor and many of the Src oncogene products (Ullrich et al., 1985). EGF's binding to the epidermoid carcinoma A431 cell line led to autophosphorylation of a portion of the receptor macromolecule that extended through the cytoplasmic side of the plasma membrane. EGF has been shown to enhance Ca uptake and phosphatidyl-inositol (PI) turnover, as well, in these cells (Sawyer and Cohen, 1981). Moreover, Sahai et al. (1982) demonstrated a two- to threefold increase in activity of the calcium-activated phospholipid-dependent kinase, protein kinase C, upon exposure of A431 cells to EGF. When applied to mitotically quiescent BSC-1 monkey kidney cells (Fig. 1b), EGF produced a 10-mV transient depolarization with a latency of only a few seconds (Rothenberg et al., 1982). In A431 cells, application of EGF caused a marked stimulation of an electrically neutral amiloride-sensitive $^{22}Na^+$ entry, which has been associated with the Na–H exchange mechanism in other cell types (Owen, 1984; Villereal et al., 1985) including heart (Piwnica-Worms et al., 1985). The resulting increase in intracellular Na has been invoked to explain the enhanced Na–K pump activity caused by EGF and a number of other peptide hormones. From measurements of ouabain-sensitive ^{86}Rb influx, Rozengurt et al. (1981) have proposed that growth factors stimulate the Na–K pump by increasing the availability of Na to the Na–K transport site. This would be a hyperpolarizing effect, because in most cells the Na–K pump is electrogenic and produces a net outward current (Glitsch, 1982; Gadsby, 1984).

The action of EGF as a calcium-mobilizing hormone was confirmed by Moolenaar et al. (1984). When human fibroblast cells loaded with the fluorescent Ca indicator Quin-2 were superfused with 8 nM EGF, the cytosolic free-Ca level rose rapidly from approximately 150 nM to a peak of 300 nM in approximately 20 sec (Moolenaar et al., 1984). This response was not prevented by removal of external Ca or by membrane depolarization in high extracellular K. The authors concluded that EGF caused the release of Ca from intracellular stores.

C.   Nerve Growth Factor

The discovery of NGF in the early 1950s by Levi-Montalcini and Hamburger (see Levi-Montalcini, 1966) was a landmark in the field of PGF function (for reviews, see Greene and Shooter, 1980; Yankner and Shooter, 1982). Isolation of the polypeptide from the mouse submaxillary gland (Cohen, 1960) and determination of its amino-acid sequence (Angeletti and Bradshaw, 1971) led to the recognition of the homologies between this molecule and the insulin family of polypeptides. Active NGF consists of two noncovalently linked, identical peptide chains, each chain consisting of 118 amino-acid residues that exhibit substantial homology with the proinsulin peptide. A cDNA sequence corresponding to murine preproNGF has been reported, and a major portion of the human beta-NGF gene has been determined (reviewed in James and Bradshaw, 1984). There are two forms of NGF receptors (Schechter and Bothwell, 1981) that clearly do not result from cooperative interactions.

The earliest described effects of NGF's binding to its receptors are a Na-dependent uptake of amino acids and sugars (Horii and Varon, 1977: Skaper and Varon, 1979a) and the extrusion of Na (Skaper and Varon, 1979b). In the absence of NGF intracellular levels of Na rise, but, upon exposure to the factor, Na efflux is stimulated rapidly and the internal concentration falls. Na extrusion began with a latency of less than 1 min, whereas several minutes preceded the onset of hexose uptake (Skaper and Varon, 1979b). Whether this stimulation of Na pumping is associated with a shift in membrane potential is not known.

D. Platelet-Derived Growth Factor

PDGF is a large multichain polypeptide whose structure is not yet well characterized. Initial reports suggested that it consists of four or five chains, but it appears more likely that the native factor comprises two peptides of 136 and 165 residues and that activity is associated primarily with the longer chain (James and Bradshaw, 1984). Binding of PDGF to its receptor evokes tyrosine-specific protein phosphorylation (Cooper et al., 1984), increased turnover of phosphatidylinositol and intracellular liberation of diacylglycerol (Habenicht et al., 1981), and activation of the Na–H exchange pump (Moolenaar et al., 1983; Owen, 1984). Moolenaar et al. (1984) applied PDGF to human fibroblast cells loaded with the fluorescent Ca-indicator Quin-2. They observed a rapid rise in fluorescence with a latency of only a few seconds, a response which resembled that to EGF and signaled a transient increase in intracellular free Ca. As with EGF, the authors concluded that PDGF caused a release of Ca from intracellular stores.

IV. MECHANISM OF PEPTIDE HORMONE ACTION

We have seen that peptides can evoke several electrophysiologically relevant responses in target cells: (1) depolarizing or hyperpolarizing shifts in membrane potential, with excitatory or depressive effects on the generation of action potentials; (2) modulation of intracellular stores of Ca and changes in the cytosolic concentration of this ion; (3) stimulation of an amiloride-sensitive Na entry, in association with the Na–H exchange mechanism; (4) stimulation of the Na–K pump; and (5) activation of ion-selective channels. The Ca-mobilizing, depolarizing action of most of the brain–gut peptides appears to be shared by two of the peptide growth factors, EGF and PDGF. Insulin's actions, in most cells where it has been applied, appear to stand in contrast to those of the other peptides. It usually causes membrane hyperpolarization, a reduction in cytosolic Ca, slowing of the cardiac beat rate, and depression of excitability. Just as with the other peptides, however, these responses are produced by cAMP-independent pathways, and insulin's ability to stimulate Na–H exchange and the Na–K pump is shared with the other peptide hormones. In this section, we explore some of the mechanisms of these effects.

A.   Brain–Gut Peptides Increase Intracellular Calcium

The peptide-induced depolarization and conductance changes that result from occupancy of cAMP-independent receptors are associated with a rise in intracellular calcium (as reviewed extensively in Petersen, 1981; Rasmussen and Barrett, 1984). CCK and bombesin secretagogues caused uptake of ^{45}Ca from the extracellular fluid and release of the ion from prelabeled cells, with a dose–response curve similar to that for agonist-induced depolarization (Matthews *et al.*, 1973; Gardner *et al.*, 1975). Many of the peptide-evoked bioelectric effects could be mimicked by increasing cytosolic Ca. Intracellular injection of calcium into pancreatic acinar cells evoked depolarization and a decrease in membrane resistance that was indistinguishable from the secretagogue-induced response (Iwatsuki and Petersen, 1977), whereas injection of the calcium chelator EGTA blocked the response (Petersen and Laugier, 1980). Initially, peptide-evoked electrophysiological changes in acinar cells were independent of extracellular Ca; however, if Ca was removed after prolonged exposure to a secretagogue when internal stores were depleted, external ions became the source of the increase in cytosolic Ca (Petersen, 1981). The acinar cell membrane can be made more permeable by Ca removal. In such cells, Streb *et al.* (1983) found that activation of the ACh receptor caused the release of Ca from an intracellular nonmitochondrial Ca store. Interestingly, a number of transportable L-amino acids (alanine, valine, serine, proline) also evoked acinar membrane depolarization and increases in conductance that were independent of external Ca. The null potential for the action of L-alanine was approximately $+40$ mV, near the sodium equilibrium potential (E_{Na}), suggesting that the conductance increased by the amino acid was selectively permeable to sodium (Iwatsuki and Petersen, 1980). This contrasts with a null potential of approximately -15 mV for the peptide-evoked depolarization.

In the liver, absence of Ca from the incubation medium prevented the activation of glycogen phosphorylation activity by VP (Keppens *et al.*, 1977), whereas the Ca ionophore A23187 mimicked VP action when extracellular Ca was present; however, on the basis of studies of Ca movements by atomic absorption, Ca-electrode, and other techniques, Exton (1981) argued that hormonal stimulation mobilizes Ca mainly from nonmitochondrial intracellular sources. As noted above, Ca removal or Ca blockers prevented the vasomotor effects of neuropeptide Y and the neuronal excitatory effects of substance P (Konishi and Otsuka, 1974; Edvinsson *et al.*, 1983), and suppressed the AHPs produced by CRF in hippocampal cells (Siggins *et al.*, 1985) and by substance P in rat parotid (Petersen, 1981).

The noninsulin growth-promoting peptides also require an early Ca-mobilization step to have a depolarizing action. Studies of Ca-tracer fluxes indicated that EGF and PDGF produced rapid alterations in cytosolic Ca and stimulation of phosphatidylinositol turnover (Sawyer and Cohen, 1981; Villereal *et al.*, 1985). By loading human fibroblast cells with Quin-2, Moolenaar *et al.* (1984) were able to show that sudden superfusion with EGF or PDGF caused an immediate doubling in cytosolic Ca concentration. The effect was detectable within 1–2 sec of peptide addition and occurred even in the absence of external Ca, leading to the conclusion that it resulted from Ca release from intracellular stores. Interestingly, neither insulin (5 μg/ml) nor the phorbol ester TPA had a similar effect. It is on the basis of such evidence that many workers have concluded that the brain–gut peptides and some of the polypeptide growth factors cause depolarization of target cells by acting as Ca-releasing hormones.

B. Calcium Release Is Mediated by Phosphoinositol Derivatives

The link between ligand binding to surface receptors and calcium release was not understood until the recent discovery that a primary action of peptide hormones is to cause breakdown of polyphosphoinositide membrane components to form soluble inositol phosphates (Michell, 1975; Creba *et al.*, 1983; Berridge, 1983). An important insight was the recognition that hormone occupancy of the peptide receptors activates phospholipase C (Michell *et al.*, 1981), which converts a minor membrane component, phosphatidylinositol-4,5-bisphosphate, into the water-soluble trisphosphate form, *myo*-inositol-1,4,5-trisphosphate (IP_3), and releases simultaneously a molecule of 1,2-diacyl-glycerol (DG). DG was discovered by Nishizuka and co-workers to be an endogenous activator of protein kinase C (PK-C) (for reviews, see Nishizuka, 1984; Nishizuka *et al.*, 1984). Moreover, IP_3 itself caused the release of intracellular Ca when applied to pancreatic acinar cells made leaky by incubation in Ca-free solution (Streb *et al.*, 1983) or when applied to isolated endoplasmic reticulum (Streb *et al.*, 1984), strongly suggesting that this phosphoinositide serves as the intracellular mediator for hormone-induced mobilization of Ca. Recent experiments confirm that IP_3 causes the mobilization of intracellular Ca from a specialized subpopulation of the endoplasmic reticulum and is thus responsible for the rapid rise of cytosolic free Ca (Burgess *et al.*, 1984; Williamson *et al.*, 1985). Protein kinase C is present in a wide variety of tissues, normally in an inactive form. Occupancy of peptide-hormone receptors activates phospholipase C and produces a transient surge of DG. Activation of PK-C requires Ca, but DG greatly increases the Ca affinity of the enzyme, rendering it active in the physiological range of cytosolic Ca concentrations. Different aspects of the phosphoinositol-related Ca-messenger system have been reviewed recently (Rasmussen and Barrett, 1984; Nishizuka, 1984; Macara, 1985; Hokin, 1985).

C. Possible Mechanisms of Insulin-Induced Hyperpolarization

There are at least four mechanisms of insulin action that could produce, or contribute to, the observed rapid IIH of heart and other tissues. Insulin occupancy of its receptor could cause (1) stimulation of an electrogenic Na–K pump, (2) mobilization and insertion into the membrane of preformed ion channels from an intracellular store, (3) transformation of a receptor macromolecule into an ion-selective channel, or (4) activation of an outward (or inactivation of an inward) background current through a mediator or second messenger system.

1. Stimulation of an Electrogenic Na–K Pump

There is ample evidence that insulin stimulates the Na–K pump in heart and other tissues (see Moore, 1983, for an extensive review) and that it enhances the activity of Na–K ATPase. These effects occur through the mediation of the insulin receptor (Hougen et al., 1978; Resh et al., 1980) and by direct binding of the hormone to the purified enzyme (McGeoch, 1983). In HTC rat hepatoma cells, insulin increased Na–K pump activity rapidly, as measured by ouabain-sensitive influx of ^{86}Rb (Gelehrter et al., 1984). Increased influx was observed with a latency of 1–2 min and was maximal (70% above control) in approximately 1 hr. The effect appeared to be mediated by insulin receptors, because (1) its concentration dependence was identical to that for insulin's induction of tyrosine aminotransferase and stimulation of 2-aminoisobutyric acid transport and (2) it was blocked by anti-receptor antibodies. The pump stimulation could be blocked by amiloride, and it could be mimicked by the Na ionophore, monensin. Insulin increases ^{22}Na influx rapidly, also, suggesting that part of its effect on the Na–K pump is secondary to an increase in intracellular Na concentration.

Pump stimulation resulted in the expected extrusion of Na and rise in cytosolic K in heart cells (Elsas et al., 1975), but as Moore (1983) has noted, these concentration changes followed the onset of IIH and therefore could not have caused it. Nonetheless, the Na–K pump is electrogenic in heart and most other tissues, transferring two K ions into the cell for every three Na ions it extrudes (Glitsch, 1982; Gadsby, 1984). Because of the net outward pump current, insulin activation would have a hyperpolarizing effect that would add to other hyper-polarizing actions. Activation at physiological (nanomolar) insulin concentrations has been demonstrated convincingly by measurement of one-way Na efflux (Moore, 1973; Clausen and Kohn, 1977), one-way K or Rb influx (Hougen et al., 1978; Flatman and Clausen, 1979; Fehlmann and Freychet, 1981; Gelehrter et al., 1984), and net fluxes (Clausen and Kohn, 1977; Elsas et al., 1975). Numerous studies have been done to test whether ouabain blocks the hyperpolarizing action of insulin by inhibiting the Na–K pump. But because the ions leak rapidly down their respective electrochemical gradients, the timing of such experiments is critical and the results have been variable and difficult to interpret (see Zierler, 1985).

2. Mobilization of Preformed Ion Channels

An alternative way that peptide hormones might induce an outward current is by causing the translocation of functional channels from an intracellular store to the plasma membrane, that is, a mechanism analogous to the way insulin stimulates glucose transport in muscle and adipose tissue (for reviews, see Gliemann and Rees, 1983; Kono, 1984). Glucose transport occurs via a facilitated diffusion system (Taylor and Holman, 1981; Whitesell and Gliemann, 1979). To accelerate the rate of glucose transport, insulin could either increase the turnover number (i.e., activity) of individual transporters or cause an increase in the number of functional transporter molecules in the membrane. Recently, it has been demonstrated that cytochalasin B binds tightly to hexose transporters. With this ligand, it has been possible to determine the number of transporter molecules in subcellular fractions, prepared by differential centrifugation, from isolated cells. Insulin acts by increasing the number of functional transporters in the plasma membrane roughly fivefold, while reducing their concentration in the low-density microsomal fraction by approximately 60% (Wardzala et al., 1978; Suzuki and Kono, 1980). These effects of insulin are rapid, with a half-time of 2–3 min, fully reversible, concentration dependent (half-maximal insulin concentration = 0.11 nM), and dependent on energy metabolism but not on protein synthesis (Karnieli et al., 1981; Kono et al., 1981, 1982; Cushman et al., 1984). These results suggest that insulin stimulates glucose transport activity through the translocation of glucose transporters from an intracellular pool, associated with the low-density microsomal fraction, to the plasma membrane. This mechanism of insulin stimulation of glucose transport appears to be applicable to both adipocytes (Gorga and Lienhard, 1984; Cushman et al., 1984; Czech, 1984) and rat diaphragm (Wardzala and Jeanrenaud, 1983).

Recent results from Czech's lab suggest that insulin modulates another membrane component—the IGF-II receptor—by a similar mechanism. Exposure of adipocytes to insulin increased the binding of ^{125}I-labeled IGF-II to a plasma membrane fraction prepared from these cells and decreased the binding to the low-density membrane fraction. Moreover, binding of an anti-IGF-II receptor antibody to the surface of insulin-exposed cells was increased also (Oka et al., 1984; Czech, 1984). It is perhaps relevant in this regard that exposure of adipocytes to insulin caused an increase in the number of integral membrane proteins per unit surface area in both leaflets of the plasma membrane (Carpentier et al., 1976).

There is no evidence whatsoever for the speculation that ion channels may be translocated from an intracellular pool to the plasma membrane in a manner that resembles the insertion of glucose transporters and IGF-II receptors. Indeed, some other proteins that have been examined are not translocated in this manner. Normally, both insulin receptors and marker enzymes, such as 5'-nucleotidase and isoproterenol-stimulated adenylate cyclase, are found primarily in the plasma membrane fraction. Exposure of cells to insulin does not alter detectably the distribution of either marker enzyme (Cushman et al., 1984), and it decreases the insulin receptor density in the plasma membrane fraction as a result of down regulation (Serravezza et al., 1983); however, the concentration of a putative channel protein in the plasma membrane before and after insulin treatment has not been investigated. Thus, a channel translocation mechanism remains an interesting hypothesis that has not been tested.

3. Insulin Activation of a Membrane Ionic Channel

Zierler (1972) attributed the IIH to a decrease in the ratio of Na permeability (P_{Na}) to K permeability (P_K), that is, to a direct effect on ionic conductances. Our results with embryonic heart cell aggregates (Lantz et al., 1980) suggest that insulin increased a K conductance, although in other preparations the hormone appears to decrease P_K (DeMello, 1967; Zierler, 1972).

Recently, we have succeeded in measuring membrane conductance of isolated 7-day ventricle cells directly by using the patch-electrode technique developed by Neher and Sakmann (for review, see Sakmann and Neher, 1983). With this technique, a glass pipette 1–2 μm in tip diameter is pressed against the surface of a cell, forming a high-resistance seal (5–50 GΩ) between the inside of the pipette and the bath. When the patch of membrane within the pipette is ruptured by suction, a voltage-clamp circuit can be used to record membrane potential or to control the voltage of the cell interior. This whole-cell recording configuration (Hamill et al., 1981) permits analysis of current–voltage relations of single cells or small cell clusters with a negligibly small access resistance. This technique has been used to record voltage-sensitive and agonist-activated currents in heart cells (Reuter, 1984) and a wide variety of other cell types (for reviews, see Hille, 1984; Auerbach and Sachs, 1984; Fischmeister et al., 1986).

The steady-state net background current across the membrane of a single 7-day ventricle cell is dominated by a strongly rectifying current that resembles the inward rectifier I_{K1} of adult cardiac cells (Noble and Tsien, 1968; Reuter, 1984). As shown in a current–voltage curve (Fig. 6a, control), over the entire voltage range positive to approximately −80 mV, there is a small, outward background current of 2 pA/pF or less. In early experiments (Fischmeister et al., 1983), we found that if the pipette solution did not contain ATP, a large, outward background current developed soon after the membrane patch was broken in cells

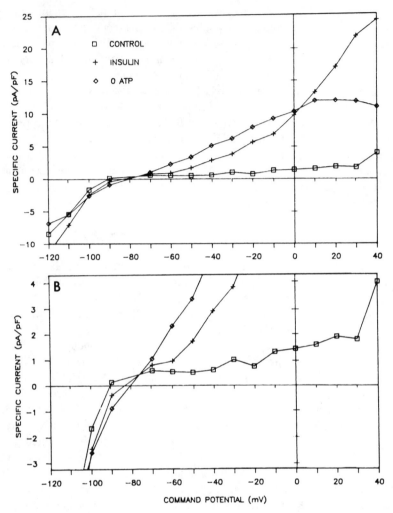

Fig. 6. Steady-state background currents from 7-day chick ventricle cells, measured with patch electrodes in whole-cell recording mode. The patch pipette contained a high-K, low-Ca intracellular-like solution. Net current was determined at the end of 400-msec command potentials, stepped in 10-mV increments sequentially from −120 to +40 mV. Cells bathed in balanced salt (control) showed a typical inward rectifier I–V curve. When the pipette solution lacked ATP (0 ATP), a characteristic ATP-depletion current developed. With 3 mM ATP in the pipette and the cell bathed in buffer containing 8 nM porcine insulin (insulin), the background outward current was progressively larger at potentials positive to approximately −80 mV. The entire curves are shown in (a) and at an expanded vertical scale in (b). [From R. K. Ayer, Jr., R. Fischmeister, and R. L. DeHaan, unpublished.]

bathed in a simple balanced salt solution (Fig. 6a, 0 ATP). This proved to be an ATP-depletion current similar to those described in adult heart preparations (Noma, 1983; Bechem and Pott, 1984; Trube and Hescheler, 1984). Such a current would have made it impossible to see any additional insulin-activated current upon superfusion with the hormone. With adequate ATP in the pipette solution, exposure of some (but not all) cells resulted in the development of an outward current with a characteristically upward concave $I–V$ curve that was readily distinguishable from the ATP-depletion current (Fig. 6a, insulin). The insulin-activated current tended toward zero at approximately -80 mV, near E_K, suggesting that it was carried mainly by K ions. Even in the pacemaker range of potentials (about -80 to -50 mV), however, the insulin-activated current was large enough (Fig. 6b) to account for the observed hyperpolarization and slowing of beat rate described above.

The neurotransmitter literature is replete with examples of ion channels that, when activated by extracellular ligands, can serve as models for the variety of mechanisms to be expected when we examine hormone-activated currents. Agonists such as ACh, glutamate, and GABA can act directly on receptor-channel macromolecules to cause them to switch from a nonconducting to an ion-selective conducting state (for reviews, see Auerbach and Sachs, 1984; Hille, 1984). The nicotinic ACh channel is perhaps the most thoroughly understood example of such a mechanism (Popot and Changeux, 1984). Alternatively, agonist binding to its receptor can modulate the opening of a distant channel by a sequence of postreceptor steps mediated by one or more diffusible intracellular second messengers. There is no evidence to suggest that the insulin receptor may be a putative channel. Moreover, with only one short lipophilic region in each alpha subunit to cross the membrane (Ullrich *et al.*, 1985), it is hard to imagine how a conformational change could lead to its conversion into a hydrophilic pore. On the other hand, it is well known that insulin causes the production of intracellular mediators (Jarett *et al.*, 1985). But the effect that is most likely related to channel activation is insulin's role in modulating intracellular Ca.

Regulation of cytosolic Ca concentration has been proposed by many workers (Clausen *et al.*, 1979; McDonald *et al.*, 1976) as an important mechanism of insulin action. An insulin-sensitive, high-affinity [Ca,Mg]-ATPase that subserves the Ca pump has been described in the plasma membrane of rat adipocytes (Pershadsingh *et al.*, 1980; Pershadsingh and McDonald, 1980). Exposure of intact adipocytes or isolated plasma membranes to 0.65 nM insulin caused dephosphorylation and a decrease in activity of the enzyme (Pershadsingh and McDonald, 1981; Jarett *et al.*, 1982). In contrast, when concentrations of insulin greater than 2 nM were added to plasma membrane preparations, enzyme activity increased. Thus, exposure to low insulin concentrations would result in intracellular Ca accumulation, whereas higher hormone concentrations would enhance active extrusion of the ion. Nonetheless, the net effect that insulin would have on actual cytosolic levels of free Ca is not clear, because in both skinned muscle fibers (Brautigan et al., 1980) and rat adipocytes (McDonald et al., 1978), 0.65 nM insulin stimulated uptake of the ion into the microsomal or sarcoplasmic reticulum fraction.

Three well-documented conductance mechanisms are regulated by intracellular Ca. (1) Many cells exhibit Ca-activated K-selective (I_{K-Ca}) channels (Schwarz and Passow, 1983; Latorre et al., 1985). Such currents have been observed with conventional microelectrodes in cardiac Purkinje fibers (Isenberg, 1977; Siegelbaum and Tsien, 1980) and in ventricular muscle (Beeler and Reuter, 1977; Siegal and Hoffman, 1980). Moreover, they are present in a variety of other cell types (Meech, 1978; Clusin and Bennett, 1977). Ca-sensitive K fluxes were measured in inside-out vesicles prepared from human red blood cell membranes (Garcia-Sancho et al., 1982) and in sarcolemmal vesicles from dog heart (Caroni and Carafoli, 1982). Agonist-stimulated single-channel currents through Ca-activated K channels have been observed directly with patch electrodes in chromaffin cells (Hamill et al., 1981), cultured rat skeletal muscle (Barrett et al., 1982), smooth muscle (Singer and Walsh, 1984), pancreatic acinar cells (Petersen and Maruyama, 1984), clonal pituitary cells (Dubinsky and Oxford, 1985), and human macrophages (Gallin, 1984). Activation of I_{K-Ca} by elevation of cytosolic Ca would hyperpolarize cells. (2) An alternative Ca-activated current was seen first in neonatal rat ventricle (Colquhoun et al., 1981). This channel is permeable to monovalent cations, but almost wholly nonselective for Na and K. Channel opening increases as a function of intracellular Ca at concentrations above approximately 500 nM. It is probably this conductance that underlies the arrhythmogenic transient inward current in glycoside-poisoned heart tissue (Lederer and Tsien, 1976). Because the reversal potential for this current is near 0 mV, an insulin-induced increase in cytosolic Ca would result in membrane depolarization. As noted above, this channel is activated by the CCK peptides in pancreatic acinar cells (Petersen and Maruyama, 1983). (3) Ca channels in some excitable cells are inactivated by intracellular Ca (Tsien, 1983). Ca current has a positive reversal potential and is thus a depolarizing current. An increase in cytosolic free Ca that inactivated a steady-state Ca current would cause hyperpolarization. Further experiments are needed to determine whether the insulin-activated current seen in embryonic heart cells is mediated by a Ca-regulated channel.

D.   Are Peptide-Induced Changes of V_m Merely Side Effects?

The depolarization induced in pancreatic acinar cells by peptide secretagogues does not itself stimulate enzyme secretion. A similar depolarizing shift in membrane potential, produced by elevated extracellular K, caused no secretion of pancreatic enzymes, and the response to CCK of K-depolarized cells was similar to that of controls (Case, 1978). On the other hand, Zierler and Rogus (1981a) have suggested that the voltage change that constitutes the IIH is itself part of the postreceptor signal mechanism. They based their hypothesis on the finding that the stimulation of glucose uptake that followed IIH could be mimicked by electrically produced hyperpolarization; however, recent experiments, in which muscle was treated with insulin while being bathed in high-K solution (to block IIH), revealed that glucose uptake was not blocked entirely, as predicted by the hypothesis (Zierler et al., 1985). Thus, it is not clear at present whether peptide-evoked potential changes play an important role in postreceptor mechanisms.

E.   Do Peptides Regulate the Cardiac Beat Rate?

The concept that peptide hormones may act in mammals as long-duration, long-range mimics of the short-acting neurotransmitters was introduced at least three decades ago (Welsh, 1955). With the discovery of peptidergic neurons and the broad distribution of peptide hormones in the central and peripheral nervous systems, the idea that these substances may serve as neurotransmitters or modulators of neural or cardiac function has achieved wide currency in recent years (Krieger, 1983; Gardner and Jensen, 1983). Observations such as those of Gu et al. (1983, 1984) that neuropeptide Y may regulate autonomic control of coronary arteries or heart rate and of Voorhees et al. (1978) that insulin suppresses the stimulation of heart rate by epinephrine lend strength to the idea. During embryonic development, cardiac tissue is sensitive to bath-applied regulator substances well before autonomic innervation of the heart is complete (for reviews, see Pappano, 1977; Creazzo et al., 1985). Functional vagal elements reach the embryonic chick heart during incubation days 5–7, whereas acetylcholine receptors are present, and the heart responds to cholinergic agonists by at least day 4 (Halvorsen et al., 1983). Even at 3 days of development, the chick heart shows an inotropic response to epinephrine (Hoffman and Van Mierop, 1971), although adrenergic fibers are not seen in the myocardium until days 10–12 (Pappano, 1977). Thus, during active morphogenesis, when the heart changes from a primitive peristaltic tube to a definitive 4-chambered pump, cardiac function would appear to be mainly under neurohumeral rather than neuronal control. The nanomolar dose range observed for insulin to cause its effects on 7-day and 14-day chick heart cell aggregates suggests that this hormone could play a role in the normal physiological regulation of the developing heart. Immunoassayable insulin reactivity is present in unfertilized and newly fertilized chicken eggs (Trenkle and Hopkins, 1971) and in embryonic tissues at all stages, even before islet cells appear in the forming pancreas at approximately 3.5 days of incubation (Przybylski, 1967; Swenne and Lundqvist, 1980). By days 6–8, embryonic tissues contain insulin at concentrations of 1–2 nM (DePablo et al., 1982). As shown in Fig. 4, this concentration of insulin available to the heart would cause 50–70% of the maximal slowing response if it were applied suddenly in a short-term exposure. Its effect at a steady-state hormone level is not known, but it could have a role in regulating insulin receptor density as well as beat rate during development. Both 7-day and 14-day chick embryo heart cells exhibited down regulation of receptors, i.e., the number of insulin binding sites decreased upon prolonged exposure to the hormone (Serravezza et al., 1981, 1983). Thus it is reasonable to propose that the embryonic heart beat may be regulated in part by insulin. Much work is required to test the validity of this working hypothesis.

V. CONCLUSIONS AND FUTURE RESEARCH DIRECTIONS

We have seen that the action of a wide range of peptide hormones includes an early effect on membrane potential or other electrical properties of the target cell. The significance of such bioelectric effects is not known and probably differs from one cell–hormone system to another, but such a ubiquitous phenomenon raises a host of questions. In every case, we need to know more about the sequence of events between receptor occupancy and the change in membrane potential or ion flux. For each system, what ion channels or pumps are activated? Are these effects all mediated by the phosphoinositide/C-kinase/Ca-release mechanism? Why is the amiloride-sensitive Na–H exchanger involved in such a large number of examples? In which cell types is the bioelectric effect an end in itself (for example, in altering the excitability or firing frequency of the target cell)? Alternatively, does modulation of membrane voltage or conductance serve as an early step in a causal sequence leading to other metabolic or behavioral changes in some target cells? Are hormone-evoked bioelectric effects simply epiphenomena in some cells, playing no role in the cell's physiology?

With specific regard to the heart, does the insulin-induced hyperpolarizing current shown here play an important role in regulating the beat rate in the embryonic heart, before autonomic control is fully developed? Do insulin or other peptides serve as subtle neuromodulators during postembryonic life? What channel carries the insulin-activated current? What is the significance of insulin's action in stimulating Ca uptake into the endoplasmic reticulum? What mediators or second messengers are activated after insulin binds to its receptor in the heart? What role does autophosphorylation of the beta subunit play in this system? What is the significance of these questions to diabetics or individuals with other insulin-related diseases?

These are some of the questions that provide the impetus for the newly developing field of electrophysiological endocrinology. The search for their answers will have an expanding impact on research in cardiovascular function in future years.

ACKNOWLEDGMENTS

I want to thank L. J. Elsas, R. K. Ayer, Jr., and R. Fischmeister for their collaboration in the experimental aspects of the work described here, B. J. Duke for preparation of all heart cell cultures that were used, and W. M. Scherer for editing and processing the manuscript. This work was supported by Grant P01-HL27385 from the National Institutes of Health.

REFERENCES

Allen, J. M., Polak, J. M., Rodrigo, J., Darcy, K., and Bloom, S. R. (1985). Localization of neuropeptide Y in nerves of the rat cardiovascular system and the effect of 6-hydroxydopamine. *Cardiovasc. Res.* **19**, 570–577.

Angeletti, R. H., and Bradshaw, R. A. (1971). Nerve growth factor from mouse submaxillary gland: Amino acid sequence. *Proc. Natl. Acad. Sci. USA* **68**, 2417–2410.

Auerbach, A., and Sachs, F. (1984). Patch clamp studies of single ionic channels. *Ann. Rev. Biophys. Bioeng.* **13**, 269–302.

Avruch, J., Alexander, M. C., Palmer, J. L., Pierce, M. W., Nemenoff, R. A., Blackshear, P. J., Tipper, J. P., and Witters, L. A. (1982a). Role of insulin-stimulated protein phosphorylation in insulin action. *Fed. Proc.* **41**, 2629–2633.

Avruch, J., Nemenoff, R. A., Blackshear, P. J., Pierce, M. W., and Osathanondh, R. (1982b). Insulin stimulated tyrosine phosphorylation of the insulin receptor in detergent extracts of human placental membranes. *J. Biol. Chem.* **257**, 15102–15106.

Ayer, R. K., Jr., Fischmeister, R. and DeHaan, R. L. (1986). In preparation.

Barker, J. L., and Smith, T. G. (1980). Bursting pacemaker activity in a peptidergic and peptide sensitive neuron. *In* "The Role of Peptides in Neuronal Function" (J. L. Barker and T. G. Smith, eds.), pp. 189–228. Marcel Dekker, New York.

Barker, J. L., Dufy, B., Owen, D. G., and Segal, M. (1983). Excitable membrane properties of cultured central nervous system neurons and clonal pituitary cells. *Cold Spring Harb. Symp. Quant. Biol.* **48**, 259–268.

Barrett, J. N., Magleby, K. L., and Pallotta, B. S. (1982). Properties of single calcium-activated potassium channels in cultured rat muscle. *J. Physiol.* **331**, 211–230.

Bayliss, W. M., and Starling, E. H. (1902). The mechanism of pancreatic secretion. *J. Physiol.* **28**, 325–353.

Bechem, M., and Pott, L. (1984). K-channels activated by loss of intracellular ATP in guinea-pig atrial cardioballs. *J. Physiol.* **348**, 50P.

Beeler, G. W., and Reuter, H. (1977). Reconstruction of the action potential of ventricular myocardial fibres. *J. Physiol.* **268**, 177–210.

Beigelman, P. M., and Hollander, P. B. (1965). Effect of insulin and insulin antibody upon rat adipose tissue membrane resting electrical potential. *Acta Endocrin.* **50**, 648–656.

Belardinelli, L., and Isenberg, G. (1983). Isolated atrial myocytes: Adenosine and acetylcholine increase potassium conductance. *Am. J. Physiol.: Heart and Circ. Physiol.* **244**, H734–H737.

Berridge, M. J. (1983). A novel cellular signalling system based on the integration of phospholipid and calcium metabolism. *In* "Calcium and Cell Function: (W. Y. Cheung, ed.), Vol. 3, pp. 1–36. Academic Press, New York.

Blackshear, P. J., Nemenoff, R. A., and Avruch, J. (1984). Characteristics of insulin and epidermal growth factor stimulation of receptor autophosphorylation in detergent extracts of rat liver and transplantable rat hepatomas. *Endocrinology* **114**, 141–152.

Blundell, T. L., Bedarkar, S., and Humbel, R. E. (1983). Tertiary structures, receptor binding, and antigenicity of insulin-like growth factors. *Fed. Proc.* **42**, 2592–2597.

Bousfield, D. (1985). *"Neurotransmitters in Action,"* Elsevier, New York.

Bradshaw, R. A., and Niall, H. D. (1978). Insulin-related growth factors. *Trends in Biochem. Sci.* **3**, 274–279.

Bradshaw, R. A., and Rubin, J. S. (1980). Polypeptide growth factors: Some structural and mechanistic considerations. *J. Supramolec. Struct.* **14**, 183–199.

Brautigan, D. L., Glenn, W., Kerrick, L., and Fischer, E. H. (1980). Insulin and glucose 6-phosphate stimulation of Ca^{2+} uptake by skinned muscle fibers. *Proc. Natl. Acad. Sci. USA* **77**, 936–939.

Brooks, P. A., and Kelly, J. S. (1985). Cholecystokinin as a potent excitant of neurons of the dentate gyrus. *Ann. N.Y. Acad. Sci.* **448**, 361–374.

Burgess, G. M., Godfrey, P. P., McKinney, J. S., Berridge, M. J., Irvine, R. F., and Putney, J. W., Jr. (1984). The second messenger linking receptor activation to internal Ca release in liver. *Nature* **309**, 63–66.

Caroni, P., and Carafoli, E. (1982). Modulation by calcium of the potassium permeability of dog heart sarcolemmal vesicles. *Proc. Natl. Acad. Sci. USA* **79**, 5763–5767.

Carpenter, G., King, L., and Cohen, S. (1978). Epidermal growth factor stimulates phosphorylation in membrane preparations *in vitro*. *Nature* **276**, 409–410.

Carpentier, J. L., Perrelet, A., and Orci, L. (1976). Effects of insulin, glucagon and epinephrine on the plasma membrane of the white adipose cell: A freeze-fracture study. *J. Lipid Res.* **17**, 335–342.

Case, R. M. (1978). Synthesis, intracellular transport, and discharge of exportable proteins in the pancreatic acinar cell and other cells. *Biol. Rev.* **53**, 211–354.

Chang, M. M., Leeman, S. E., and Niall, H. D. (1971). Amino acid sequence of substance P. *Nature* **232**, 86–87.

Chvatchko, Y., Gazzano, H., Van Obberghen, E., and Fehlmann, M. (1984). Subunit arrangement of insulin receptors in hepatoma cells. *Mol. and Cell. Endocrin.* **36**, 59–65.

Clapham, D. E., and Neher, E. (1984). Substance P reduces acetylcholine-induced currents in isolated bovine chromaffin cells. *J. Physiol.* **347**, 255–277.

Clausen, T., and Kohn, P. G. (1977). The effect of insulin on the transport of sodium and potassium in rat soleus muscle. *J. Physiol.* **265**, 19–42.

Clausen, T., Dahl-Hansen, A. B., and Elbrink, J. (1979). The effect of hyperosmolarity and insulin on resting tension and calcium fluxes in rat soleus muscle. *J. Physiol.* **292**, 505–526.

Clusin, W. T., and Bennett, M. V. L. (1977). Calcium-activated conductance in skate electroreceptors. Voltage clamp experiments. *J. Gen. Physiol.* **69**, 145–182.

Cohen, S. (1960). Purification of nerve growth promoting protein from the mouse salivary gland and its neurocytotoxic antiserum. *Proc. Natl. Acad. Sci. USA* **46**, 302–311.

Cohen, S. (1962). Isolation of a mouse submaxillary gland protein accelerating incisor eruption and eyelid opening in the newborn animal. *J. Biol. Chem.* **237**, 1555–1562.

Colquhoun, D., Neher, E., Reuter, H., and Stevens, C. F. (1981). Inward current channels activated by intracellular Ca in cultured cardiac cells. *Nature* **294**, 752–754.

Cooper, J. A., Sefton, B. M., and Hunter, T. (1984). Diverse mitogenic agents induce the phosphorylation of two related 42,000 dalton proteins on tyrosine in quiescent chick cells. *J. Mol. Cell. Biol.* **4**, 30–37.

Creazzo, T., Titus, L., and Hartzell, H. C. (1985). Neural regulation of the heart: A model for modulation of voltage-sensitive channels and regulation of cellular metabolism *In* "Neurotransmitters in Action" (D. Bousfield, ed.), pp. 74–80. Elsevier-North Holland, Amsterdam.

Creba, J. A., Downes, C. P., Hawkins, P. T., Brewster, G., Michell, R. H., and Kirk, C. J. (1983). Rapid breakdown of phosphatidylinositol-4-phosphate and phosphatidylinositol-4,5-bisphosphate in rat hepatocytes stimulated by vasopressin and other Ca^{2+}-mobilizing hormones. *Biochem. J.* **212**, 733–747.

Creed, K. E. (1979). Functional diversity of smooth muscle. *Brit. Med. Bull.* **35**, 243–247.

Crim, J. W., and Vigna, S. R. (1983). Brain, gut and skin peptide hormones in lower vertebrates. *Am. Zool.* **23**, 621–638.

Cuatracasas, P. (1971). Insulin–receptor interactions in adipose tissue cells: Direct measurement and properties. *Proc. Natl. Acad. Sci. USA* **68**, 1264–1268.

Cuatracasas, P. (1972). Properties of the insulin receptor isolated from liver and fat cell membranes. *J. Biol. Chem.* **247**, 1980–1991.

Cushman, S. W., Wardzala, L. J., Simpson, I. A., Karnieli, H., Hissin, P. J., Wheeler, T. J., Hinkle, P. C., and Salans, L. B. (1984). Insulin-induced translocation of intracellular glucose transporters in the isolated rat adipose cell. *Fed. Proc.* **43**, 2251–2255.

Czech, M. P. (1984). New perspectives on the mechanism of insulin action. *Rec. Prog. Horm. Res.* **40**, 347–377.

Czech, M. P. (1985). The nature and regulation of the insulin receptor: Structure and function. *Ann. Rev. Physiol.,* **47**, 357–382.

Czech, M. P., and Massague, J. (1982). Subunit structure and dynamics of the insulin receptor. *Fed. Proc.* **41**, 2719–2723.

Czech, M. P., Oppenheimer, C. L., and Massague, J. (1983). Interrelationship among receptor structure for insulin and peptide growth factors. *Fed. Proc.* **42**, 2598–2601.

Das, M. (1983). Epidermal growth factor receptor and mechanisms for animal cell division. *Cur. Top. Memb. Transp.* **18**, 381–405.

DeHaan, R. L., Goodrum, G., Strumlauf, E., and Elsas, L. J. (1984). Insulin-specific receptor-mediated slowing of beat rate in embryonic heart cells. *Am. J. Physiol.: Cell Physiol.* **246**, C347–C359.

DeMello, W. C. (1967). Effect of insulin on the membrane resistance of frog skeletal muscle. *Life Sci.* **6**, 959–963.

DeMeyts, P., and Roth, J. (1975). Cooperativity in ligand binding: A new graphic analysis. *Biochem. Biophys. Res. Comm.* **66**, 1118–1126.

DePablo, F., Roth, J., Hernandez, E., and Pruss, R. M. (1982). Insulin is present in chicken eggs and early chick embryos. *Endocrinology* **111**, 1909–1916.

Deutsch, P. J., Wan, C. F., Rosen, O. M., and Rubin, C. S. (1983). Latent insulin receptors and possible receptor precursors in 3T3-Li adipocytes. *Proc. Natl. Acad. Sci. USA* **80**, 133–136.

Dicker, P., Pohjanpelto, P., Pettican, P., and Rozengurt, E. (1981). Similarities between fibroblast-derived growth factor and platelet-derived growth factor. *Exp. Cell Res.* **135**, 221–227.

Dodd, J., and Kelly, J. S. (1981). The actions of cholecystokinin and related peptides on pyramidal neurones of the mammalian hippocampus. *Brain Res.* **205**, 337–350.

Dreifuss, J. J., Muhlethaler, M., and Gahwiler, B. H. (1982). Electrophysiology of vasopressin in normal rats and in Brattleboro rats. *Ann. N. Y. Acad. Sci.* **394**, 689–702.

Dubinsky, J. M., and Oxford, G. S. (1985). Dual modulation of potassium channels by thyrotropin releasing hormone in clonal pituitary cells. *Proc. Natl. Acad. Sci. USA* **82**, 4282–4286.

Edvinsson, L. (1985). Characterization of the contractile effect of neuropeptide Y in feline cerebral arteries. *Acta Physiol. Scand.* **125**, 33–41.

Edvinsson, L., Emson, P., McCulloch, J., Tatemoto, K., and Uddmann, R. (1983). Neuropeptide Y: Cerebrovascular innervation and vasomotor effects in the cat. *Neurosci. Let.* **43**, 79–84.

Ehlers, C. L., Henriksen, S. J., Wang, M., River, J., Vale, W., and Bloom, F. E. (1983).

162   Robert L. DeHaan

Corticotropin releasing factor produces increases in brain excitability and convulsive seizures in rats. *Brain Res.* **270**, 363–367.

Elsas, L. J., Wheeler, F. B., Danner, D. J., and DeHaan, R. L. (1975). Amino acid transport by aggregates of cultured chicken heart cells. *J. Biol. Chem.* **250**, 9381–9390.

Endo, F., and Elsas, L. J. (1984). Structural analysis and subunit interaction of insulin receptor from membranes of cultured embryonic chick heart cells. *Endocrinology* **115**, 1828–1837.

Exton, J. H. (1981). Molecular mechanisms involved in alpha-adrenergic responses. *Mol. Cell. Endocrinol.* **23**, 233–264.

Fehlmann, M., and Freychet, P. (1981). Insulin and glucagon stimulation of (Na$^+$–K$^+$) ATPase transport activity in isolated rat hepatocytes. *J. Biol. Chem.* **256**, 7449–7452.

Fischmeister, R., Ayer, R. K., Jr., and DeHaan, R. L. (1983). Insulin regulates the ionic conductance of the embryonic heart cell membrane. *Biophys. J.* **41**, 75a.

Fischmeister, R., Ayer, R. K., Jr., and DeHaan, R. L. (1986). Some limitations of the cell-attached patch clamp technique: A two-electrode analysis. *Pflüg. Arch.* **406**, 73–82.

Flatman, J. A., and Clausen, T. (1979). Combined effects of adrenaline and insulin on active electrogenic Na$^+$–K$^+$ transport in rat soleus muscle. *Nature* **281**, 580–581.

Fontaine-Perus, J., Chanconie, M., and LeDouarin, N. (1985). Embryonic origin of substance P containing neurons in cranial and spinal sensory ganglia of the avian embryo. *Dev. Biol.* **107**, 227–238.

Frol'kis, V. V. (1977). Hormonal regulation of electrical properties of cell membrane. *Problemy Endokrinologii* **23**, 86–93.

Fujita-Yamaguchi, Y., Choi, S., Sakamoto, Y., and Itakura, K. (1983). Purification of insulin receptor with full binding activity. *J. Biol. Chem.* **258**, 5045–5049.

Gadsby, D. C. (1982). Hyperpolarization of frog skeletal muscle fibers and of canine cardiac Purkinje fibers during enhanced Na$^+$–K$^+$ exchange: Extracellular K$^+$ depletion or increased pump current? *Curr. Top. Membr. Transp.* **16**, 17–34.

Gadsby, D. C. (1984). The Na–K pump of cardiac cells. *Ann. Rev. Biophys. Bioeng.* **13**, 373–398.

Gallacher, D. V., and Petersen, O. H. (1980). Substance P increases membrane conductance in parotid acinar cells. *Nature* **283**, 393–395.

Gallin, E. K. (1984). Calcium- and voltage-activated potassium channels in human macrophages. *Biophys. J.* **46**, 821–825.

Galper, J. B., Dziekan, L. C., Miura, S., and Smith, T. W. (1982). Agonist-induced changes in the modulation of K$^+$ permeability and beating rate by muscarinic agonists in cultured heart cells. *J. Gen. Physiol.* **80**, 231–256.

Gammeltoft, S. (1984). Insulin receptors: Binding kinetics and structure–function relationship of insulin. *Physiol. Rev.* **64**, 1321–1378.

Garcia-Sainz, J. A., and Fain, J. N. (1980). Effect of insulin, catecholamines and calcium ions on phospholipid metabolism in isolated white fat-cells. *Biochem. J.* **186**, 781–789.

Garcia-Sancho, J., Sanchez, A., and Herreros, B. (1982). All-or-none response of the Ca^{++}-dependent K$^+$-channel in inside-out vesicles. *Nature* **296**, 744–746.

Gardner, J. D., and Jensen, R. T. (1983). Gastrointestinal peptides: The basis of action at the cellular level. *Rec. Prog. Horm. Res.* **39**, 211–243.

Gardner, J. D., Conlon, T. P., Klaevman, H. L., Adams, T. D., and Ondetti, M. A. (1975). Action of cholecystokinin and cholinergic agents on calcium transport in isolated pancreatic acinar cells. *J. Clin. Invest.* **56**, 366–375.

Gavryck, W. A., Moore, R. D., and Thompson, R. C. (1975). Effect of insulin upon membrane-bound (Na$^+$ + K$^+$)-ATPase extracted from frog skeletal muscle. *J. Physiol.* **252**, 43–58.

Gelehrter, T. D., Shreve, P. D., and Dilworth, V. M. (1984). Insulin regulation of Na–K pump activity in rat hepatoma cells. *Diabetes* **33**, 428–434.

Gliemann, J., and Rees, W. D. (1983). The insulin-sensitive hexose transport system in adipocytes. *Curr. Top. Memb. Transp.* **18**, 339–379.

Glitsch, H. G. (1982). Electrogenic sodium pumping in the heart. *Ann. Rev. Physiol.* **44**, 389–400.

Gorga, J. C., and Lienhard, G. E. (1984). One transporter per vesicle: Determination of the basis of the insulin effect on glucose transport. *Fed. Proc.* **43**, 2237–2241.

Gospodarowicz, D. (1981). Growth factor for animal cells in culture: A nonimmunologist's view of mitogenic factors other than lymphokines. *In* "Lymphokines" (E. Pick, ed.), Vol. 4, pp. 1–33. Academic Press, New York.

Greenberg, M. J., and Prince, D. A. (1983). Invertebrate neuropeptides: Native and naturalized. *Ann. Rev. Physiol.* **45**, 271–288.

Greene, L. A., and Shooter, E. M. (1980). The nerve growth factor: Biochemistry, synthesis and mechanism of action. *Ann. Rev. Neurosci.* **3**, 353–402.

Gu, J., Adrian, T. E., Tatemoto, K., Polak, J. M., Allen, J. M., and Bloom, S. R. (1983). Neuropeptide tyrosine (NPY)—A major cardiac neuropeptide. *Lancet* (May 7) 1008–1010.

Gu, J., Polak, J. M., Allen, J. M., Huang, W. M., Sheppard, M. N., Tatemoto, K., and Bloom, S. R. (1984). High concentrations of a novel peptide, Neuropeptide Y, in the innervation of mouse and rat heart. *J. Histochem. Cytochem.* **32**, 467–472.

Habenicht, A. J. R., Glomset, J. A., King, W. C., Nist, C., Mitchell, D., and Ross, R. (1981). Early changes in phosphatidylinositol and arachidonic acid metabolism in quiescent Swiss 3T3 cells stimulated to divide by platelet-derived growth factor. *J. Biol. Chem.* **256**, 12329–12335.

Haddas, R. A., Landis, C. A., and Putney, J. W. (1979). Relationship between calcium-release and potassium-release in rat parotid gland. *J. Physiol.* **291**, 457–465.

Halvorsen, S. W., Engel, B., Hunter, D. D., and Nathanson, N. M. (1983). Development and regulation of cardiac muscarinic acetylcholine receptor number, function and guanyl nucleotide sensitivity. *In* "Myocardial Injury" (J. J. Spitzer, ed.), pp. 143–158. Plenum Publishing, New York.

Hamill, O. P., Marty, A., Neher, E., Sakmann, B., and Sigworth, F. J. (1981). Improved patch-clamp techniques for high-resolution current recording from cells and cell-free membrane patches. *Pflüg. Arch.* **391**, 85–100.

Hedo, J. A., Harrison, L. C., and Roth, J. (1981). Binding of insulin receptors to lectins: Evidence of common carbohydrate determinants on several membrane receptors. *Biochemistry* **20**, 3385–3393.

Helman, S. I., Els, W. J., Cox, T. C., and Van Driessche, W. (1981). Hormonal control of the Na entry process at the apical membrane of frog skin. *In* "Membrane Biophysics, Structure and Function in Epithelia" (M. A. Dinno and A. B. Callahan, eds.), pp. 47–56. Alan R. Liss, New York.

Herzberg, V., Boughter, J. M., Carlisle, S., and Hill, D. E. (1980). Evidence for two insulin receptor populations on human erythrocytes. *Nature* **286**, 270–280.

Hille, B. (1984). "Ionic Channels of Excitable Membranes." Sinauer Assoc., Sutherland, Mass.

Hoekfelt, T., Johansson, O., Ljungdahl, A., and Schultzberg, T. (1980). Peptidergic neurones. *Nature* **284**, 515–521.

Hoekfelt, T., Skirboll, L., Everitt, B., Meister, B., Brownstein, M., Jacobs, T., Faden, A., Kuga, S., Goldstein, M., Markstein, R., Dockray, G., and Reheld, J. (1985). Distribution of cholecystokinin-like immunoreactivity in the nervous system. *Ann. N.Y. Acad. Sci.* **448**, 255–274.

Hoffman, L. E., and Van Mierop, L. H. S. (1971). Effects of epinephrine on heart rate and arterial blood pressure of the developing chick embryo. *Ped. Res.* **5**, 474–477.

Hokin L. E. (1985). Receptors and phosphoinositide-generated second messengers. *Ann. Rev. Biochem.* **54**, 205–235.

Horii, Z. I., and Varon, S. (1977). Nerve growth factor action on membrane permeation to exogenous substrates in dorsal root ganglion dissociates from the chick embryo. *Brain Res.* **124**, 121–133.

Hougen, T. J., Hopkins, B. E., and Smith, T. W. (1978). Insulin effects on monovalent cation and Na$^+$-K$^+$ ATPase activity. *Am. J. Physiol.* **234**, 659–663.

Isenberg, G. (1977). Cardiac purkinje fibers: Ca^{2+}$_i$ controls the potassium permeability via the conductance components g_{K1} and $\bar{g}_{K2}$. *Pflüg. Arch.* **371**, 77–85.

Iwatsuki, N., and Petersen, O. H. (1977). Acetylcholine-like effects of intracellular calcium application in pancreatic acinar cells. *Nature* **268**, 147–149.

Iwatsuki, N., and Petersen, O. H. (1978). In vitro action of bombesin on amylase secretion, membrane potential and membrane resistance in rat and mouse pancreatic acinar cells. *J. Clin. Inv.* **61**, 41–46.

Iwatsuki, N., and Petersen, O. H. (1980). Amino-acids evoke short-latency membrane conductance increase in pancreatic acinar cells. *Nature* **283**, 492–494.

Iwatsuki, N., Kato, K., and Nishigama, A. (1977). The effects of gastrin and gastrin analogues on pancreatic acinar cell membrane potential and resistance. *Brit. J. Pharmacol.* **60**, 147–154.

Jacobs, S., and Cuatracasas, P. (1983). Insulin receptors. *Ann. Rev. Pharmacol. Toxicol.* **23**, 461–479.

Jacobs, S., Hazum, E., and Cuatracasas, P. (1980). The subunit structure of rat liver insulin receptor: Antibodies directed against the insulin-binding subunit. *J. Biol. Chem.* **255**, 6937–6940.

James, R., and Bradshaw, R. A. (1984). Polypeptide growth factors. *Ann. Rev. Biochem.* **53**, 259–292.

Jard, S. (1983). Vasopressin isoreceptors in mammals: Relation to cyclic AMP-dependent and cyclic AMP-independent transduction mechanisms. *Curr. Top. Memb. Transp.* **18**, 255–285.

Jarett, L., Kiechle, F. L., and Parker, J. C. (1982). Chemical mediator or mediators of insulin action: Response to insulin and mode of action. *Fed. Proc.* **41**, 2736–2741.

Jarett, L., Wong, E. H. A., Macauley, S. L., and Smith, J. A. (1985). Insulin mediators from rat skeletal muscle have differential effects on insulin-sensitive pathways of intact adipocytes. *Science* **227**, 533–535.

Jensen, R. T., Lemp, G. F., and Gardner, J. D. (1980). Interaction of cholecystokinin with specific membrane receptors on pancreatic acinar cells. *Proc. Natl. Acad. Sci. USA* **77**, 2079–2083.

Kahn, C. R., and Baird, K. L. (1978). The fate of insulin bound on adipocytes: Evidence for compartmentalization and processing. *J. Biol. Chem.* **253**, 4900–4906.

Karnieli, E., Zarnowski, M. J., Hissin, P. J., Simpson, I. A., Salans, L. B., and Cushman, S. W. (1981). Insulin-stimulated translocation of glucose transport systems in the isolated rat adipose cell: Time course, reversal, insulin concentration dependency, and relationship to glucose transport activity. *J. Biol. Chem.* **256**, 4772–4777.

Kasuga, M., Zick, Y., Blithe, D. L., Crettaz, M., and Kahn, C. R. (1982). Insulin stimulates tyrosine phosphorylation of the insulin receptor in a cell-free system. *Nature* **298**, 667–669.

Katzen, H. M., Soderman, D. D., and Green, B. C. (1981). Evidence that insulin and concanavalin A can co-bind to solubilized receptors without inhibiting each other. *Biochem. Biophys. Res. Comm.* **98**, 410–416.

Kelly, K. L., Kiechle, F. L., and Jarett, L. (1984). Insulin stimulation of phospholipid methylation in isolated rat adipocyte plasma membranes. *Proc. Natl. Acad. Sci. USA* **81**, 1089–1092.

Keppens, S., Vandenheede, J. R., and DeWulf, H. (1977). On the role of calcium as second messenger in liver for the hormonally induced activation of glycogen phosphorylase. *Biochim. Biophys. Acta* **496**, 448–457.

Kessler, J. A., Spray, D. C., Saez, J. C., and Bennett, M. V. L. (1984). Determination of synaptic phenotype: Insulin and cAMP independently initiate development of electrotonic coupling between cultured sympathetic neurons. *Proc. Natl. Acad. Sci. USA* **81**, 6235–6239.

Kidokoro, Y. (1975). Spontaneous calcium action potentials in a clonal pituitary cell line and their relationship to prolactin secretion. *Nature* **258**, 741–742.

Konishi, S., and Otsuka, M. (1974). Excitatory action of hypothalamic substance P on spinal motoneurones of newborn rats. *Nature* **252**, 734–735.

Kono, T. (1984). Translocation hypothesis of insulin action on glucose transport. *Fed. Proc.* **43**, 2256–2257.

Kono, T., Suzuki, K., Dansey, L. E., Robinson, F. W., and Blevins, T. L. (1981). Energy-dependent and protein synthesis-independent recycling of the insulin-sensitive glucose transport mechanism in fat cells. *J. Biol. Chem.* **256**, 6400–6407.

Kono, T., Robinson, F. W., Blevins, T. L., and Ezaki, O. (1982). Evidence that translocation of the glucose transport activity is the major mechanism of insulin action on glucose transport in fat cells. *J. Biol. Chem.* **257**, 10942–10947.

Krieger, D. T. (1983). Brain peptides: What, where and why? *Science* **222**, 975–985.

Kuriyama, H., and Suzuki, H. (1976). Changes in electrical properties of rat myometrium during gestation and following hormonal treatments. *J. Physiol.* **260**, 315–333.

LaManna, V. R., and Ferrier, G. R. (1981). Electrophysiological effects of insulin on normal and depressed cardiac tissues. *Am. J. Physiol.: Heart and Circ. Physiol.* **240**, H636–H644.

Lantz, R. C., Elsas, L. J., and DeHaan, R. L. (1980). Ouabain-resistant hyperpolarization induced by insulin in aggregates of embryonic heart cells. *Proc. Natl. Acad. Sci. USA* **77**, 3062–3066.

Latorre, R., Alvarez, O., Cecchi, X., and Vergara, C. (1985). Properties of reconstituted ion channels. *Ann. Rev. Biophys. Biophys. Chem.* **14**, 79–111.

Lederer, W. J., and Tsien, R. W. (1976). Transient inward current underlying arrhythmogenic action of cardiotonic steroids in Purkinje fibres. *J. Physiol.* **263**, 73–100.

Lembeck, F. (1953). Zur frage der zentralen ubertragung afferenter impulse. III. Mitteilung das vorkommen und die bedeutung der substanz P in den dorsalen wurzeln des ruckenmarks. *Naunyn Schmiedebergs Arch. Pharmakol.* **219**, 197–213.

Levi-Montalcini, R. (1966). The nerve growth factor, its mode of action on sensory and sympathetic nerve cells. *Harvey Lect.* **60**, 217–259.

Lewis, S. A., Hanrahan, J. W., and Van Driessche, W. (1984). Channels across epithelial layers. *Curr. Top. Membr. Transp.* **21**, 253–293.

Li, J. H. Y., Palmer, L. G., Edelman, I. S., and Lindermann, B. (1982). The role of sodium-channel density in the Natriferic response of the toad urinary bladder to an antidiuretic hormone. *J. Membr. Biol.* **64**, 77–89.

Livett, B. G. (1984). Adrenal medullary chromaffin cells *in vitro*. *Physiol. Rev.* **64**, 1103–1161.

Macara, I. G. (1985). Oncogenes, ions and phospholipids. *Am. J. Physiol. Cell. Physiol.* **248**, C3–C11.

McDonald, J. M. Bruns, D. E., and Jarett, L. (1976). The ability of insulin to alter the stable calcium pools of isolated adipocyte subcellular fractions. *Biochem. Biophys. Res. Comm.* **71**, 114–121.

McDonald, J. M., Bruns, D. E., and Jarett, L. (1978). Ability of insulin to increase calcium uptake by adipocyte endoplasmic reticulum. *J. Biol. Chem.* **253**, 3504–3508.

McGeoch, J. E. M. (1983). Specific insulin binding to purified Na, K-ATPase associated with rapid activation of the enzyme. *Curr. Top. Membr. Transp.* **19**, 977–983.

Malinow, M. R. (1958). The effect of insulin on the electrical activity of isolated ventricular muscle of the rat. *Acta Physiol. Lat. Am.* **8**, 125–128.

Marquardt, H., Hunkapiller, M. W., Hood, L. E., Twardzik, D. R., De Larco, J. L., Stephenson, J. R., and Todaro, G. J. (1983). Transforming growth factors produced by retrovirus-transformed rodent fibroblasts and human melanoma cells: Amino acid sequence homology with epidermal growth factor. *Proc. Natl. Acad. Sci. USA* **80**, 4684–4688.

Maruyama, Y., and Petersen, O. H. (1982). Cholecystokinin activation of single-channel is mediated by internal messenger in pancreatic acinar cells. *Nature* **300**, 61–63.

Massague, J., and Czech, M. P. (1982). The subunit structures of two distinct receptors for insulin-like growth factors I and II and their relationship to the insulin receptor. *J. Biol. Chem.* **257**, 5038–5045.

Matthews, E. K., Petersen, O. H., and Williams, J. A. (1973). Pancreatic acinar cells: Acetylcholine-induced membrane depolarization, calcium efflux and amylase release. *J. Physiol.* **234**, 689–701.

Meech, R. W. (1978). Calcium-dependent potassium activation in nervous tissue. *Ann. Rev. Biophys. Bioeng.* **7**, 1–18.

Mendoza, S. A., Wigglesworth, N. M., and Rozengurt, E. (1980). Vasopressin rapidly stimulates Na entry and Na–K pump activity in quiescent cultures of mouse 3T3 cells. *J. Cell. Physiol.* **105**, 153–162.

Michell, R. H. (1975). Inositol phospholipids and cell surface receptor function. *Biochim. Biophys. Acta* **415**, 81–147.

Michell, R. H., Kirk, C. J., and Billah, M. M. (1979). Hormonal stimulation of phosphatidylinositol breakdown, with particular reference to the hepatic effects of vasopressin. *Biochem. Soc. Trans.* **7**, 861–865.

Michell, R. H., Kirk, C. J., Jones, L. M., Downes, C., and Creba, J. A. (1981). The stimulation of inositol lipid metabolism that accompanies calcium mobilization in stimulated cells: Defined characteristic and unanswered questions. *Phil. Trans. R. Soc. Ser. B.* **296**, 123–127.

Moolenaar, W. H., Tsien, R. W., van der Saag, P. T., and deLaat, S. W. (1983). Na^+/H^+ exchange and cytoplasmic pH in the action of growth factors in human fibroblasts. *Nature* **304**, 645–648.

Moolenaar, W. H., Tertoolen, L. G. J., and deLaat, S. W. (1984). Growth factors immediately raise cytoplasmic free Ca^{2+} in human fibroblasts. *J. Biol. Chem.* **259**, 8066–8069.

Moore, R. D. (1973). Effect of insulin upon the sodium pump in frog skeletal muscle. *J. Physiol.* **232**, 23–45.

Moore, R. D. (1981). Stimulation of Na–H exchange by insulin. *Biophys. J.* **33**, 203–210.

Moore, R. D. (1983). Effects of insulin upon ion transport. *Biochim. Biophys. Acta* **737**, 1–49.

Moore, R. D., and Rabovsky, J. L. (1979). Mechanisms of insulin action on resting membrane potential of frog skeletal muscle. *Am. J. Physiol.: Cell Physiol.* **236**, C249–C259.

Muhlethaler, M., Dreifuss, J. J., and Gahwiler, B. H. (1982). Vasopressin excites hippocampal neurones. *Nature* **296**, 749–751.

Muhlethaler, M., Sawyer, W. H., Manning, M. M., and Dreifuss, J. J. (1983). Characterization of a uterine-type oxytocin receptor in the rat hippocampus. *Proc. Natl. Acad. Sci. USA* **80**, 6713–6717.

Muhlethaler, M., Raggenbass, M., and Dreifuss, J. J. (1984). Peptides related to vasopressin in invertebrates. *Experientia* **40**, 777–782.

Myrdal, S. E., and DeHaan, R. L. (1983). Concanavalin A increases spontaneous beat rate of embryonic chick heart cell aggregates. *J. Cell. Physiol.* **117**, 319–325.

Nishizuka, Y. (1984). Turnover of inositol phospholipids and signal transduction. *Science* **225**, 1365–1370.

Nishizuka, Y., Takai, Y., Kishimoto, A., Kikkawa, U., and Kaibuchi, K. (1984). Phospholipid turnover in hormone action. *Rec. Prog. Horm. Res.* **40**, 301–345.

Noble, D., and Tsien, R. W. (1968). The kinetics and rectifier properties of the slow potassium current in cardiac Purkinje fibres. *J. Physiol. (London)* **195**, 185–214.

Noma, A. (1983). ATP-regulated K^+ channels in cardiac muscle. *Nature* **305**, 147–148.

Oka, Y., Mottola, C., Oppenheimer, C. L., and Czech, M. P. (1984). Insulin activates the appearance of insulin-like growth factor. II. Receptors on the adipocyte cell surface. *Proc. Natl. Acad. Sci. USA* **81**, 4028–4032.

Olefsky, J. M., and Chang, H. (1978). Insulin binding to adipocytes. Evidence for functionally distinct receptors. *Diabetes* **27**, 946–958.

Oomura, Y., Otita, M., Kita, H., Ishibashi, S., and Okajima, T. (1978). Hypothalamic neuron response to glucose, phlorizin and cholecystokinin. *In* "Iontophoresis and Transmitter Mechanisms in the Mammalian Central Nervous System" (R. W. Ryall and J. S. Kelly, eds.), pp. 120–123. Elsevier, Amsterdam.

Owen, N. E. (1984). Platelet-derived growth factor stimulates Na^+ influx in vascular smooth muscle cells. *Am. J. Physiol.: Cell Physiol.* **247**, C501–C505.

Ozawa, S., and Kimura, M. (1979). Membrane potential changes caused by thyrotropin-releasing hormone in the clonal GH3 cell and their relationship to secretion of pituitary hormone. *Proc. Natl. Acad. Sci. USA* **76**, 6017–6020.

Palmer, L. G., and Edelman, I. S. (1981). Control of apical sodium permeability in the toad urinary bladder by aldosterone. Part I. Mechanism of action of aldosterone. *Ann. N. Y. Acad. Sci.* **372**, 1–14.

Pappano, A. (1977). Ontogenetic development of autonomic neuroeffector transmission and transmitter reactivity in embryonic and fetal hearts. *Pharmacol. Rev.* **29**, 3–33.

Pershadsingh, H. A., and McDonald, J. M. (1980). A high affinity calcium-stimulated magnesium-dependent adenosine triphosphatase in rat adipocyte plasma. *J. Biol. Chem.* **255**, 4087–4093.

Pershadsingh, H. A., and McDonald, J. M. (1981). $[Ca^{2+} + Mg^{2+}]$-ATPase in adipocyte plasmalemma: Inhibition by insulin and concanavalin A on the intact cell. *Biochem. Int.* **2**, 243–248.

Pershadsingh, H. A., Landt, M., and McDonald, J. M. (1980). Calmodulin-sensitive ATP-dependent Ca^{2+} transport across adipocyte plasma membranes. *J. Biol. Chem.* **255**, 8983–8986.

Petersen, O. H. (1981). Electrophysiology of exocrine gland cells. *In* "Physiology of the Gastrointestinal Tract" (L. R. Johnson, ed.), Vol. 1, pp. 749–772. Raven Press, New York.

Petersen, O. H., and Iwatsuki, N. (1978). The role of calcium in pancreatic acinar cell stimulus–secretion coupling: An electrophysiological approach. *Ann. N.Y. Acad. Sci.* **307**, 599–617.

Petersen, O. H., and Laugier, R. (1980). Receptor mediated control via the calcium effector of membrane ion permeability in pancreatic acinar cells. *Biochem. Soc. Trans.* **8**, 268–270.

Petersen, O. H., and Maruyama, Y. (1983). Cholecystokinin and acetylcholine activation of single channel currents via second messenger in pancreatic acinar cells. *In* "Single Channel Recording" (B. Sakmann and E. Neher, eds.), pp. 425–435. Plenum, New York.

Petersen, O. H., and Maruyama, Y. (1984). Calcium-activated potassium channels and their role in secretion. *Nature* **307**, 693–696.

Petersen, O. H., and Philpott, H. G. (1979). Pancreatic acinar cells: Effects of micro-iontophoretic polypeptide application on membrane potential and resistance. *J. Physiol.* **290**, 305–315.

Petruzzelli, L. M., Ganguly, S., Smith, C. J., Lobb, M. H., Rubin, C. S., and Rosen, O. M. (1982). Insulin activates a tyrosine-specific protein kinase in extracts of 3T3-Li adipocytes and human placenta. *Proc. Natl. Acad. Sci. USA* **79**, 6792–6796.

Phillis, J. W., and Kirkpatrick, J. R. (1979). Actions of various gastrointestinal peptides on the isolated amphibian spinal cord. *Can. J. Physiol. Pharmacol.* **57**, 887–889.

Phillis, J. W., and Limacher, J. J. (1974). Substance P excitation of cerebral cortical Betz cells. *Brain Res.* **69**, 158–163.

Piwnica-Worms, D., Jacob, R., Horres, C. R., and Lieberman, M. (1985). Na–H exchange in cultured chick heart cells. pH_i regulation. *J. Gen. Physiol.* **85**, 43–64.

Popot, J.-L., and Changeux, J.-P. (1984). Nicotinic receptor of acetylcholine: Structure of an oligomeric integral membrane protein. *Physiol. Rev.* **64**, 1162–1239.

Przybylski, R. J. (1967). Cytodifferentiation of the chick pancreas. I. Ultrastructure of the islet cells and the initiation of granule formation. *Gen. Comp. Endocrinol.* **8**, 115–128.

Rasmussen, H., and Barrett, P. Q. (1984). Calcium messenger system: An integrated view. *Physiol. Rev.* **64**, 938–984.

Rechler, M. M., and Nissley, S. P. (1985). The nature and regulation of the receptors for insulin-like growth factors. *Ann. Rev. Physiol.* **47**, 425–442.

Rehfeld, J. F., Hansen, H. F., and Marley, P. D. (1985). Molecular forms of cholecystokinin in the brain and the relationship to neuronal gastrins. *Ann. N.Y. Acad. Sci.* **448**, 11–23.

Rehm, W., Schumann, H., and Heinz, E. (1961). Insulin on frog gastric mucosa. *Fed. Proc.* **20**, 193a.

Resh, M. D., Nemenoff, R. A., and Guidotti, G. (1980). Insulin stimulation of (Na^+, K^+)-

adenosine triphosphatase-dependent Rb^+ uptake in rat adipocytes. *J. Biol. Chem.* **255**, 10938–10945.

Reuter, H. (1984). Ion channels in cardiac cell membranes. *Ann. Rev. Physiol.* **46**, 473–484.

Reznik, V. M., Shapiro, R. J., and Mendoza, S. A. (1985). Vasopressin stimulates DNA synthesis and ion transport in quiescent epithelial cells. *Am. J. Physiol.: Cell Physiol.* **249**, C267–270.

Roberts, M. L., Iwatsuki, N., and Petersen, O. H. (1978). Parotid acinar cells: Ionic-dependence of acetylcholine-evoked membrane potential changes. *Pflüg. Arch.* **376**, 159–167.

Ronnett, F. V., Knutson, V. P., Kohanski, R. A., Simpson, T. L., and Lane, M. D. (1984). Role of glycosylation in the processing of newly translated insulin proreceptor in 3T3-L1 adipocytes. *J. Biol. Chem.* **259**, 4566–4575.

Rosenzweig, S. A., Madison, L. D., and Jamieson, J. D. (1984). Analysis of cholecystokinin-binding proteins using endo-beta-N-acetylglucosaminidase F. *J. Cell Biol.* **99**, 1110–1116.

Rothenberg, P., Reuss, L., and Glaser, L. (1982). Serum and epidermal growth factor transiently depolarize quiescent BSC-1 epithelial cells. *Proc. Natl. Acad. Sci. USA* **79**, 7783–7787.

Rozengurt, E., Gelehrter, T. D., Legg, A., and Pettican, P. (1981). Melittin stimulates Na entry, Na–K pump activity and DNA synthesis in quiescent cultures of mouse cells. *Cell* **23**, 781–788.

Sahai, A., Smith, K. B., Panneerselvam, M., and Salomon, D. S. (1982). Activation of calcium-and phospholipid-dependent protein kinase by epidermal growth factor (EGF) in A431 cells: Attenuation by 12-o-tetradecanoylphorbol-13-acetate (TPA). *Biochem. Biophys. Res. Comm.* **109**, 1206–1214.

Sakmann, B., and Neher, E. (1983). "Single Channel Recording." Plenum, New York.

Sawyer, S. T., and Cohen, S. (1981). Enhancement of calcium uptake and phosphatidylinositol turnover by epidermal growth factor in A-431 cells. *Biochemistry* **20**, 6280–6286.

Schechter, A. L., and Bothwell, M. A. (1981). Nerve growth factor receptors on PC12 cells: Evidence for two receptor classes with differing cytoskeletal association. *Cell* **24**, 867–874.

Schwarz, W., and Passow, H. (1983). Ca^{2+}-activated K^+ channels in erythrocytes and excitable cells. *Ann. Rev. Physiol.* **45**, 359–374.

Serravezza, J. C., Wheeler, F. B., DeHaan, R. L., and Elsas, L. J. (1981). Characterization and regulation of insulin binding by embryonic chick heart cells. *Dev. Biol.* **84**, 417–424.

Serravezza, J. C., Endo, F., DeHaan, R. L., and Elsas, L. J., II (1983). Insulin-induced receptor loss reduces responsiveness of chick heart cells to insulin. *Endocrinology* **113**, 497–505.

Shipley, S. E., and DeHaan, R. L. (1981). Regulation of spontaneous beat rate in heart cell aggregates: Antagonistic cell effects of insulin and concanavalin A. *Fed. Proc.* **40**, 367a.

Siegal, M. S., and Hoffman, B. A. (1980). Effects of calcium on canine Purkinje fiber action potential duration in the presence of agents affecting potassium permeability. *Circ. Res.* **46**, 227–236.

Siegelbaum, S. A., and Tsien, R. W. (1980). Calcium-activated transient outward current in calf cardiac Purkinje fibres. *J. Physiol.* **299**, 485–506.

Siggins, G. R., Gruol, D., Aldenhoff, J., and Pittman, Q. (1985). Electrophysiological actions of corticotropin-releasing factor in the central nervous system. *Fed. Proc.* **44**, 237–242.

Simpson, I. A., and Hedo, J. A. (1984). Insulin receptor phosphorylation may not be a prerequisite for acute insulin action. *Science* **223**, 1301–1304.

Singer, J., and Walsh, J. (1984). Large-conductance Ca^{++}-activated potassium channels in smooth muscle membranes. Reduction in unitary currents due to internal Na^+ ions. *Biophys. J.* **45**, 68–69.

Skaper, S. D., and Varon, S. (1979a). Sodium dependence of nerve growth factor-regulated hexose transport in chick embryo sensory neurons. *Biochem. Biophys. Res. Comm.* **88**, 563–568.

Skaper, S. D., and Varon, S. (1979b). Nerve growth factor action on 2-deoxy-D-glucose transport in dorsal root ganglionic dissociates from chick embryo. *Brain Res.* **163**, 89–100.

Sladek, J. R., and Sladek, C. D. (1985). Neurological control of vasopressin release. *Fed. Proc.* **44**, 66–71.

Snyder, S. H., Bruns, R. F., Daly, J. W., and Innis, R. B. (1981). Multiple neurotransmitter receptors in the brain: Amines, adenosine and cholecystokinin. *Fed. Proc.* **40**, 142–145.

Stark, R. J., and O'Doherty, J. (1982). Intracellular Na^+ and K^+ activities during stimulation of rat soleus muscle. *Am. J. Physiol.: Endocrinol.* **242**, E193–E200.

Starling, E. H. (1905). On the chemical correlations of the functions of the body. *Lancet* **2**, 339–341.

Streb, H., Irvine, R. F., Berridge, M. J., and Schulz, I. (1983). Release of Ca^{2+} from a non-mitochondrial intracellular store in pancreatic acinar cells by inositol-1,4,5-trisphosphate. *Nature* **306**, 67–69.

Streb, H., Bayerdorffer, E., Haase, W., Irvine, R. F., and Schulz, I. (1984). Effect of inositol-1,4,5-trisphosphate on isolated subcellular fractions of rat pancreas. *J. Membr. Biol.* **81**, 241–253.

Suzuki, K., and Kono, T. (1980). Evidence that insulin causes translocation of glucose transport activity to the plasma membrane from an intracellular storage site. *Proc. Natl. Acad. Sci. USA.* **77**, 2542–2545.

Swenne, I., and Lundqvist, G. (1980). Islet structure and pancreatic hormone content of the developing chick embryo. *Gen. Comp. Endocrinol.* **41**, 190–198.

Tatemoto, K., Carlquist, M., and Mutt, V. (1982). Neuropeptide Y—A novel brain peptide with structural similarities to peptide YY and pancreatic polypeptide. *Nature* **296**, 659–660.

Taylor, L. P., and Holman, G. D. (1981). Symmetrical kinetic parameters for 3-O-methyl-D-glucose transport in adipocytes in the presence and absence of insulin. *Biochim. Biophys. Acta* **642**, 325–335.

Trenkle, A., and Hopkins, K. (1971). Immunological investigation of an insulin like substance in the chicken embryo. *Gen. Comp. Endocrinol.* **16**, 493–497.

Trube, G., and Hescheler, J. (1984). Inward-rectifying channels in isolated patches of heart cell membrane: ATP-dependence and comparison with cell-attached patches. *Pflüg. Arch.* **401**, 178–184.

Tsien, R. W. (1983). Calcium channels in excitable cell membranes. *Ann. Rev. Physiol.* **45**, 341–358.

Ullrich, A., Bell, J. R., Chen, E. Y., Herrera, R., Petruzzelli, L. M., Dull, T. J., Gray, A., Coussens, L., Liao, Y.-C., Tsubokawa, M., Mason, A., Seeburg, P. H., Grunfield, C., Rosen, O. M., and Ramachandran, J. (1985). Human insulin receptor and its relationship to the tyrosine kinase family of oncogenes. *Nature* **313**, 756–761.

Vale, W., Speiss, J., River, C., and River, J. (1981). Characterization of a 41-residue ovine hypothalamic peptide that stimulates secretion of corticotropin and β-endorphin. *Science* **231**, 1394–1397.

Valentino, R. J., Foote, S. L., and Aston-Jones, G. (1983). Corticotropin-releasing factor activates noradrenergic neurons of the locus coeruleus. *Brain Res.* **270**, 363–367.

Villereal, M. L., Owen, N. E., Vincentini, L. M., and Mix, L. L. (1985). Regulation of Na^+/H^+ exchange in cultured human fibroblasts. *In* "Regulation and Development of Membrane Transport Processes" (J. S. Graves, ed.), pp. 21–42. John Wiley, New York.

von Euler, U. S., and Gaddum, J. H. (1931). An unidentified depressor substance in certain tissue extracts. *J. Physiol.* **72**, 74–87.

Voorhees, W., Dunn, A., and Hiatt, N. (1978). Insulin alteration of epinephrine action on the heart. *Gen. Pharmacol.* **9**, 433–436.

Walsh, J. H. (1981). Hormones and peptides. *In* "Physiology of the Gastrointestinal Tract" (L. R. Johnson, ed.), pp. 59–144. Raven Press, New York.

Wardzala, L. J., and Jeanrenaud, B. (1983). Identification of the D-glucose-inhibitable cytochalasin

B binding site as the glucose transporter in rat diaphragm plasma and microsomal membranes. *Biochim. Biophys. Acta* **730**, 49–56.

Wardzala, L. J., Cushman, S. W., and Salans, L. B. (1978). Mechanism of insulin action on glucose transport in the isolated rat adipose cell. Enhancement of the number of functional transport systems. *J. Biol. Chem.* **253**, 8002–8005.

Welsh, J. H. (1955). Neurohormones. *In* "The Hormones" (G. Pincus and K. V. Thimann, eds.), pp. 98–151. Academic Press, New York.

Wheeler, F. B., Santora, A. C., Danner, D. J., DeHaan, R. L., and Elsas, L. J. (1978). Developmental control of 2-aminoisobutyric acid transport by 7- and 14-day chick heart cell aggregates: Roles of insulin and amino acids. *Dev. Biol.* **67**, 73–89.

Wheeler, F. B., Santora, A. C., and Elsas, L. C. (1980). Evidence supporting a two-receptor model for insulin-binding by cultured embryonic heart cells. *Endocrinology* **107**, 195–207.

Whitesell, R. R., and Gliemann, J. (1979). Kinetic parameters of transport of 3-O-methylglucose and glucose in adipocytes. *J. Biol. Chem.* **254**, 5276–5283.

Willetts, J., Urban, L., Murase, K., and Randić, M. (1985). Actions of cholecystokinin octapeptide on rat spinal dorsat horn neurons. *Ann. N.Y. Acad. Sci.* **448**, 385–402.

Williams, P. F., Baxter, R. C., and Turtle, J. R. (1980). Receptors for insulin and insulin-like molecules. *Circ. Res.* **46**, Part II, Suppl. 1, 110–117.

Williamson, J. R., Cooper, R. H., Joseph, S. K., and Thomas, A. P. (1985). Inositol trisphosphate and diacylglycerol as intracellular second messengers in liver. *Am. J. Physiol.: Cell Physiol.* **17**, C203–C216.

Wondergem, R. (1983). Insulin depolarization of rat hepatocytes in primary monolayer culture. *Am. J. Physiol.: Cell Physiol.* **13**, C17-C23.

Woodbury, J. W., and McIntyre, D. M. (1954). Electrical activity of single muscle cells of pregnant uteri studied with intracellular ultramicroelectrodes. *Am. J. Physiol.* **177**, 355–360.

Yankner, B. A., and Shooter, E. M. (1982). The biology and mechanism of action of nerve growth factor. *Ann. Rev. Biochem.* **51**, 845–868.

Yip, C. C., Yeung, C. W. T., and Moule, M. L. (1980). Photoaffinity labeling of insulin receptor with an insulin analogue selectivity modified at the amino terminal of the β chain. *Biochemistry* **19**, 2196–2203.

Zierler, K. L. (1957). Alterations in resting membrane potential of skeletal muscle produced by insulin. *Science* **126**, 1067–1068.

Zierler, K. L. (1972). Insulin, ions and membrane potentials. *In* "Handbook of Physiology: Endocrinology," Vol. I, Sec. 7, pp. 347–368. Am. Physiol. Soc., Washington, D.C.

Zierler, K. L. (1985). Membrane polarization and insulin action. *In* "Insulin, Its Receptor and Diabetes" (M. Hollenberg, ed.), pp. 1–59. Marcel Dekker, New York.

Zierler, K. L., and Rogus, E. M. (1981a). Effects of peptide hormones and adrenergic agents on membrane potentials of target cells. *Fed. Proc.* **40**, 121–124.

Zierler, K. L., and Rogus, E. M. (1981b). Rapid hyperpolarization of rat skeletal muscle induced by insulin. *Biochim. Biophys. Acta* **640**, 687–692.

Zierler, K. L., and Rogus, E. M. (1981c). Insulin does not hyperpolarize rat muscle by means of an ouabain-inhibitable process. *Am. J. Physiol.: Cell Physiol.* **241**, C145–C149.

Zierler, K. L., Rogus, E. M., Scherer, R. W., and Wu, F. S. (1985). Insulin action on membrane potential and 2-deoxyglucose uptake: Effects of high extracellular potassium. *Am. J. Physiol.: Endocrinol.* **249**, E17–E25.

6

Sodium–Calcium Exchange and Its Role in Generating Electric Current

Denis Noble

I. INTRODUCTION

In this chapter I review the sodium–calcium exchange process in terms of its contribution to the flow of electric current. I begin by describing some of the theory of sodium–calcium exchange in general and fairly simple terms. I follow by discussing some specific predictions of its possible role in the generation of ionic current: this serves to identify certain known ionic currents in the heart as possible candidates for transport by the exchanger. Finally, I review in each case the arguments for and against the hypothesis that a current is carried by the exchange mechanism. Recently, Mullins (1979, 1981) has also analyzed this hypothesis fairly extensively. Some of this chapter owes much to a theoretical project (DiFrancesco and Noble, 1985; DiFrancesco *et al.*, 1986) that was designed in part to test the quantitative plausibility of Mullins's proposals in addition to other theories of the role of ionic exchange and concentration changes in cardiac excitation. I shall illustrate some of the conclusions by using the model developed for that project.

II. EQUILIBRIUM AND STEADY-STATE THEORY OF THE SODIUM–CALCIUM EXCHANGE PROCESS

Experimental work on the exchange process is reviewed by Fozzard in Chapter 7 of this book. Here, I summarize the main features that need to be taken into account in any theoretical treatment:

171

CARDIAC MUSCLE:
THE REGULATION OF EXCITATION AND CONTRACTION

1. The process operates close enough to equilibrium for it to be readily reversible. Depending on the experimental conditions, calcium can be *either* extruded in exchange for entering sodium ions *or* gained by the cell in exchange for loss of sodium. These two possibilities are sometimes described as two modes of operation of the exchange mechanism and in diagrams are often shown as separate movements. Presumably, however, depending on its binding of ions on each side of the membrane, any given exchanger molecule can switch at random between the two modes.

2. The process does not depend directly on energy gradients other than those provided by the Na and Ca electrochemical gradients. It should be noted, however, that although energy from ATP splitting does not seem to be used, ATP does nevertheless influence the process, perhaps by altering the affinity of the carrier for ions.

3. The stoichiometry is not settled with certainty, but a considerable amount of experimental evidence now favors the view that the stoichiometry is $3:1$ (Na:Ca). This experimental evidence has been reviewed recently by Blaustein and Nelson (1982), but see Fozzard (Chapter 7), also.

These assumptions lead directly to equations for the equilibrium state. If we define the membrane potential at which the carrier process is in exact equilibrium (*not* just a steady state near equilibrium; this distinction will become important later) as E_{NaCa}, then we can write (cf. Baker *et al.*, 1969):

$$E_{NaCa} = (nE_{Na} - 2E_{Ca}) / (n - 2) \tag{1}$$

where n is the exchange stoichiometry, and:

$$E_{Na} = (RT/F)\ln(a_{Na})_o / (a_{Na})_i \tag{2}$$

$$E_{Ca} = (RT/2F)\ln(a_{Ca})_o / (a_{Ca})_i \tag{3}$$

where $(a_x)_o$ and $(a_x)_i$ are, respectively, the extracellular and intracellular activities of the xth ion species, and R, T, and F have their usual meanings. For the stoichiometry of $3:1$ assumed above, we obtain:

$$E_{NaCa} = 3E_{Na} - 2E_{Ca} \tag{4}$$

We can use this equation in either of two ways. First, if we know the sodium ion gradient, the extracellular calcium concentration, and the resting membrane potential (at equilibrium, E_{NaCa} must equal the membrane potential, E_m), we can ask what level of intracellular calcium could be maintained in the equilibrium state. With [Na]$_i$ at 10 mM (Ellis, 1977; Deitmer and Ellis, 1978; Sheu and Fozzard, 1982; Eisner *et al.*, 1983), [Na]$_o$ at 140 mM, and equal ionic activity coefficients inside and outside the cell, we can calculate E_{Na} to be +70 mV. If the resting potential were set at −90 mV, the equilibrium level of E_{Ca} would be $(3\ E_{Na} - E_{NaCa})/2$, i.e., (210 + 90 mV)/2 = +150 mV. With extracellular calcium at 2 mM, we would obtain approximately 12 nM as the free level of intracellular calcium that could be maintained by the energy of the sodium gradient. If the activity coefficient were approximately 0.3, the free activity $(a_{Ca})_i$ would be only 4 nM. This concentration is *extremely* small compared to experimental measurements, which tend to give activity values nearer to 100 nM; therefore, the first conclusions would be:

1. There *is* enough energy in the sodium gradient to allow a 3 : 1 exchange process to maintain calcium at least as low as observed experimentally and possibly much lower. This conclusion would be strongly reinforced if the stoichiometry were assumed to be 4 : 1 or even higher.

2. If the assumptions made thus far are correct, then the exchange process cannot be in true equilibrium in the resting state, because the resting level of $[Ca]_i$ is thought to be considerably higher than 12 nM.

The second conclusion leads us to another use for Eq. (4): given an estimated value of $(a_{Ca})_i$, we can ask how far from equilibrium the exchange process might be, that is, we can calculate E_{NaCa}. If $(a_{Ca})_i$ is 30 nM, we obtain $E_{Ca} = 30 \log (2/0.0003) = +115$ mV. Then $E_{NaCa} = 3 \times 70 - 2 \times 115 = -20$ mV, i.e., the equilibrium potential for the exchange process falls approximately midway between the resting potential and the peak plateau of the action potential. For $(a_{Ca})_i = 50$ nM we obtain $E_{NaCa} = -6$ mV.

This conclusion is similar to that of Mullins (1981). Mullins used a 4 : 1 stoichiometry in Eq. (1), but assumed much larger levels of intracellular sodium than have been measured experimentally. These two differences largely cancel each other for the purpose of this particular calculation.

For such a conclusion to be correct, there must be, and indeed there is (Niedergerke, 1963), a permeability during rest that allows calcium to enter the cell and drive E_{NaCa} positive to the resting potential. If this resting flux carries a background current, it must be inward. Moreover, such a current would likely be larger than that carried by the exchange process itself, which, with E_{NaCa} positive to the resting potential, would also carry an inward current. I return to this question later, but, for the moment, we may draw the following additional conclusions:

3. The exchange process may carry a steady inward current even at rest.

4. To this current one must also add any current generated by the background calcium leak.

There must exist a background inward current in the heart because, except at levels of $[K]_o$ larger than approximately 12–20 mM, the resting potential does not lie exactly at the potassium equilibrium potential (E_K). In ventricular and Purkinje tissues, it can lie 10–20 mV positive to the expected value of E_K. In spontaneously beating sinus node cells, the deviation is even larger (Noma and Irisawa, 1976), with a difference of at least 30 mV. This inward background current has been of fundamental importance in nearly all electrical models of pacemaker activity in the heart.

The first current that might therefore be identified with the sodium–calcium exchange process is the background inward current. Later in the chapter, I try to answer the question of how large a fraction of the background inward current might be associated with the exchange and the accompanying calcium leak.

III. THEORY OF TRANSIENT CHANGES IN THE SODIUM–CALCIUM EXCHANGE PROCESS

The uncertainties in giving an equilibrium account of the exchange process are negligible compared to the problems that arise in attempting to describe its behavior during transient changes in $[Ca]_i$. Yet these may be of the greatest importance. One activator of the exchange carrier, intracellular calcium, varies from a resting concentration of approximately 100 nM (or maybe even less: some estimate a level closer to 50 nM) to approximately 5–10 μM (i.e., 10,000 nM) during the peak of the calcium transient that activates contraction. There is, therefore, a variation in $[Ca]_i$ of approximately two orders of magnitude during every cardiac cycle. Even if the current carried by the exchanger in the resting state should prove to be very small, it might become substantial during activity.

We encountered several problems in formulating a satisfactory theoretical description that would allow us effectively to test the hypothesis that some of the currents during activity are attributable directly to electrogenic activity of the carrier. I discuss these briefly in turn and indicate both how we have dealt with the problems in our own modeling work and how this work might be developed.

1. First, we need to know how the exchange rate varies with the ionic concentrations. The sodium-dependent efflux of calcium from a variety of tissues (for review, see Blaustein and Nelson, 1982) shows a sigmoid dependence on external sodium, consistent with evidence that three or more sodium ions are required to bind to the external site to activate transport. The simplest approach would be, therefore, to use the same value of n for both the overall stoichiometry and the activation by sodium, with activation by calcium depending on occupation of a single cation binding site. Even with this information, there remain a large number of unknown parameters in any plausible model. This is well illustrated by the model developed by Mullins (1977). To incorporate equations for the carrier transport into our model of electrical activity (DiFrancesco and Noble, 1985), we decided to make some simplifying assumptions. A substantial number of the unknown parameters should remain constant, provided that large variations in sodium concentrations do not occur. This *is* a reasonable assumption, at least during a single action potential. Some of the possible sodium dependence is incorporated into a scaling factor, k_{NaCa}, that determines the magnitude of the current that may be transported. In the absence of a membrane potential, this

would give rise to an equation of the form:

$$i_{NaCa} = k_{NaCa} \{(a_{Na})_i^n \cdot (a_{Ca})_o - (a_{Na})_o^n \cdot (a_{Ca})_i\} \tag{5}$$

2. If the process is electrogenic, then it is likely to be voltage dependent. There is experimental evidence that this is the case. Sodium-dependent efflux of calcium from squid axons is, for example, reduced by membrane depolarization (Blaustein et al., 1974; Mullins and Brinley, 1975) and increased by hyperpolarization (Mullins and Brinley, 1975). Nelson and Blaustein (1981) observed a small depolarization (approximately 2 mV) in giant barnacle muscle fibers that may be associated with activation of the exchange by intracellular calcium. In heart muscle, Mentrard and Vassort (1982) have observed a small component of current that could be attributed to voltage dependence of the exchange current. Other studies of heart muscle that consider current flow that may be generated by the exchange process are described later in the chapter.

If we accept for the moment that the process is voltage dependent, we must still decide how to describe it. This problem is familiar to membrane electrophysiologists who encounter nonlinear current–voltage relations, and a large number of possible approaches now exist (see, e.g., Jack et al., 1975, Chapter 8, for a review of some of them). One of the simplest approaches is based on the assumption that the effect of the electric field is partitioned between the outward and inward movements of the charged species in a way that depends in part on the position of the peak energy barrier for movement in the electric field. The partition parameter, which I call γ, can then vary from 0 (when the peak energy barrier is located at one configuration of the carrier, e.g., when the excess sodium charge lies at the outside surface) to 1 (when the peak occurs on the other membrane surface). A value of 0.5 would reflect the symmetric case. A development of Eq. (5) then would be (DiFrancesco and Noble, 1985):

$$\begin{aligned} i_{NaCa} = k_{NaCa} \{&(a_{Na})_i^n \cdot (a_{Ca})_o \cdot \exp[(n-2)\gamma EF/RT] \\ &- (a_{Na})_o^n \cdot (a_{Ca})_i \cdot \exp[-(n-2)(1-\gamma)\,EF/RT]\} \end{aligned} \tag{6}$$

[This equation is the same as that used by DiFrancesco and Noble (1985) except for the fact that their denominator term, which depends on sodium concentration, has been incorporated into the constant k_{NaCa}.]

Before we use this equation, I must reemphasize some of its limitations. First, as explained above, the scaling factor k_{NaCa} is not independent of ion concentrations. A simple way of appreciating this point is to note that if all the ion concentrations were to be reduced, even with their transmembrane ratios remaining fairly constant, the activity of the carrier would be reduced almost certainly. In Eq. (6) this effect would be partially reproduced, but some of the change would occur also in k_{NaCa}, which is not, therefore, a simple constant. Because, at present, we have little experimental evidence, DiFrancesco and I opted to ignore this problem. It might not be possible, however, to ignore it in work that tries to assess theoretically the effects of large variations in sodium concentration (e.g., when considering the important case of sodium pump block, when $[Na]_i$ increases greatly). We can only hope that Eq. (6) will yield at least a plausible description of the behavior of the carrier during substantial variations in calcium concentration. Second, we do not know whether the activation by calcium is linear, nor at what level it saturates (this is to say that there must be some maximal value for i_{NaCa}). Finally, even with this simplified model, we do not know precisely what value to use for γ, nor whether the current level saturates at some level of electrical gradient (which again might depend on a maximal transport rate). One particular case of interest is the symmetric one, when $\gamma = 0.5$. This produces an interesting result when the carrier system is close to equilibrium: the current then becomes a hyperbolic sine function of the membrane potential (see also Mullins, 1977). Simple as this case may be, its description is not likely to be realistic for many cases. In particular, when $[Ca]_i$ varies by nearly two orders of magnitude, the conditions that allow Eq. (6) to reduce to a hyperbolic sine are seriously violated. It is worth emphasizing this point because most of the conditions of physiological interest cannot be described well by a hyperbolic sine function.

IV. THE CALCIUM TRANSIENT

Without a description of the changes in $[Ca]_i$ that may activate the exchange carrier, the value of Eq. (6) is very limited in practice; therefore, the DiFrancesco–Noble model incorporates a representation of these changes, also. In Chapter 11 of this book, Fabiato discusses the experimental evidence for intracellular calcium movements during activity. The main hypothesis from this work is that release of calcium during depolarization is itself triggered by a rise of intracellular calcium. Such an increase may be generated by either the entry of calcium via sarcolemmal calcium channels or the effect of depolarization on the Na–Ca exchange process. We have chosen to represent this process by a simple model in which one or more (usually two) calcium ions are required to bind to the release-activating site to facilitate the release of stored calcium. Figure 1 shows the general assumptions involved, whereas detailed equations can be found in DiFrancesco and Noble (1985). Here, I comment on some of the main problems we encountered.

When we began this modeling work, we used the equations for calcium current proposed originally in the McAllister *et al.* (1975) or Beeler and Reuter (1977) model. They were based on current kinetics measured experimentally in multicellular preparations. Although these were in fact highly variable (for reviews, see Coraboeuf, 1980; Noble and Powell, 1985), the majority of measurements described a current that was activated and inactivated much more slowly than the fast sodium current. In the Beeler and Reuter equations, for example,

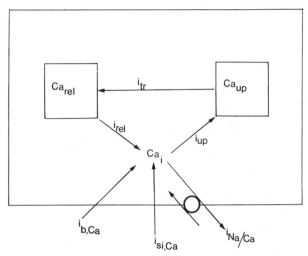

Fig. 1. Diagram summarizing the processes assumed in the DiFrancesco–Noble (1985) model to control Ca ion movements. An energy-consuming pump is assumed to transport Ca into the sarcoplasmic reticulum (represented by the uptake flux i_{up}), which then reprimes a releasable store. Release (i_{rel}) is activated by cytoplasmic free calcium. Ca leaves the cell via the Na–Ca exchange and may enter the cell through voltage-dependent Ca channels or through a background (leak) channel. Rarely, it may enter the cell through the exchanger, when [Ca]$_i$ is very low and the voltage very positive. These were the minimum assumptions required to model the [Ca]$_i$ transient and to model oscillatory variations in [Ca]$_i$ when [Ca]$_i$ is raised. The model is being developed further to incorporate other calcium buffering and transport processes.

the activation time constant is approximately 22 msec, whereas the inactivation time constant is approximately 300 msec. DiFrancesco and I found it quite difficult to formulate a plausible model of calcium-induced release of calcium that would exhibit such slow current kinetics and yet reproduce the time course of the intracellular calcium transient as measured with aequorin (see, e.g., Allen and Kurihara, 1980). The problem arises because this transient is quite fast: changes are detectable within a few milliseconds, and the time to peak is only approximately 50 msec. It was, therefore, a matter of great importance to learn, from recent work on the calcium current in isolated cells (see review by Noble and Powell, 1985), that the main component of the current is both very much faster and significantly larger than the multicellular work suggested. The time to peak current is now estimated to be 2–3 msec, and the inactivation time constant lies in the range of 10–20 msec. When we incorporated these new kinetic parameters into our model, DiFrancesco and I found it much easier to reproduce a rapid initial rise of intracellular calcium and a more rapid, subsequent release from stores in the reticulum.

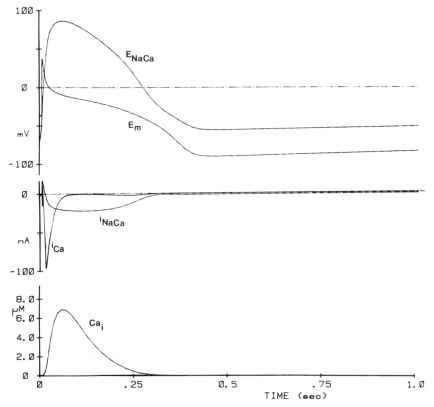

Fig. 2.   Computed time course of the reversal potential (E_{NaCa}) and exchange current (i_{NaCa}) for the sodium–calcium exchange process in a model of the Purkinje fiber action potential (DiFrancesco and Noble, 1985). The exchange stoichiometry was assumed to be $3:1$. The resting value of E_{NaCa} lies at approximately -40 mV, which is less negative than the resting potential because there is a small calcium leak that drives the exchange process away from strict equilibrium. During a calcium transient rising to approximately 6 μM, E_{NaCa} swings positive to approximately $+80$ mV. A calcium transient of approximately 1 μM (Wier and Isenberg, 1982) would give a peak value of $+30$ mV for E_{NaCa}. In either case, the membrane potential during activity lies positive to E_{NaCa} for only a very brief time (e.g., 10 msec) so that the exchange process should generate net inward current (corresponding to *outward* movement of calcium) fairly early during the plateau, when it could contribute to slower components of the second inward current. Whether it does this in fact should depend on the steepness of the voltage dependence of the exchange process (see a later section of this chapter). [From DiFrancesco *et al.* (1986).] The computations shown in this and other figures were obtained using the computer program OXSOFT HEART.

The second problem remains unresolved. This is that the calcium-induced process of Ca release is regenerative, yet release is known to be graded. The resolution of this problem probably lies in the Fabiatos' observation (personal communication) that calcium can inhibit as well as activate release. This feature has not yet been incorporated into the modeling, but this deficiency does not matter greatly in this discussion.

What does matter is that a reasonably accurate description of the time course of the calcium transient should be obtained. Figure 2 shows the time course given by the model. The time to peak and the time constant of decay are roughly comparable to experimental results, but the model does not reproduce some of the fine details, such as the double peak observed in Purkinje fibers by Wier and Isenberg (1982).

V. THE SODIUM–POTASSIUM EXCHANGE PROCESS

A plausible description of the sodium–calcium exchange process in the cell as a whole cannot be complete without a description of the process that generates the sodium gradient, i.e., the sodium–potassium exchange pump. Fortunately, considerable progress has been made in characterizing this process in the heart (Ellis, 1977; Deitmer and Ellis, 1978; Gadsby, 1980; Eisner and Lederer, 1980; Daut, 1983), and this information has been incorporated into the model, also. This enables the model to reproduce accurately those changes in both ionic currents and ion concentrations that are attributable to variations in the rate of the sodium–potassium exchange pump. In particular, it is plausible that the model could not only generate a steady-state pump current equal to that observed experimentally but also maintain intracellular sodium in the range of 8–10 mM. An important assumption required to achieve this degree of correspondence was that the great majority of the resting (background) inward current is attributable to a sodium leak. This assumption gives an accurate reconstruction of the speed with which internal sodium concentration changes when the Na–K exchange pump is blocked. Later in this chapter, I discuss the significance of this finding in assessing how much of the background current might be attributable to sodium–calcium exchange. The details are given in DiFrancesco and Noble (1985).

VI. VARIATION OF E_{NaCa} DURING ACTIVITY

We are now in a position to answer one of the important questions, which is how might the value of E_{NaCa} vary during each cardiac cycle. Because we know $[Ca]_o$, $[Na]_o$, $[Na]_i$, and E_m and have a plausible mathematical description of the variation in $[Ca]_i$, we have all the information required. Figure 2 shows the result for the Purkinje fiber model in which the resting level of E_{NaCa} lies at -40 mV. This is more negative than the value of -20 mV calculated above largely because the resting value of $[Ca]_i$ in the model is lower (approximately 50 nM as opposed to 100 nM). This difference is not significant in the question of what happens to E_{NaCa} when $[Ca]_i$ rises to values observed typically during an action potential. In Figure 2, $[Ca]_i$ rises to 7 μM within approximately 50 msec. This is sufficient to displace E_{NaCa} rapidly to approximately +80 mV. Consequently, except for a *very brief* period during the upstroke of the action potential, E_{NaCa} lies positive to E_m; hence, the exchanger generates *inward* current associated with the outward movement of calcium ions. On the basis of this hypothesis, the exchange process is not a quantitatively significant contributor to net entry of calcium during the action potential.

It is important to ask how reliable this calculation might be. There are several possible sources of error. First, in Purkinje fibers, the calcium transient does not usually rise as high as 7 μM, even though this would be typical of values in ventricular muscle. A peak of 1 μM would increase the peak value of E_{Ca} by 25 mV. Hence, E_{NaCa} would be 50 mV lower, i.e., approximately +30 mV. In the Purkinje fiber, this potential is still considerably positive to the plateau. In ventricular muscle, in which the plateau occurs at approximately +40 mV, the peak value of E_{NaCa} would also be positive to the plateau because, in this case, E_{NaCa} would be expected to peak at approximately +80 mV. Hence, in both Purkinje fibers and ventricular muscle, the exchanger process should carry inward current during most of the action potential.

The second possible source of error is that the stoichiometry of the exchange process might not be 3 : 1. It is easy to show that a lower value (e.g., 2.5 : 1—see Sheu and Fozzard, 1982; Fozzard, Chapter 7) would give rise to an even larger positive swing in E_{NaCa} (because in this case $E_{NaCa} = 5 E_{Na} - 4 E_{Ca}$). If a ratio of 4 : 1 is used, the swing is less ($E_{NaCa} = 2 E_{Na} - E_{Ca}$). But in this case, we must assume *also* that either the resting level of $[Ca]_i$ is *much* lower (so that the net change in E_{Ca} is much larger) or the process is even further away from equilibrium at rest (i.e., the resting value of E_{NaCa} is more positive, requiring a smaller swing in E_{Ca} to keep E_{NaCa} positive to E_m). It is not likely, therefore, that the general conclusion about the position of E_{NaCa} relative to E_m is strongly dependent on the stoichiometry used.

This means that *outward* current carried by the exchange process should be very brief. Only when the $[Ca]_i$ transient is much less than 1 μM would the exchanger be expected to carry a significant outward current for a lengthy period in comparison to the duration of the action potential.

VII. HOW MUCH CURRENT SHOULD THE CARRIER GENERATE?

If all the calcium removed from the cell were attributable to the exchange process, there would be in the steady state a fixed relationship between the time integral of current flowing through calcium channels and the time integral of current carried by the exchange process. For a 3 : 1 stoichiometry, we obtain:

$$\int i_{NaCa} \, dt = 0.5 \int i_{Ca} \, dt \tag{7}$$

For a 4 : 1 stoichiometry, the two integrals would be equal. Thus, the integral of the current carried by the exchange process could be as much as 50–100% of the time integral of the current carried by the calcium channels. This would be an upper limit because, if any calcium were removed by other means (e.g., a calcium pump), less calcium would need to be removed by the exchange process.

Equation (7) needs to be developed a little further because it must apply also during the resting state. We can then distinguish between *background* and *transient* currents that may be carried by the exchange process. For the background current we can write:

$$(i_{NaCa})_b = 0.5(i_{Ca})_b \tag{8}$$

Here, I have omitted integral signs because, in the resting state, there would be no time variations; thus, the relation between the two current amplitudes should apply at all times.

For the transient case, although we will still need an integral equation like Eq. (7), we can restrict our consideration to transient *changes* in both currents. This distinction will prove important later in the chapter.

VIII. TIME CONSTANT FOR EXCHANGE PROCESS

Finally, it would be helpful to have some idea of how rapid changes in carrier current might be. There might, of course, be several time constants:

(i) that for the speed with which alterations in ion concentration (even if instantaneous) would change the activity of the carrier (This would depend on the speed of the relevant ion binding processes, about which we know very little. For simplicity, I shall assume that they are fast compared to the duration of the cardiac cycle. I shall return later to the question of whether any of the conclusions about ionic current carried by the exchange process set some limits on this speed.)

(ii) that for the rate of change of intracellular calcium

(iii) that for the rate of change of intracellular sodium.

Over time scales relevant to a single cardiac cycle, the third process would be very slow; therefore, we can concentrate on the rate of change of [Ca].

Furthermore, for simplicity, we shall consider sodium–calcium exchange as the rate-limiting process for changes in $[Ca]_i$. In this case, we can write:

$$d[Ca]_i/dt = k_2 \cdot i_{NaCa} \tag{9}$$

where k_2 is a constant dependent on, among other factors, the intracellular volume and the surface/volume ratio of the cell. If we consider the case in which the product of terms including $[Ca]_i$ in Eq. (6) is dominant (i.e., when $(a_{Ca})_i \cdot (a_{Na})_o{}^n >> (a_{Ca})_o \cdot (a_{Na})_i{}^n$), we can write:

$$d[Ca]_i/dt = -k_2 \cdot k_{NaCa} \cdot [Na]_o{}^3 \cdot [Ca]_i \cdot \exp(-EF/2RT) \qquad (10)$$

(I have set γ equal to 0.5 and n equal to 3), or

$$d[Ca]_i/dt = -k_3 \cdot [Ca]_i \cdot \exp(-EF/2RT) \qquad (11)$$

where k_3 is a new constant dependent on k_{NaCa}, k_2, and $[Na]_o$. From Eq. (11) we can obtain an equation for the time constant:

$$\tau_{NaCa} = \exp(EF/2RT)/k_3 \qquad (12)$$

from which it is clear that the time constant should be a function of potential. How steep this function will be depends on the value of γ, assumed to be 0.5 in Eq. (12), and on the significance of the $[Ca]_o$-dependent flux (at high $[Ca]_i$, it will be negligible). With $\gamma = 0.5$, τ_{NaCa} would be expected to fall by approximately one-third for every 50 mV of hyperpolarization. This would have several important consequences:

1. If we were to set τ_{NaCa} at approximately 100 msec near 0 mV so that the carrier could transport a sizable proportion of calcium out of the cell during the calcium transient (if the carrier is the main route by which calcium leaves the cell, it must, in the steady state, remove as much calcium as it allows to enter through calcium channels), the time constant would be only a few milliseconds (approximately 30 msec) at the resting potential. This would place restrictions on the speed of current changes in the pacemaker range that might be attributable to the carrier current. In the DiFrancesco–Noble (1985) model, the inward transients attributable to i_{NaCa} near the resting potential are indeed very fast. This feature of the model does depend, however, on assumptions about other calcium-dependent processes. For example, if an internal calcium buffer were to release calcium fairly slowly during diastole, a small, longer-lasting transient exchange current could occur.

2. If the cell is not voltage-clamped, then the speed with which calcium is removed from the cell can accelerate as a result of activity of the exchange system because the cell hyperpolarizes as i_{NaCa} is reduced, thereby reducing the time constant for the process progressively. This effect can lead to some curious alterations in the predicted time courses of the current, causing i_{NaCa} to terminate in a fairly abrupt manner as $[Ca]_i$ returns to its resting level. In this connection, it is worth noting that Nakatani and Yau (personal communication; see Nakatani and Yau, 1984) have observed time courses of this kind in experiments measuring the sodium–calcium exchange current in retinal rods loaded with calcium.

It is worth discussing these conclusions a little more fully because of their pertinence to the role assigned to the sodium–calcium exchange process and the current it may generate in the DiFrancesco–Noble (1985) model. The exchange process is sometimes thought of as a mechanism by which calcium may be pumped out of the cell *after* the action potential has repolarized (see, e.g., Mullins, 1981, p. 2). It is already evident that I favor the alternative view: that apart from a very small background current to balance a resting calcium leak, the exchange current and the calcium movement it generates will be greatest when the calcium transient is largest, i.e., during the action potential itself.

This view depends, however, on two assumptions that may not always apply:

1. The voltage dependence of the $[Ca]_i$-activated mode of the exchange is not so steep as to produce a negligible response to changes in $[Ca]_i$ during the action potential. If the voltage dependence were steep enough to make the change in i_{NaCa} negligible, the exchange current might become larger after repolarization than during depolarization.

2. The exchange mechanism's response to variations in [Ca]i is sufficiently fast. At present, there are no direct measurements of this, but it is worth noting that if, as argued later in this chapter, the sodium–calcium exchange process is responsible for at least a large part of the transient inward current (i_{TI}), it would have to respond to changes in $[Ca]_i$ with a delay of not more than a few tens of milliseconds. This would be fast enough to respond to the $[Ca]_i$ transient during an action potential.

IX.   IONIC CURRENTS THAT MIGHT BE ATTRIBUTED TO SODIUM–CALCIUM EXCHANGE

We are now in a position to review the various candidates for current mechanisms that may be attributed to the exchange process.

A.   Background Inward Current

I have shown already that a background inward current does exist in the heart and that it is of great importance in pacemaker activity. Could it be attributed to the exchange process? There are two kinds of evidence relevant to this question, one theoretical, the other experimental.

The theoretical argument is based on DiFrancesco and Noble's observation (1985) that to reproduce the speed with which $[Na]_i$ rises after Na–K pump inhibition, nearly all (at least 75%) of the background inward current must be carried by sodium. They attributed this to a simple Na leak that would carry approximately -25 nA in a typical multicellular Purkinje strand used for volt-

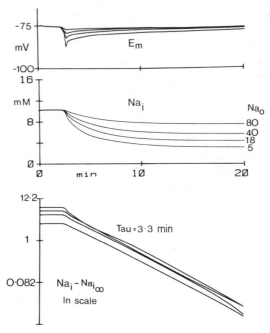

Fig. 3.   Influence of $[Na]_o$ on membrane potential and intracellular sodium, $[Na]_i$. $[Na]_o$ was reduced from 140 mM at 2 min to 80, 40, 18, or 5 mM at 2.5 min (i.e., a mixing time of 30 sec was assumed in the model). This produced a transient hyperpolarization similar in amplitude and duration to that observed experimentally (Ellis, 1977). In the model, the hyperpolarization was generated by a reduction in i_{NaCa} while the new equilibrium was being approached. Note that the effect was largely transient. This is because the exchange current must eventually return to the value required to balance the calcium leak.

The bottom diagram shows the computed changes in $[Na]_i$ plotted on a semilogarithmic scale. $[Na]_i$ falls exponentially with a mean time constant of 3.3 min, also very close to the experimental value. [From DiFrancesco and Noble (1985).]

age-clamp work. By comparison, the exchange current was calculated to carry approximately only −4 nA at rest (see DiFrancesco and Noble, 1985, Fig. 7). (These values would have to be divided by at least 10 to yield estimates relevant to a single-cell preparation.) By itself, this argument is not conclusive because, if a larger fraction of the background current were attributed to the exchange process, it would be generated nonetheless by sodium entry and thus contribute to the rise in intracellular sodium when the Na–K pump was blocked. A better question is whether the assumptions lead to accurate predictions of how the exchange current might contribute to the resting potential. One way to answer this question is to see how well the model reproduces the small changes in resting potential that occur when extracellular sodium is varied. Ellis (1977) observed a *transient* hyperpolarization of a few millivolts when Purkinje fibers were placed in low sodium. Figure 3 shows that the model reproduces this effect, as well as the speed of change in intracellular sodium, quite nicely. We may conclude, therefore, that an analysis of the background current and of changes in membrane potential during variations of external sodium is quantitatively plausible if we can assume that the exchange process carries no more than 10–20% of the net background inward current.

The second argument is based on experimental evidence. To measure resting current that might be carried by the exchange process, Mentrard and Vassort (1982) used blockers and ion substitution to try to eliminate all other currents that might vary when external sodium was changed. The current they have dissected in this way is indeed small compared to the net leak current.

More recently, Kimura *et al.* (1986) have measured a "background" current attributable to sodium–calcium exchange using whole cell patch-clamp recording in single ventricular cells. Their results show nearly exponential current–voltage relations similar to those expected from the theory discussed in this chapter. The results are also consistent with a 3 : 1 stoichiometry for the exchange process.

B.   Transient Outward Current

There are now known to be at least two components of transient outward current in the heart (Coraboeuf and Carmeliet, 1982). One is blocked by a 4-aminopyridine (4-AP) and is almost certainly a transient potassium current. The other is resistant to 4-AP, but is blocked by intracellular injection of EGTA (Siegelbaum and Tsien, 1980). Thus this component may be activated by the calcium transient. Its speed and amplitude (approximately 20 nA) are not dissimilar to those of the transient outward current carried by the exchange process in the DiFrancesco–Noble model. Further experimentation may, therefore, reveal that the exchange mechanism contributes significantly to the 4-AP-insensitive, transient outward current, but at present this can be considered only tentative conjecture.

C.   The Pacemaker Current, i_f

This current is activated on hyperpolarization into the pacemaker range of potentials (negative to -50 mV). It has a reversal potential near -20 mV and carries an inward current in the pacemaker range that is eliminated by removal of extracellular sodium ions. It is the latter property that led Mullins (1981) to suggest that it may be carried by the sodium–calcium exchange process. This idea can be excluded for several reasons:

1. At first, it might seem that a reversal potential near -20 mV makes this current, with its external sodium dependence, an ideal candidate for an exchange current. This assumption relies, however, on a misconception about the nature of the sodium–calcium exchange reversal potential, E_{NaCa}. Because the nature of E_{NaCa} is of more general importance than its application to the present issue, it bears further elaboration. As defined earlier, it is a thermodynamic quantity representing the potential at which the exchange process would be in equilibrium. If for brief periods (e.g., during an action potential) all relevant ion concentrations except $[Ca]_i$ are constant, the *only* way in which the exchange current, i_{NaCa}, can display time dependence in the relevant time range is by responding to variations in $[Ca]_i$. Thus, only by virtue of a change in its reversal potential can the exchange current display a time dependence that allows it to be identified with time-dependent currents during electrical activity that might otherwise be taken as evidence for a channel current. Hence, because E_{NaCa} is not constant, it cannot be measured as an experimentally determined reversal potential in the way that the reversal potential for i_f, or any other time-dependent channel current, can be measured (i.e., as a parameter independent of the process that generates the time dependence of the current).

For a similar reason, the exchange current cannot behave exactly like the nonspecific channel current identified in patch-clamp studies by Colquhoun *et al.* (1981), even though this current, too, depends on $[Ca]_i$ and extracellular sodium and shows a reversal potential near -20 mV.

In fact, if $[Ca]_i$ always increases on depolarization, the time-dependent *change* in i_{NaCa} will *always* be in the inward direction, even when the voltage lies positive to E_{NaCa}. In the latter case, the time-dependent inward change would be attributable to the reduction of an outward current. Later in this chapter, I return to the question of the current–voltage relation that would be generated when the exchange current is activated by $[Ca]_i$.

2. The time-dependent change in i_f is in the opposite direction to that expected. Upon hyperpolarization, it increases gradually, whereas the exchange current should *decrease* with time as it pumps out the calcium that activates it.

3. This leads to the next difficulty, that the time constant of this process is likely to be much shorter than the time constant (approximately 1–2 sec) of i_f in the pacemaker range.

4. Finally, it is extremely difficult to see how the exchange process could be responsible for the gating characteristics of i_f (DiFrancesco, 1984) or explain its pharmacology (such as its sensitivity to low levels of cesium).

D.   The Second Inward Current, i_{si}

By far the most important and far-reaching of Mullins's (1979, 1981) suggestions concerning currents that may be carried by the exchange process is that it may generate at least part of the second inward current in the heart. Because the following is the longest section under this heading, I subdivide it, discussing separately the range of relevant evidence for each of various cardiac preparations.

1. Purkinje Fibers

Figure 2 shows the predicted time course of the exchange current during a Purkinje fiber action potential computed with the DiFrancesco–Noble model. The peak inward current in this case is approximately -20 nA and lasts approximately 200 msec. It is, therefore, considerably smaller and slower than the fast calcium current, i_{Ca}. Thus, if it does contribute to i_{si}, it should contribute a relatively slow and small component. Figure 4 shows the expected behavior during voltage-clamp steps. Several additional conclusions may be drawn:

1. There is a fairly narrow voltage range (between -50 and -30 mV in this case) over which the slow inward current is dominated by the computed exchange current. At stronger depolarizations, the exchange current appears only as a slow tail on the inward current record and may be masked easily by other components (such as the delayed K current and the transient outward current).

2. The computed threshold for the inward current attributed to i_{NaCa} depends critically on the value assumed for the level of $[Ca]_i$ at which Ca is released from stores in the sarcoplasmic reticulum. In the computer model, if this level is raised (e.g., from its standard value of 1 μM to 1.5 μM), it becomes difficult to distinguish i_{NaCa} within any range of potentials.

3. If a component resembling that attributed to i_{NaCa} in the model occurs experimentally, it should be sensitive to procedures that change the quantity of Ca released.

Does such a component of current occur in experimental records? The answer is yes. Over just this voltage range, Eisner et al. (1979) and Lederer and Eisner (1982) recorded a slow inward current in sheep Purkinje fibers that:

(a) activates within approximately 100 msec
(b) lasts approximately 300–400 msec
(c) is abolished by agents (such as caffeine and tetracaine) that are thought to interfere with release of Ca
(d) is increased by procedures (such as sodium-pump inhibition) that produce a positive inotropic effect.

At that time, we attributed the current simply to i_{si} and made no attempt to dissect this current into a genuine calcium current and other components of slow inward current. Clearly, it would now be worthwhile to reinvestigate such very slow currents in Purkinje fibers, preferably under conditions that increase the current magnitude (such as sodium-pump inhibition or adrenergic stimulation).

188   Denis Noble

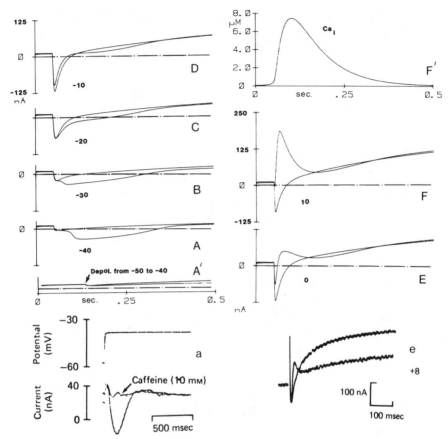

Fig. 4. Voltage-clamp currents (including the exchanger current) computed from the DiFrancesco–Noble (1985) model or recorded in some Purkinje fiber experiments chosen for comparison. In records (A) to (F), the voltage was stepped from −80 mV to the potentials indicated, first with the sodium current blocked and then with the [Ca]ᵢ-dependent current changes removed also. Record F′ shows the intracellular calcium transient computed during record F. Record A′ shows the effect of changing the holding potential to −50 mV to inactivate Ca release from the sarcoplasmic reticulum. (The contractile repriming process in the model is assumed to be voltage dependent.)

The sodium–calcium exchange current is most evident during depolarizations to −40 and −30 mV and then becomes much smaller at stronger depolarizations. Record (a) shows experimental records from Eisner *et al.* (1979) for comparison with the model. Note that a much slower time scale was used in the experimental record. Apart from this, the current amplitude and time course are not dissimilar to those computed in the model.

The records at 0 and +10 mV show how easily the inward currents (calcium current and exchange current) can be masked by the outward current transient. Record (e) shows an experimental result from Siegelbaum and Tsien (1980) to compare with record (E). Siegelbaum and Tsien removed the calcium transient by injecting EGTA intracellularly. In their experimental records and in the model, this produced a much simpler current trace. For further details see DiFrancesco and Noble (1985).

Reuter's (1967) original work on the slow inward current in Purkinje fibers also describes a current that is very slow compared to the calcium current identified in more recent work. Some of this current may be attributable to i_{NaCa}, but we cannot be sure of this because there exists in some cardiac cells, too, a very slow calcium channel (Hume and Giles, 1983; Lee *et al.*, 1984a,b) that inactivates very slowly and only partially. It should not be assumed that *all* very slow inward currents are generated by the sodium–calcium exchange process. Moreover, it is unlikely that the exchange process would have generated the substantial long-lasting inward current that Reuter recorded even at positive potentials (see Reuter, 1967).

2. Rat Ventricle

Preparations of rat ventricular cells are particularly important and useful because the action potentials therefrom show three distinct phases of repolarization: a very rapid phase attributable to inactivation of the TTX-sensitive sodium current and activation of a 4-AP-sensitive, transient outward current (Mitchell *et al.*, 1984b); a fairly short, early plateau attributable to the calcium current (Mitchell *et al.*, 1984b); and a low-level, long-lasting final phase whose properties are very distinctive.

The third phase is abolished when contraction is abolished by *either* exposure to 1 μM ryanodine (see Fig. 5b), a drug that is thought to inhibit release of Ca from the reticulum stores, *or* intracellular application of the calcium chelator EGTA (Mitchell *et al.*, 1984a). In contrast, the second phase is not abolished. These observations are consistent with the hypothesis that the inward current, which generates the third phase, is activated by calcium ions.

The third phase can be abolished also by replacement of sodium ions by choline. The second phase is not affected by this procedure either. This observation suggests that the current activated by intracellular calcium carries sodium into the cell. There are two possible candidates for such a process. The first is the nonspecific cation channel that has been recorded in patch-clamp studies of cardiac cell membranes (Colquhoun *et al.*, 1981) and in a variety of other tissues. The second is activation by calcium of the sodium–calcium exchange process, which would carry sodium into the cell in exchange for calcium leaving the cell.

One way to distinguish between these two mechanisms is to use lithium as the sodium substitute (see Fig. 5a). Lithium cannot support the calcium efflux from nerve axons, which is dependent on external sodium (Baker *et al.*, 1967), whereas the nonspecific channels seem, as expected, to carry lithium as well as sodium (Yellen, 1982). In the third phase of repolarization in rat ventricle, lithium does *not* support the current responsible (Mitchell *et al.*, 1984a; Schouten and ter Keurs, 1985), which suggests that the sodium–calcium exchange mechanism (rather than the Ca-activated nonspecific channels) is involved.

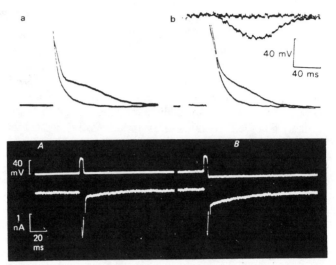

Fig. 5. The late plateau current in the rat ventricular action potential and the slow inward current underlying it. Upper traces: (a) Superimposed action potentials in normal solution and in a solution in which 89% of sodium ions have been replaced by lithium ions (shortened action potential). (b) Abolition of late phase of action potential (lower traces) and of contraction (upper traces) by 3-min exposure to 1 μM ryanodine. [From Mitchell *et al.* (1984a).] Lower traces: Currents recorded on depolarization from −40 to 0 mV followed by repolarization to −40 (A) or −60 mV (B). This slowly decaying inward current, recorded on repolarizing into the range of the late plateau, was abolished by ryanodine, intracellular injection of EGTA, or low extracellular Na. [From Mitchell *et al.* (1984c).]

Finally, voltage-clamp experiments (Mitchell *et al.*, 1984c) show that the inward current underlying the third phase can be recorded *negative* to the potential range of activation of the calcium current (see Fig. 5, lower panels). In fact, the current becomes greater as the membrane potential is made more negative in this range, whereas the calcium current would be expected to deactivate rapidly. As with the late plateau, this slow component of current is abolished by ryanodine or intracellular injection of EGTA, but is not sensitive to TTX (10 μM) or, initially, to nifedipine (but see below for the slower progressive effects of calcium-channel blockers on this current).

In summary, then, the rat ventricular action potential shows a very slow phase that might be attributed to activation of inward sodium current via the sodium–calcium exchange mechanism and that cannot be attributed to the nifedipine-sensitive, fast calcium current.

3. Guinea Pig Ventricle

The guinea pig ventricular cell shows an action potential that is more typical, i.e., the initial rapid depolarization is followed, at positive potentials, by a very long-lasting plateau that is terminated eventually by a more rapid phase of repolarization. There is, therefore, no neat separation into three phases as in rat ventricle. Nevertheless, nearly all the observations described in Section IX,D,2 have clear parallels in recent work on guinea pig cells.

First, sodium substitution by either choline or lithium shortens the plateau considerably (Mitchell et al., 1984a). This effect cannot be caused by the sodium-mediated, TTX-sensitive current, because TTX has a much smaller effect on the duration of the action potential. Nevertheless, the result is not, in itself, conclusive because removal of sodium raises intracellular calcium, which could activate a K^+ current that would speed repolarization. It is necessary therefore to use voltage-clamp experiments to determine whether an inward current with an appropriate time course can be found.

This has been done by Lee et al. (1983), who showed that depolarization from -80 to -40 mV in isolated guinea pig cells activates the calcium current (the sodium current being blocked by TTX), which is then followed by a fairly rapid inactivation and a much slower and smaller inward current (see Fig. 6, top panels). Like the slow current found in the rat, this current is not affected initially by calcium-current blockers. It is therefore possible to abolish the rapid calcium-channel current (Lee et al., 1983, used 0.2 mM cadmium to do this) and then record the slow current alone.

The properties of this current, which E. W. Lee et al. (1983) and K. S. Lee et al. (1984a,b) called $i_{si,2}$, suggest that, like that in rat ventricle, it is activated by intracellular calcium. Thus, it is largely absent in cells that are perfused with EGTA (K. S. Lee, D. Noble, and A. J. Spindler, unpublished observations) by the suction electrode technique. Moreover, in response to a calcium-current blocker, both $i_{si,2}$ and the contraction amplitude diminish gradually over 3–5 min. A similar progressive change occurs in the contraction and slow inward current in rat ventricular cells after the addition of nifedipine to block the fast calcium current (Mitchell et al., 1984b). The obvious interpretation here is that as the sarcoplasmic reticulum becomes depleted of calcium after blockade of the calcium channel, the amount of calcium released during each depolarization diminishes, as does the contraction and any calcium-activated current. Finally, when the cell is clamped to approximately -30 mV, the initial twitch is sometimes followed by a slow oscillatory contraction. This phenomenon is accompanied by oscillations of $i_{si,2}$ (Lee et al., 1984b).

The existence of an inward current that responds to, rather than generates, the intracellular [Ca] transient may be of great importance in relation to the dynamic response of cardiac muscle to variations in frequency of stimulation, in which the progressive changes in electrical response follow closely the progressive changes in inotropic state (see review by Boyett and Jewell, 1980). In single, guinea pig ventricular cells, the slow component of i_{si} that might be attributed to the exchange process does indeed change during long trains of stimuli precisely in the

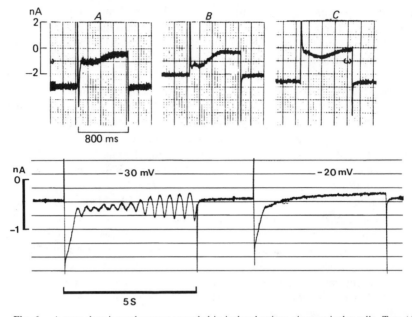

Fig. 6. A very slow inward current recorded in isolated guinea pig ventricular cells. Top: (A) Currents recorded on depolarization from −80 to −40 mV in the presence of 40 μM TTX. Note slow inward current of approximately 1 nA after the fast calcium current (which on this time scale is compressed into a brief spike). (B, C) Current records 20 and 60 sec after adding 1 mM cadmium. Bottom: In some cells, over a certain range of potentials, the slow component shows oscillatory behavior. These oscillations in current are accompanied by small oscillatory movements. In this case, oscillatory current was observed at −30 mV, but the current became monotonic at −20 mV. In other cells, the oscillations occurred over a wider range of potentials. The time course and amplitude of these oscillations resemble strongly those of the transient inward current, i_{TI}, occurring during sodium-pump blockade.

manner that would explain the variations in the duration of the action potential (Fedida *et al.*, 1985).

4.   Rabbit Sinoatrial Node

Brown *et al.* (1983, 1984a,b) have reported two components of second inward current in small preparations of rabbit sinoatrial node. There are several different voltage-clamp protocols that can reveal the slower component.

One method is to apply a voltage clamp at various times during the natural pacemaker depolarization. If this is done toward the end of the pacemaker potential (near −40 mV), there occurs an inward current that activates very slowly (over 50–100 msec) and then inactivates over a similar period. This time course resembles strongly that of the current $i_{si,2}$ in the guinea pig cell when clamped at a similar potential (Lee *et al.*, 1983), and Brown *et al.* (1984a,b) suggested that it may be attributable to activation of the sodium–calcium exchange mechanism. This suggestion was based on extensive computer modeling of ionic currents and pacemaker activity in the sinoatrial node.

A second method is to apply voltage-clamp steps to −40 mV from various holding potentials. This protocol is the standard one used to measure the inactivation curve for the calcium current. In many experiments, this gives the expected result: the current recorded at −40 mV increases monotonically as the holding potential becomes more negative. In a significant number of experiments, however, the results are more complex. Either the time course of the inward current changes markedly (from being very slow on clamping from the less negative holding potentials to becoming much faster on clamping from the more negative potentials) or the current may show two quite separate peaks (Brown *et al.*, 1984a). In the latter case, the second peak is very slow, and the time course of the current resembles strongly that obtained by applying a voltage clamp at the end of the pacemaker depolarization. As the holding potential is made more negative, the slow peak activates more rapidly and fuses eventually with the fast current peak so that it then appears only as a slow tail on the fast current record. This behavior corresponds well to the computed behavior of the sodium–calcium exchange process in a model of sinus node activity.

5. Ferret Ventricle

Arlock and Noble (1985) have described the current $i_{si,2}$ in ferret ventricle. It can be distinguished from the calcium current, i_{Ca}, by using rapid block of this current with Mn^{2+} or other blockers. Initially, $E_{si,2}$ and the contraction are unaffected. Only after some minutes do $i_{si,2}$ and the contraction decrease. This resembles the behavior in guinea pig cells described in Fig. 6.

X. RELATION BETWEEN SLOW COMPONENTS OF i_{si} AND THE TRANSIENT INWARD CURRENT, i_{TI}

There is a strong resemblance between the time course of the presumed Ca-activated component of i_{si} ($i_{si,2}$) and the transient inward current (i_{TI}) first recorded in Purkinje fibers treated with cardiac glycosides (Lederer and Tsien, 1976). This resemblance may not be at all accidental. After all, i_{TI} is already well established as a $[Ca]_i$-activated current, and the same hypotheses (sodium–calcium exchange current and nonspecific cation channel current) have been formulated for the mechanism of i_{TI} (Kass *et al.*, 1978). Although i_{TI} has often been thought of as an *additional* current induced by sodium-pump blockade, it is

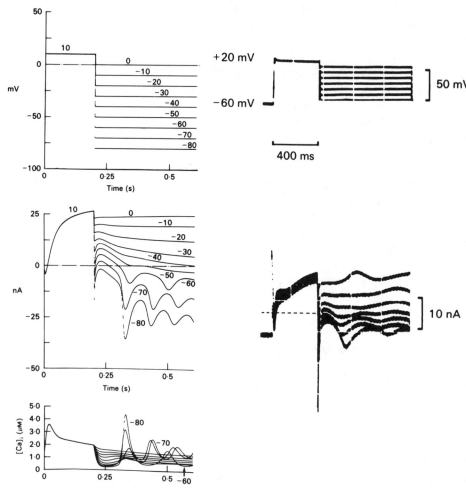

Fig. 7. Reconstruction of oscillatory changes in [Ca]$_i$ and membrane current when the Na–K exchange pump is partially blocked. In this particular set of computations, the pump was reduced to 25% of its normal capacity, which allowed [Na]$_i$ to rise from its normal value of 8 mM to approximately 20 mM. In the model, this condition is sufficient to generate oscillatory currents that reproduce i_{TI}. Top: Voltage-clamp steps. Middle: Net membrane currents. The oscillatory variations in i_{NaCa} are superimposed on a monotonic current relaxation caused by the decay of i_K and onset of i_f. The peak amplitude of the inward current oscillation is strongly voltage dependent in this version of the model so that the oscillation becomes almost negligible positive to -30 mV. Bottom: Computed variations in [Ca]$_i$. Right: experimental results from the rabbit sinoatrial node after 5-min exposure to 0.3 mM K$^+$. [From Brown *et al.* (1986).]

possible that it may be instead an oscillatory form of a current (i.e., $i_{si,2}$) that is activated also during normal electrical activity. In the sinoatrial node (Brown *et al.*, 1984c) and in single, guinea pig ventricular cells (K. S. Lee, D. Noble, and A. J. Spindler, unpublished observations), the time course and amplitude of i_{TI} are virtually indistinguishable from those of $i_{si,2}$, and envelope tests show a strong correlation between the behavior of the very slow inward current during depolarization and the time course of i_{TI} on repolarization (Brown *et al.*, 1984c, 1986).

All the elements thought to be necessary to generate i_{TI} are present in the DiFrancesco–Noble model, i.e., the sodium–potassium exchange pump, the sodium–calcium exchange process, and Ca-induced release of Ca from the sarcoplasmic reticulum. It is therefore worth determining whether sodium-pump blockade is sufficient in the model to produce oscillatory current variations like those recorded experimentally. Figure 7 shows the results of such a calculation (Brown *et al.*, 1986). Clearly, the model does reproduce transient inward currents of amplitude and time course similar to those observed experimentally. In this case, the current perturbations are attributable to variations in the activity of the sodium–calcium exchange process, but the fact that the equations can succeed in reproducing the phenomenon in this way does not necessarily mean that calcium activation of nonspecific channels does not occur also. For a more extensive discussion of this question, see Noble (1984).

Fast Extracellular Calcium Transients

If $i_{si,2}$ is carried by the sodium–calcium exchange process, then it should correspond to a net *outward* flux of calcium from the cell during the later phases of the action potential. This idea has recently been tested by applying the computer model to results on fast extracellular calcium transients using tetramethylmurexide. In rabbit atrium, extracellular calcium does indeed show two opposite changes during the action potential; an initial rapid fall attributable to calcium entry at the beginning of the action potential, followed after 30–40 msec by an increase attributable to calcium exit from the cells. The correspondence between the experimental results and the behavior of the computer model is very close (see Hilgemann and Noble, 1986).

XI. ARTIFICIALLY INDUCED SLOW INWARD CURRENT

So far, we have dealt with slow inward currents that occur naturally. But, if one of these currents is activated by the $[Ca]_i$ transient, it should be possible to generate such currents artificially by inducing release of calcium. Clusin *et al.*

(1983) have done this by using caffeine to induce release of Ca in clusters of embryonic heart cells. This generates an inward current that has a voltage dependence consistent with its being carried by the sodium–calcium exchange process, i.e., there is no reversal potential in the range of -100 to $+50$ mV. A similar approach has been described recently for outer segments of retinal rods by Nakatani and Yau (1984), who recorded an inward current that was stimulated by intracellular loading of calcium and that flowed only in the presence of external sodium.

XII. CURRENT–VOLTAGE RELATIONS FOR [Ca]$_i$-INDUCED VARIATIONS IN i_{NaCa}

This is a suitable point at which to discuss the nature of the current–voltage relation expected for variations in i_{NaCa} induced by changes in [Ca]$_i$. There has been some confusion on this issue, largely because of misapplication of the simplified hyperbolic sine function for the voltage dependence of the exchange process. As I showed in Section III, conclusion 2 of this chapter, large variations in intracellular calcium are precisely the condition under which the hyperbolic sine function would *not* be expected to hold. If, in Eq. (6), the product of terms including [Ca]$_o$ was presumed not to change when [Ca]$_i$ is varied, then the *difference* in current caused by changes in intracellular calcium would be determined entirely by the product of terms including [Ca]$_i$, which is a simple exponential function of the membrane potential. Interestingly enough, this is similar to the current–voltage relation for the Ca-activated current studied by Clusin *et al.* (1983). It is also the current–voltage relation that Arlock and Katzung (1985) found for i_{TI} in ventricular muscle.

The precise shape of the current–voltage relation is important because it determines whether significant transient inward current caused by the exchange process would be observed during depolarizations. If the current–voltage $(I–V)$ relation is steep (i.e., γ near 0), the exchange process would carry little current during a depolarization to near 0 mV. Its role in carrying calcium out of the cell then becomes significant only when the membrane has repolarized to a sufficiently negative potential. Such a steep voltage dependence might explain the kind of $I–V$ relations for i_{TI} that have been reported by Henning and Vereecke (1983) in Purkinje fibers, in which the current falls fairly steeply toward zero as the membrane is depolarized toward -30 mV and then stays at zero over a considerable voltage range. When such a current–voltage relation occurs, currents like $i_{si,2}$ would also be expected to be small or negligible. Certainly, currents of this kind do not occur in all voltage-clamp experiments on the second inward current in the heart. Thus, the precise characterization of the voltage dependence of [Ca]$_i$-dependent flux through the exchanger is of great importance. Measurements of the current–voltage relations for the sodium–calcium exchange have recently been achieved in some elegant patch clamp recordings on single ventricular cells by Kimura *et al.* (1986). They find that the difference current induced by changing sodium or calcium concentrations is well-approximated by exponentials of the kind described in the theory used here. The mode of the exchanger corresponding to inward sodium movement gives a voltage dependence that is about twice as steep as that for outward sodium movement. In the theory described here, this would require a value of γ of about 0.35.

XIII. CONCLUSIONS

For cardiac muscle, the consequences of the electrogenicity of sodium–calcium exchange are clearly profound—a fact that has been emphasized by quite a number of reviews in the last 5 or 6 years. I hope this chapter shows the probability that a component of i_{si} in at least some cardiac tissues is attributable to the exchange process, that this component has properties similar to those of i_{TI}, and that it may carry a peak current of approximately 10–20% of the maximum amplitude of the calcium current. In the resting state, the current carried by the exchange process may be quite small, as also shown experimentally by Mentrard and Vassort (1982).

A major theoretical problem arises because some of the important conclusions depend on the steepness of the voltage dependence of the exchanger's $[Ca]_i$-dependent mode. Depending on how the electric field is partitioned between this mode and the reverse mode, depolarization to zero or to positive potentials could either make the $[Ca]_i$-dependent flux negligible until very late in the action potential or allow it to carry a substantial proportion of the slower phases of the second inward current, i_{si}. It is particularly worth bearing this problem in mind when trying to extrapolate from results in one cardiac preparation to another. So far, the best experimental evidence that the exchange current contributes to i_{si} comes from work with some mammalian cardiac preparations, there being little or no relevant evidence in amphibian preparations. It is not impossible that there is a genuine difference here, and that this may also apply to different mammalian preparations or even to the same type of cells prepared in different ways, because the extent to which the exchange process operates away from its equilibrium state depends on the leakiness of the cells to calcium.

The major experimental problem in this area arises because, as yet, we have no specific blocker of the sodium–calcium exchange process. At present, the only manipulation that may help to distinguish between $[Ca]_i$-dependent carrier fluxes and $[Ca]_i$-dependent channel activation is to replace external sodium with lithium. But in isolated cells, it is not yet possible to make such replacement complete without generating an intolerably large increase in the concentration of intracellular calcium. With these experimental limitations, progress in this field has so far depended on a combination of fairly indirect experimental work and theoretical work designed to test the quantitative plausibility of some of the hypotheses suggested by these experiments. Nevertheless, the accumulated evidence does now strongly suggest that the exchange mechanism carries a small inward background current at rest and a much larger inward current during the action potential in mammalian cardiac muscle. This current forms a small part of the slower phase of the "second inward current," i_{si}, and corresponds to a net outward flow of calcium from the cell. On this view, the exchange mechanism contributes both to electrical activity and to the maintenance of calcium balance during rhythmic activity of the heart.

REFERENCES

Allen, D. G., and Kurihara, S. (1980). Calcium transients in mammalian ventricular muscle. *Eur. Heart J.* **1** (Suppl. A), 5–15.

Arlock, P., and Katzung, B. G. (1985). Effects of replacement of extracellular sodium on transient inward current and contractions in papillary muscle. *J. Physiol.* **360,** 105–120.

Arlock, P., and Noble, D. (1985). Two components of 'second inward current' in ferret papillary muscle. *J. Physiol.* **369,** 88P.

Baker, P. F., Blaustein, M. P., Hodgkin, A. L., and Steinhardt, R. A. (1967). The effect of sodium concentration on calcium movements in giant axons of *Loligo. J. Physiol.* **192,** 43P.

Baker, P. F., Blaustein, M. P., Hodgkin, A. L., and Steinhardt, R. A. (1969). The influences of calcium on sodium efflux in squid axons. *J. Physiol.* **200,** 431–458.

Beeler, G. W., and Reuter, H. (1977). Reconstruction of the action potential of ventricular myocardial fibres. *J. Physiol.* **268,** 177–210.

Blaustein, M. P., and Nelson, M. T. (1982). Sodium–calcium exchange: Its role in the regulation of cell calcium. *In* "Membrane Transport of Calcium" (E. Carafoli, ed.), pp. 217–236. Academic Press, London.

Blaustein, M. P., Russell, J. M., and DeWeer, P. (1974). *J. Supramolec. Structure* **2,** 558–581.

Boyett, M. R., and Jewell, B. R. (1980). Analysis of the effects of changes in rate and rhythm upon electrical activity in the heart. *Prog. Biophys.* **36,** 1–52.

Brown, H. F., Kimura, J., Noble, D., Noble, S. J., and Taupignon, A. I. (1983). Two components of 'second inward current' in the rabbit sinoatrial node. *J. Physiol.* **334,** 56P.

Brown, H. F., Kimura, J., Noble, D., Noble, S. J., and Taupignon, A. I. (1984a). The slow inward current, i_{si}, in the rabbit sino-atrial node investigated by voltage clamp and by computer simulation. *Proc. R. Soc. London Ser. B.* **222,** 305–328.

Brown, H. F., Kimura, J., Noble, D., Noble, S. J., and Taupignon, A. I. (1984b). The ionic currents underlying pacemaker activity in rabbit sino-atrial node: Experimental results and computer simulation. *Proc. R. Soc. London Ser. B.* **222,** 329–347.

Brown, H. F., Noble, D., Noble, S. J., and Taupignon, A. I. (1984c). Transient inward current and its relation to the very slow inward current in the rabbit SA node. *J. Physiol.* **349,** 47P.

Brown, H. F., Noble, D., Noble, S. J., and Taupignon, A. I. (1986). Relationship between the transient inward current and slow inward currents in the sino-atrial node of the rabbit. *J. Physiol.* **370,** 299–315.

Clusin, W. T., Fischmeister, R., and DeHaan, R. L. (1983). Caffeine-induced current in embryonic heart cells: Time course and voltage dependence. *Am. J. Physiol.* **245**, H528–H532.

Colquhoun, D., Neher, E., Reuter, H., and Stevens, C. F. (1981). Inward channels activated by intracellular Ca in cultured heart cells. *Nature* **294**, 752–754.

Coraboeuf, E. (1980). Voltage clamp studies of the slow inward current. *In* "The Slow Inward Current and Cardiac Arrhythmias" (D. P. Zipes, J. C. Bailey, and V. Elharrar, eds.), pp. 25–95. Martinus Nijhoff, The Hague.

Coraboeuf, E., and Carmeliet, E. (1982). Existence of two transient outward currents in sheep cardiac Purkinje fibres. *Pflügers Arch. Eur. J. Physiol.* **392**, 352–359.

Daut, J. (1983). Inhibition of the sodium pump in guinea-pig ventricular muscle: Inhibition of the pump current by cardiac glycosides. *J. Physiol.* **339**, 643–662.

Deitmer, J. W., and Ellis, D. (1978). The intracellular sodium activity of cardiac Purkinje fibres during inhibition and reactivation of the sodium–potassium pump. *J. Physiol.* **284**, 241–259.

DiFrancesco, D. (1984). Characterization of the pacemaker (i_f) current kinetics in calf Purkinje fibres. *J. Physiol.* **348**, 341–367.

DiFrancesco, D., and Noble, D. (1985). A model of cardiac electrical activity incorporating ionic pumps and concentration changes. *Philos. Trans. R. Soc. London Ser. B.* **307**, 353–398.

DiFrancesco, D., Hart, G., and Noble, D. (1986). In preparation.

Eisner, D. A., and Lederer, W. J. (1980). Characterization of the sodium pump in cardiac Purkinje fibres. *J. Physiol.* **303**, 441–474.

Eisner, D. A., Lederer, W. J., and Noble, D. (1979). Caffeine and tetracaine abolish the slow inward current in sheep cardiac Purkinje fibres. *J. Physiol.* **293**, 76P.

Eisner, D. A., Lederer, W. J., and Vaughan-Jones, R. D. (1983). The control of tonic tension by membrane potential and intracellular sodium activity in the sheep cardiac Purkinje fibre. *J. Physiol.* **335**, 723–743.

Ellis, D. (1977). The effects of external cations and ouabain on the intracellular sodium activity of sheep heart Purkinje fibres. *J. Physiol.* **274**, 211–240.

Fedida, D., Noble, D., and Spindler, A. J. (1985). Frequency-dependent changes in inward current in single guinea-pig ventricular cells. *J. Physiol.* (proceedings of the September 1984 meeting) **358**, 53.

Gadsby, D. C. (1980). Activation of electrogenic Na/K exchange by extracellular K$^+$ in canine cardiac Purkinje fibers. *Proc. Nat. Acad. Sci. U.S.A.* **77**, 4035–4039.

Henning, B., and Vereecke, J. (1983). Effects of Cs and Ba on the transient inward current of sheep cardiac Purkinje fibers. *J. Physiol.* **345**, 149P.

Hilgemann, D., and Noble, D. (1986). Simulation of extracellular calcium transients in rabbit cardiac muscle. *J. Physiol.* **371**, 195P.

Hume, J. R., and Giles, W. R. (1983). Ionic currents in single bullfrog atrial cells. *J. Gen. Physiol.* **81**, 153–194.

Jack, J. J. B. J., Noble, D., and Tsien, R. W. (1975). "Electric Current Flow in Excitable Cells." The Clarendon Press, Oxford (paperback edition, 1983).

Kass, R. S., Lederer, W. J., Tsien, R. W., and Weingart, R. (1978). Role of calcium ions in transient inward current and after contractions induced by strophanthidin in cardiac Purkinje fibres. *J. Physiol.* **281**, 187–208.

Kimura, J., Noma, A., and Irisawa, H. (1986). Na–Ca exchange current in mammalian heart cells. *Nature (London)* **319**, 596–597.

Lederer, W. J., and Eisner, D. A. (1982). The effects of sodium pump activity on the slow inward current in sheep cardiac Purkinje fibres. *Proc. R. Soc. London Ser. B.* **214**, 249–262.

Lederer, W. J., and Tsien, R. W. (1976). Transient inward current underlying arrhythmogenic effects of cardiotonic steroids in Purkinje fibres. *J. Physiol.* **263**, 73–100.

Lee, E. W., Lee, K. S., Noble, D., and Spindler, A. J. (1983). A very slow inward current in single ventricular cells. *J. Physiol.* **345**, 6P.

Lee, K. S., Lee, E. W., Noble, D., and Spindler, A. J. (1984a). Further properties of the very slow inward currents in isolated single guinea-pig ventricular cells. *J. Physiol.* **349,** 48P.

Lee, K. S., Noble, D., Lee, E., and Spindler, A. J. (1984b). A new calcium current underlying the plateau of the cardiac action potential. *Proc. R. Soc. London Ser. B.* **223,** 35–48.

McAllister, R. E., Noble, D., and Tsien, R. W. (1975). Reconstruction of the electrical activity of cardiac Purkinje fibres. *J. Physiol.* **251,** 1–59.

Mentrard, D., and Vassort, G. (1982). The Na–Ca exchange generates a current in frog heart cells. *J. Physiol.* **334,** 55P.

Mitchell, M. R., Powell, T., Terrar, D. A., and Twist, V. W. (1984a). The effects of ryanodine, EGTA, and low-sodium on action potentials in rat and guinea-pig ventricular myocytes: Evidence for two inward currents during the plateau. *Br. J. Pharmacol.* **81,** 543–550.

Mitchell, M. R., Powell, T., Terrar, D. A., and Twist, V. W. (1984b). Strontium, nifedipine and 4-amino-pyridine modify the time course of the action potential in cells from rat ventricular muscle. *Br. J. Pharmacol.* **81,** 551–556.

Mitchell, M. R., Powell, T., Terrar, D. A., and Twist, V. W. (1984c). Possible association between an inward current and the late plateau of action potentials in ventricular cells isolated from rat heart. *J. Physiol.* **351,** 40P.

Mullins, L. J. (1977). A mechanism for Na/Ca transport. *J. Gen. Physiol.* **70,** 681–695.

Mullins, L. J. (1979). The generation of electric currents in cardiac fibers by Na/Ca exchange. *Am. J. Physiol.* **236,** C103–C110.

Mullins, L. J. (1981). "Ion Transport in Heart." Raven Press, New York.

Mullins, L. J., and Brinley, F. J., Jr. (1975). The sensitivity of calcium efflux from squid axons to changes in membrane potential. *J. Gen. Physiol.* **65,** 135–152.

Nakatani, K., and Yau, K.-W. (1984). Measurement of Na–Ca exchange in toad retinal rod after Ca loading. *J. Physiol.* **353,** 77P.

Nelson, M. T., and Blaustein, M. P. (1981). Effect of Na_o-dependent calcium efflux on the membrane potential of internally perfused barnacle muscle fibers. *Biophys. J.* **33,** 61a.

Niedergerke, R. (1963). Movements of Ca in beating ventricles of the frog. *J. Physiol.* **167,** 551–580.

Noble, D. (1984). The surprising heart: A review of recent progress in cardiac electrophysiology. *J. Physiol.* **353,** 1–50.

Noble, D., and Powell, T. (1985). Calcium currents and calcium-dependent inward current. *In* "Control and Manipulation of Calcium Movement" (J. Parratt, ed.), pp. 29–49. Raven Press, New York.

Noma, A., and Irisawa, H. (1976). A time and voltage dependent potassium current in the rabbit sinoatrial node cell. *Pflügers Arch. Ges. Physiol.* **366,** 251–258.

Reuter, H. (1967). The dependence of slow inward current in Purkinje fibres on the extracellular calcium concentration. *J. Physiol.* **192,** 479–492.

Schouten, V. J. A., and ter Keurs, H. E. D. J. (1985). The slow repolarization phase of the action potential in rat myocardium. *J. Physiol.* **360,** 13–25.

Sheu, S. S., and Fozzard, H. A. (1982). Transmembrane Na^+ and Ca^2 electrochemical gradients in cardiac muscle and their relationship to force development. *J. Gen. Physiol.* **80,** 325–351.

Siegelbaum, S. A., and Tsien, R. W. (1980). Calcium-activated transient outward current in calf cardiac Purkinje fibres. *J. Physiol.* **299,** 485–506.

Wier, W. G., and Isenberg, G. (1982). Intracellular Ca transients in voltage clamped cardiac Purkinje fibres. *Pflügers Arch. Eur. J. Physiol.* **392,** 284–290.

Yellen, G. (1982). Ca-activated non-selective channels in neuroblastoma. *Nature* **296,** 357–359.

7

Some Experimental Studies of Na–Ca Exchange in Heart Muscle

Harry A. Fozzard

I. INTRODUCTION

Contraction of striated muscle requires an increase in the activity of intracellular Ca^{2+} (a^i_{Ca}) (e.g., the review by Ebashi and Endo, 1968). In cardiac muscle, a multiplicity of factors, including pH (Fabiato and Fabiato, 1978) and phosphorylation of protein (e.g., Winegrad *et al.*, 1983), may modify this Ca-dependent event; however, the key feature in control of muscle contraction is the regulation of a^i_{Ca}. The source of the Ca^{2+} needed for the contraction in skeletal muscle and in mammalian cardiac muscle is the terminal cisternae of the sarcoplasmic reticulum (SR), from which Ca^{2+} is released to produce the phasic contraction (twitch) and to which it returns to permit relaxation (Fig. 1). It is important to remember that the normal physiological stimulus for contraction of striated muscle is the action potential. The triggering of contraction by the action potential is clearly related to transmembrane depolarization, because other interventions such as high external potassium (K_o) solutions or voltage clamp also trigger contraction. An important unresolved problem is what couples depolarization to the release of Ca^{2+} from the SR.

Depolarization-dependent contraction was first examined in detail by taking advantage of the K^+-electrode property of the membrane. Raising K_o produced tension that depended critically on membrane potential (Niedergerke, 1956, for heart muscle; Hodgkin and Horowicz, 1960, for skeletal muscle). Although K contractures continue to be useful in studying regulation of contraction (e.g.,

CARDIAC MUSCLE:
THE REGULATION OF EXCITATION AND CONTRACTION

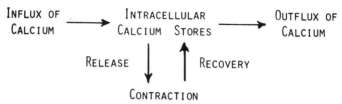

Fig. 1. Schematic illustration of the regulation of cellular Ca^{2+}. Entry of Ca^{2+} into the cell occurs largely via the Ca channel (i_{si}), which is voltage dependent. Ca^{2+} is sequestered in the sarcoplasmic reticulum, from which it is released to produce contraction. The trigger for release of Ca^{2+} from the sarcoplasmic reticulum is not yet completely identified, but it appears to be closely related to the transsarcolemmal Ca^{2+} current. Relaxation is by reuptake of Ca^{2+} into the sarcoplasmic reticulum. With each action potential, a small amount of Ca^{2+} is added to the cell, so in the steady state there must be an equivalent efflux. A major candidate for that efflux mechanism is Na–Ca exchange.

Gibbons and Fozzard, 1971b; Chapman and Tunstall, 1981), a better way to control membrane voltage as an experimental variable is by voltage clamp. This was first studied systematically in heart muscle by Fozzard and Hellam (1968) and Morad and Trautwein (1968). They and others showed a complex relationship between membrane voltage, time, and contraction (e.g., Gibbons and Fozzard, 1971a, 1975a; Beeler and Reuter, 1970).

A.   Calcium Current and Tension

Heart muscle has a voltage-dependent Ca^{2+} current (Reuter, 1973), and this current (usually called i_{si}) is a good candidate for explaining the voltage dependence of contraction. According to this explanation, depolarization triggers i_{si}, and this in turn causes a rise in a^i_{Ca} to activate the contraction. Beeler and Reuter (1970), Gibbons and Fozzard (1975b), and many others have found poor correlation between the size of i_{si} and the temporally associated contraction (reviewed by Fozzard, 1977), although almost everyone finds that the occurrence of i_{si} is essential as a trigger. Thus, i_{si} appears to be only a part of the mechanism coupling depolarization to contraction.

The concept of i_{si} as a trigger can be expressed in the following way. Upon depolarization, Ca^{2+} enters the cell through i_{si} and triggers release of Ca^{2+} from the SR (Fig. 1). This model then predicts that the size of the resulting contraction depends on the amount of Ca^{2+} in the SR available to be released, and perhaps also on the size of the trigger Ca^{2+}. Considerable evidence supporting this phenomenon (called Ca-induced Ca^{2+} release) has been developed by the Fabiatos (e.g., Fabiato, 1981, 1983) in heart muscle, although evidence of the role of Ca-generated release of Ca is less clear in skeletal muscle. In addition to serving as a trigger, i_{si} is also hypothesized to load the SR with more Ca^{2+}, which is released with subsequent contractions. Thus, i_{si} may have two functions in the mechanical activation of mammalian heart muscle: triggering release of Ca^{2+} from the SR and loading the SR with more Ca^{2+} for subsequent contractions (Fabiato, 1983).

Under some conditions, action potentials or voltage-clamp steps can cause first a twitch and then a slowly developing steady tension. This steady-state tension occurs, according to this model, because activation and inactivation voltages for i_{si} overlap and produce a voltage-dependent steady Ca^{2+} current (Reuter, 1973; Gibbons and Fozzard, 1975b). Whether this steady Ca^{2+} current is a significant factor in causing steady tension is not yet clear, because Ca-induced release of Ca^{2+} requires a pulse rather than a steady level of Ca^{2+} (Fabiato, 1983).

B. Discovery of Na–Ca Exchange

If a finite Ca^{2+} current occurs with each action potential, then some Ca^{2+} enters the cell with each depolarization (Fig. 1). If there were no mechanism to extrude Ca^{2+} from the cell against its electrochemical gradient, the cardiac cell would quickly turn to stone. Indeed, the steady state requires that Ca^{2+} influx by i_{si} be matched exactly by Ca^{2+} efflux. Alteration of the intracellular content of Ca^{2+} could be accomplished by either a change in influx or a change in efflux. It was while seeking the mechanism of Ca^{2+} efflux that Reuter and Seitz (1968) discovered its dependence on Na^+, leading them to propose the process called Na–Ca exchange.

Research on the interaction between the effects of Na_o and Ca_o on cardiac contraction has a considerable history, with key contributors including Wilbrandt and Koller (1948) and Lüttgau and Niedergerke (1958). In 1968, while searching for a Ca pump, Reuter and Seitz found Na-dependent influx and efflux of Ca in cardiac muscle. They proposed that it was caused by Na–Ca countertransport and that the energy for Ca efflux came from the movement of Na^+ down its electrochemical gradient. Shortly thereafter, Baker *et al.* (1969) observed a dependence of Ca influx on Na^+ in squid axons, and they too suggested that it might be related to control of cardiac contraction. Squid nerve and barnacle muscle are amenable to internal perfusion, and that has made them particularly good tissues in which to study Na–Ca exchange. Much of what we know about the Na–Ca exchange system comes from those tissues, rather than from cardiac cells. Although it is plausible to extrapolate from squid axon and barnacle to heart muscle, the conditions are not likely to be identical, and direct studies in heart are very desirable.

The original model proposed by Reuter and Seitz (1968) involved an exchange of 2 Na^+ for 1 Ca^{2+}, an electroneutral exchange. Data from squid showed, however, a $3:1$ or higher coupling (Blaustein and Hodgkin, 1969). This coupling ratio could mean that the exchange is voltage dependent, and flux studies by Mullins and Brinley (1975) and Baker and McNaughton (1976) showed that Na–Ca exchange was indeed dependent on the membrane potential. All of these studies may be called kinetic, because they measured unidirectional fluxes. They included the assumptions that the ionic conditions were in a steady state and that all of the ionic flux was by Na–Ca exchange. Mullins (1979) explored the implications of a voltage-dependent Na–Ca exchange in cardiac muscle and showed that it could be a powerful factor in controlling contraction strength.

Another kinetic method that has contributed to our understanding has used isolated sarcolemmal vesicles. Reeves and Sutko (1979) and Pitts (1979) were able to show that these vesicles contain a Na–Ca exchange transporter. Reeves and Sutko (1980), Philipson and Nishimoto (1980), and Caroni et al. (1980) were able to show also that a potential difference could be generated by the transport. Kadoma et al. (1982) reported measurements of initial velocities of Ca^{2+} efflux that are consistent with a coupling ratio greater than 2 (values varied from 2.44 to 3.17) and observed an effect of ATP. Recently Caroni and Carafoli (1983) reported a striking effect of ATP on the affinity of the exchanger's intracellular binding site for Ca^{2+}, via the activity of a calmodulin-dependent protein kinase. It is important to characterize this effect, because to regulate resting a_{Ca}^i, Na–Ca exchange must have a K_m somewhere in the range of resting a_{Ca}^i. Perhaps it will soon be possible to compare the apparent affinities in intact cells with those measured in isolated sarcolemmal preparations. The use of sarcolemmal vesicles to study Na–Ca exchange will no doubt contribute much to our understanding, but there remain problems with quantitative studies of the transport system in vesicles, whose small and variable sizes lead to such rapid changes in ion gradients.

C.   Model of Na–Ca Exchange

One concept of Na–Ca exchange is illustrated in Fig. 2. The level of intracellular Na^+ is understood as a balance between the passive leak into the cell, mostly through channels, and the active extrusion by the Na–K pump that uses ATP to move Na^+ against its gradient. The actual level of a_{Na}^i is determined by the extent to which the pump is activated by a_{Na}^i. The Na–Ca exchanger balances the electrochemical gradients for these two ions. Operating in the Ca efflux mode, it moves Ca^{2+} out of the cell by the energy derived from the movement of Na^+ down its gradient into the cell. If there is a significant passive leak of Ca^{2+} into the cell through Ca channels, then the level of a_{Ca}^i is influenced by the leak. There is also an ATP-dependent Ca pump (Caroni and Carafoli, 1980). This system is reported to have a K_m of approximately 100 nM a_{Ca}^i, but its V_{max} is apparently much less than that of Na–Ca exchange. Its role in regulating a_{Ca}^i is not yet clear. A further curiosity already mentioned about Na–Ca exchange is

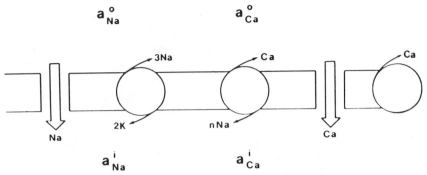

Fig. 2.   Schematic illustration of the regulation of intracellular Na^+ and Ca^{2+} by the sarcolemma. Intracellular Na^+ is regulated by a balance between passive Na^+ leakage into the cell and Na^+ efflux by the Na–K pump. The pump uses ATP and is activated by intracellular Na^+. This pump-leak model is balanced with intracellular Na^+ activity near 7 mM, but the balance point can be easily changed by altering either the leak or the pump. The energy present in the Na^+ electrochemical gradient is used to drive the Na–Ca exchanger, which transports more than 2 Na^+ into the cell while moving 1 Ca^{2+} out of the cell. This model of Ca^{2+} control could be influenced, however, by Ca^{2+} leakage or by a separate Ca pump.

that its K_m for a^i_{Ca} appears to be ATP dependent. Very little ATP is required; it appears not to provide energy for the Ca efflux, but, instead, to maintain some transport protein in a phosphorylated state (Caroni and Carafoli, 1983).

Steady-state methods for study of Na–Ca exchange are based on the equilibrium equation describing the way the a^i_{Ca} depends on the Na gradient and membrane potential (Blaustein, 1974):

$$a^i_{Ca} = a^o_{Ca} \left(\frac{a^i_{Na}}{a^o_{Na}} \right)^n \exp\frac{(n-2)FV_m}{RT}$$

where n is the Na–Ca exchange coupling ratio. This equation is valid only at energetic equilibrium. With the advent of ion-sensitive microelectrodes it has become possible to measure a^i_{Na} and a^i_{Ca} under steady-state conditions. Knowing V_m, a^o_{Na}, and a^o_{Ca}, one can calculate n; conversely, for any assumed n and measured a^i_{Na}, one can predict a^i_{Ca}. The validity of these values for n or a^i_{Ca} depends, of course, on how closely the Na–Ca exchange process approaches equilibrium.

II.   EXPERIMENTAL STUDIES

We (Sheu and Fozzard, 1982) have studied the predictions of this simple model of Na–Ca exchange in Purkinje strands and ventricular trabecular muscles from sheep hearts. The superfusing Tyrode solution contained, in mM: 127 NaCl, 4 KCl, 1.8 CaCl$_2$, 1.05 MgCl$_2$, 22 NaHCO$_3$, 2.5 NaH$_2$PO$_4$, and 5.5 glucose. All solutions were gassed with 95% O$_2$ and 5% CO$_2$ at 34°C. Solutions with low Na$^+$ were made by substituting sucrose for NaCl, with adjustment of the other concentrations to maintain the same activity in spite of the lower ionic strength. Membrane potential was measured with open-tipped micropipettes filled with KCl. Na$^+$- and Ca^{2+}-sensitive, liquid ion-exchanger microelectrodes were made with the neutral ligands ETH 227 (Steiner *et al.*, 1979) and ETH 1001 (Oehme *et al.*, 1976) as described previously (Sheu and Fozzard, 1982). Tension was measured by a photoelectric transducer, and the tissue was either quiescent or stimulated at a rate of 0.2 Hz, unless stated otherwise.

Intracellular a_{Na} and a_{Ca}

Levels of a^i_{Na} were 6.4 $\pm$ 1.2 mM in ventricular muscle. Lee and Fozzard (1975), who used glass ion-selective microelectrodes (ISE), found a^i_{Na} in heart muscle to be approximately 7 mM. The values reported from several labs using various types of ISE are shown in Table I. These values were from different tissues exposed to different solutions and were obtained with ISE of different constructions. Similarly, a^i_{Ca} has been measured in this lab as well as in those of several others (Lee *et al.*, 1980b; Marban *et al.*, 1980; Coray *et al.*, 1980; Sheu and Fozzard, 1982; Bers and Ellis, 1982; Lado *et al.*, 1982, 1984); we obtained values of 70–90 nM (Table II). Our results, when entered into the above equation, yield a value for n of 2.5–2.6.

TABLE I

Intracellular Sodium in Heart Muscle

Reference	Tissue	Method	a^i_{Na} (mM)
Lee and Fozzard (1975)	Rabbit ventricle	NAS 27-04 glass	5.7
Ellis (1977)	Sheep Purkinje	NAS 11-18 glass	7.2
Lee *et al.* (1980a)	Sheep Purkinje	NAS 11-18 glass	6.4 $\pm$ 1.6
Sheu *et al.* (1980)	Sheep Purkinje	K($\varnothing$-Cl)$_4\beta$	6.6 $\pm$ 0.6
Glitsch and Pusch (1980)	Sheep Purkinje	Na glass	8.1 $\pm$ 2.4
Cohen *et al.* (1982)	Sheep Purkinje	ETH 227	8.2 $\pm$ 2.0
	Guinea pig ventricle	K($\varnothing$-Cl)$_4\beta$	6.9
Sheu and Fozzard (1982)	Sheep ventricle	ETH 227	6.4 $\pm$ 1.2
	Sheep Purkinje	ETH 227	8.0 $\pm$ 0.6
Lee and Dagostino (1982)	Dog Purkinje (1 Hz)	ETH 227	7.6 $\pm$ 0.6
Wasserstrom *et al.* (1983)	Sheep Purkinje (1 Hz)	ETH 227	7.6 $\pm$ 0.6
Lado *et al.* (1984)	Sheep ventricle	ETH 227	6.9 $\pm$ 0.5
	Sheep Purkinje	ETH 227	7.9 $\pm$ 0.34

TABLE II

Intracellular Calcium in Heart Muscle

Reference	Tissue	a^i_{Ca} (nM)[a]	$[Ca]_i$ (nM)[a]
Lee *et al.* (1980b)	Rabbit ventricle	38 ± 7 (83)	—
Marban *et al.* (1980)	Ferret ventricle	—	260 ± 80
Coray *et al.* (1980)	Sheep ventricle	—	360 ± 150
	Sheep Purkinje	—	170 ± 50
Bers and Ellis (1982)	Sheep Purkinje	—	75–590
Lado *et al.* (1982)	Sheep Purkinje	93 ± 15	—
Sheu and Fozzard (1982)	Sheep ventricle	87 ± 20	—
	Sheep Purkinje	92 ± 9	—
Lado *et al.* (1984)	Sheep ventricle	70 ± 4	—
	Sheep Purkinje	98 ± 9	—

[a] $a_{Ca} = 0.32[Ca]$.

We then lowered the amount of Na^+ in the external solution, seeking to change the Na^+ gradient (Sheu and Fozzard, 1982). This has the effect of also reducing the Na^+ passive leak, so that a^i_{Na} falls, too. In each case, a^i_{Na} fell when a^o_{Na} was reduced. The fall in a^i_{Na} was not sufficient to restore the electrochemical gradient completely, and a^i_{Ca} rose. In each case, the new value of n was 2.5–2.6, not differing between normal and 40% a^o_{Na} solutions.

To investigate the effect of passive Ca leak into the cell, we changed Ca_o to 4.8 or 0.36 mM, increasing or reducing the driving force for passive influx. Perhaps because of an effect of Ca_o on the passive permeability of the membrane to Na, a^i_{Na} rose in low Ca_o solutions. Using the new values for a^i_{Na} and a^i_{Ca}, we calculated the value of n to be unchanged. This result is most consistent with a minimal effect of Ca^{2+} leakage on the level of a^i_{Ca}, because the Na^+ gradient appeared to dominate.

One of the implications of a coupling ratio that is not 2 is that the Na–Ca exchange may be voltage dependent. The most direct way to investigate this is to change V_m. We were not able to control voltage directly in these experiments, so we altered V_m by exposing the tissue to high levels of K_o. This changed the Na^+ electrochemical gradient dramatically. In experiments using both Purkinje and ventricular muscle fibers, a^i_{Ca} rose markedly, exactly to the level that was predicted by n of 2.5. While supporting the idea of a fixed coupling ratio and a Na–Ca exchange system that can control a^i_{Ca} rapidly, these results imply also that high K_o contractures are the result of an adjustment of a^i_{Ca} by Na–Ca exchange (Chapman, 1983).

An alternative approach to changing the Na^+ gradient is to concentrate or dilute a^i_{Na} by moving water out of or into the cells by exposing them to solutions of different tonicity (Lado et al., 1984). We superfused Purkinje strands and ventricular muscles with solutions having either a 25% reduction or 50% or 100% increase in tonicity. We kept a^o_{Na} constant and changed the tonicity by sucrose. During 5- to 10-min exposures to the test solutions (sufficient time to establish a new steady state), we monitored a^i_{Na} and a^i_{Ca} as well as V_m. In each case, the a^i_{Na} changed almost exactly as expected from the water movements. For example, in Purkinje strands, it rose from 6.9 ± 0.3 mM in solutions of normal tonicity to 10.8 ± 0.3 mM in solutions with double the normal tonicity; however, a^i_{Ca} rose much more than expected, from 101 ± 11 to 412 ± 43 nM. This was the increase we would have predicted had a^i_{Ca} been controlled by Na–Ca exchange with $n = 2.6$.

One of the variables influencing contraction strength in heart muscle is the frequency of its activation—the frequency–force relationship. Early studies showed a loss of tissue K^+ upon increasing stimulation rate and contraction strength (Hajdu, 1953), a loss that would be expected to accompany a gain in Na^+. Langer (1965) related a gain in Ca^{2+} to changes in intracellular Na^+ upon stimulation. A period of stimulation is followed by a transient hyperpolarization (Vassalle, 1970), apparently because of increased electrogenic Na–K pumping induced by a rise in a^i_{Na} (Cohen et al., 1981; Gadsby, 1980; Eisner et al., 1981). The stimulation-dependent rise in a^i_{Na} has been demonstrated directly with ion-sensitive microelectrodes (Cohen et al., 1982; Lee and Dagostino, 1982) and has been postulated to increase a^i_{Ca} through Na–Ca exchange. Lado et al. (1982) were able to record a stimulation-dependent increase in a^i_{Ca}, as predicted by the rise in a^i_{Na}, and the change in a^i_{Ca} was the amount predicted for $n = 2.6$. It must be recognized that the evidence that this frequency-dependent change in a^i_{Ca} and tension is caused by Na–Ca exchange is only indirect.

If the electrochemical energy gradient for Na^+ ($\Delta\bar{\mu}_{Na}$) is the driving force to establish the electrochemical energy gradient for Ca^{2+} ($\Delta\bar{\mu}_{Ca}$), then the relationship can be illustrated as in Fig. 3. This relationship was used by Sheu and Fozzard (1982) to illustrate the apparent coupling ratio between these energy gradients, because the equilibrium equation predicts the relationship as a function of the coupling ratio. Added to this figure are the data from subsequent experiments on frequency-dependent changes in a^i_{Na} (Cohen et al., 1982) and a^i_{Ca} (Lado et al., 1982), changes in a^i_{Na} and a^i_{Ca} as a consequence of altered tonicity (Lado et al., 1984), and additional details on the response to cardiac glycoside. For all conditions except late in the poisoning with digitalis, the data fit an energetic coupling ratio of approximately 2.5–2.6. Whatever the molecular events may be during Na–Ca exchange, this relationship appears to hold for a wide variety of conditions in intact cells. Any comprehensive description of Na–Ca exchange should be able to account for these results.

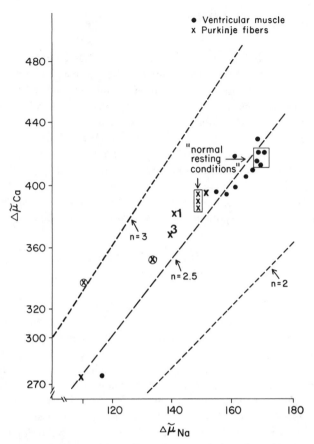

Fig. 3. The relationship between the Na$^+$ electrochemical gradient ($\Delta\tilde{\mu}_{Na}$) and the Ca^{2+} electrochemical gradient ($\Delta\tilde{\mu}_{Ca}$). Lines are drawn to illustrate the predicted equilibrium relation between these energy gradients for coupling ratios of 2.0, 2.5, and 3.0. Solid dots are measurements made in sheep ventricular muscle (Sheu and Fozzard, 1982), with normal values enclosed by the box and the other values obtained when the external solutions had altered ion concentrations. Points denoted by X are measurements in sheep Purkinje fibers, according to the same format (Sheu and Fozzard, 1982; Lado et al., 1984). The numbers 1 and 3 refer to measurements made in sheep Purkinje fibers stimulated at 1 or 3 Hz (Cohen et al., 1982; Lado et al., 1982). Symbols that are circled are measurements early and late during digitalis poisoning.

III. DISCUSSION

The possible consequences of these properties of Na–Ca exchange have been developed by Mullins (1979). He points out that the Na–Ca exchange system makes a_{Na}^i a prime regulator of intracellular Ca, and presumably tension, in heart muscle. He emphasizes also that when heart muscle is depolarized, such as during the plateau of the action potential, the Na–Ca exchange system could reverse direction and transport Ca^{2+} into the cell. He makes a good case for Na–Ca exchange as the primary determinant of the amount of Ca^{2+} within the cell. His key assumption about the transport system (other than its reversibility) is that it can move substantial amounts of Ca during the 200–300 msec of the action potential. The implications of Mullins's assumptions regarding control of cardiac contraction are sufficiently important to warrant careful testing.

A. Comparison with Na–Ca Exchange in Sarcolemmal Vesicles

It has already been noted that several investigators have been able to isolate vesicular preparations of cardiac sarcolemma and show that they will transport Ca^{2+} in the presence of a Na^+ gradient (e.g., see Langer, 1982). These studies have added greatly to our understanding of Na–Ca countertransport, and progress has been made toward purification of the exchanger complex (Hale et al., 1984). One of the measurements that can be obtained from vesicular studies is the affinity of the transporter for Na^+ and Ca^{2+}. Most investigators have found that the K_m for Ca^{2+} is 15–40 μM (e.g., Philipson and Nishimoto, 1982), a value so high as to raise doubts that Na–Ca exchange could play a significant physiological role. Others (Caroni and Carifoli, 193) have found a much higher affinity (1–2 μM Ca), which would be close enough to the resting level of a_{Ca}^i to participate in its control during diastole, as well as during the systolic phase. These studies in vesicles are complicated not only by technical problems of kinetic measurements but also by the possibility that the exchanger is modified during the isolation of the membrane. The exchanger's affinity for Na^+ is in the range of 13–26 mM (Reeves and Sutko, 1983), but this varies with the method used to measure it.

Stoichiometry of the pump can also be examined by vesicular studies. Using K^+ gradients and valinomycin to convert the vesicles into "K^+ electrodes," Reeves and Hale (1984) have found a reversal potential for Na–Ca exchange that would be expected for a coupling ratio of 3. Results from other vesicular flux studies are most consistent with a ratio of 3 or slightly less. Although these studies suffer from artificial conditions and the limitations of isotopic flux measurements, their further development promises to permit identification of individual ion binding sites and complete kinetic characterization at the molecular level.

B. Importance of the Coupling Ratio

The implication of the analysis made by Sheu and Fozzard (1982) is that a^i_{Ca} is controlled by Na–Ca exchange and that it operates close to its equilibrium. Equilibrium would be somewhat more positive than the resting potential, so that the exchange system would operate in the Ca^{2+} efflux mode. The exchanger would operate at only a fraction of its maximal velocity, but this would be sufficient to balance Ca^{2+} influx. If this interpretation is accurate, a modest depolarization (e.g., 20–30 mV) could switch the exchange system to its Ca^{2+} influx mode.

During a normal action potential, Ca^{2+} enters through i_{si} and is released from the SR, so that a^i_{Ca} rises to the several-μM level. This Ca^{2+} transient lasts 100–150 msec (Wier, 1980), during which the Na–Ca exchange system would be expected to move Ca^{2+} out of the cell, even though the membrane potential is approximately 0–20 mV. Because this depolarization usually outlasts the Ca^{2+} transient, Ca^{2+} could be brought into the cell by the Na–Ca exchange system during that period. This mechanism might explain the positive inotropic effect of prolonged depolarization (Gibbons and Fozzard, 1975a); however, the existence or extent of this entry of Ca^{2+} depends on the reversal potential of the Na–Ca exchange system, which, in turn, depends on the coupling ratio. The difference between our apparent coupling ratio values of 2.5–2.6, measured in intact cells, and the value of 3.0 obtained with sarcolemmal vesicles is consistent with reversal potentials between −80 and 0 mV, making of great physiological importance the determination of the correct value. At this stage, the studies of sarcolemmal vesicles and those of intact tissue are both subject to significant criticism. Resolution of these experimental problems will be necessary before we can decide whether Mullins's (1979) suggestions are correct. In either case, the result will have a major influence on our understanding of control of cardiac contraction.

C. a^i_{Ca} and Tension

A role of Na–Ca exchange in tonic tension, as found in high-K_o contractures, is supported by experiments of Chapman and Tunstall (1981) and Chapman et al. (1983). We monitored a^i_{Ca} directly during high-K_o contractures (Sheu and Fozzard, 1982) and found a good correlation with tension; however, the physiological contraction is a transient one, thought by most investigators to be caused by release of Ca^{2+} from the SR. We were surprised to find a good correlation between *resting* a^i_{Ca} and *twitch* contractions under a variety of conditions, and Lee and Dagostino (1982) found a correlation when a^i_{Ca} was raised by cardiac glycoside. But it remains unclear how resting, diastolic a^i_{Ca} is related to the SR's release of Ca^{2+}. It is possible that the amount of Ca^{2+} stored in the SR is influenced significantly by the cytoplasmic level. For example, if the Ca pump in the SR membrane is able to concentrate Ca^{2+} 100-fold, then raising a^i_{Ca} should raise Ca^{2+} in the SR proportionately. Upon trigger for release of Ca^{2+}, there would then be more Ca^{2+} released. Although this suggestion is plausible, it has not been tested by direct experiment.

IV. SUMMARY

Cardiac muscle controls its contraction in the steady state by regulating entry of Ca^{2+} into the cell through voltage-dependent calcium channels and Ca^{2+} efflux from the cell. Na–Ca exchange appears to be the principal transport system for Ca^{2+} efflux, although there remains the possibility that an ATP-dependent Ca^{2+} pump plays a role, also. Na–Ca exchange is a transport system that uses the movement of Na^+ down its electrochemical gradient into the cell to transport Ca^{2+} up its electrochemical gradient out of the cell. The exchange is not neutral (i.e., not $2Na^+ : 1Ca^{2+}$), but is closer to $3Na^+ : 1Ca^{2+}$. This confers on the transport system a voltage dependence.

Direct study of Na–Ca transport in cardiac muscle has been made possible by monitoring membrane potential and intracellular Na^+ and Ca^{2+} activities (with ion-sensitive microelectrodes) during changes in the Na^+ or Ca^{2+} gradient. Normal intracellular Na^+ activity at rest is near 7 mM, and intracellular Ca^{2+} activity is between 50 and 100 nM. Under a wide variety of conditions that alter the Na^+ gradient greatly, the Ca^{2+} gradient adjusts to a new value dependent on the change in intracellular Na^+. The two gradients maintain an apparent ratio of 2.5–2.6.

The Na–Ca exchange system can operate in a reverse mode, moving Na^+ out of the cardiac cell in exchange for the entry of Ca^{2+}. This might happen during the plateau phase of an action potential, but evidence in favor of this mode of operation for Na–Ca exchange is only indirect.

Na–Ca exchange appears to be important in regulating the strength of contraction in heart muscle, including the inotropic response to changes in extracellular ion concentrations and to frequency of stimulation. Additional studies are required before we can understand its role completely. To achieve this goal, investigations of intact cells must be supplemented by studies of sarcolemmal vesicles and careful modeling of the multiple interactive mechanisms in the cell.

ACKNOWLEDGMENTS

The experimental studies discussed here were done in collaboration with Charles Cohen, Shey-Shing Sheu, and Mario Lado, who also contributed greatly to the concept of Na–Ca exchange presented here. The studies were supported by a grant from USPHS HL-20592.

REFERENCES

Baker, P. F., and McNaughton, P. A. (1976). The effect of membrane potential on the calcium transport systems in squid axons. *J. Physiol. (Lond.)* **260**, 24–25P.

Baker, P. F., Blaustein, M. P., Hodgkin, A. L., and Steinhardt, R. A. (1969). The influence of calcium on sodium efflux in squid axons. *J. Physiol. (Lond.)* **200**, 431–458.

Beeler, G. W., Jr., and Reuter, H. (1970). The relation between membrane potential, membrane currents and activation of contraction in ventricular myocardial fibers. *J. Physiol. (Lond.)* **207**, 211–229.

Bers, D. M., and Ellis, D. (1982). Intracellular calcium and sodium activity in sheep heart Purkinje fibres. *Pfluegers Arch.* **393**, 171–178.

Blaustein, M. P. (1974). The interrelationship between sodium and calcium fluxes across cell membranes. *Rev. Physiol. Biochem. Pharmacol.* **70**, 33–82.

Blaustein, M. P., and Hodgkin, A. L. (1969). The effect of cyanide on the efflux of calcium from squid axons. *J. Physiol. (Lond.)* **200**, 497–527.

Caroni, P., and Carafoli, E. (1980). An ATP-dependent Ca^{2+}-pumping system in dog heart sarcolemma. *Nature (Lond.)* **283**, 765–767.

Caroni, P., and Carafoli, E. (1983). The regulation of the Na^+–Ca^{2+} exchanger of heart sarcolemma. *Eur. J. Biochem.* **132**, 451–460.

Caroni, P., Reinlib, L., and Carafoli, E. (1980). Charge movements during the Na^+–Ca^{2+} exchange in heart sarcolemmal vesicles. *Proc. Natl. Acad. Sci. USA* **77**, 6354–6358.

Chapman, R. A. (1983). Control of cardiac contractility at the cellular level. *Am. J. Physiol. (Heart Circ. Physiol.)* **245**, H535–H552.

Chapman, R. A., and Tunstall, J. (1981). The tension–depolarization relationship of frog atrial trabeculae as determined by potassium contractures. *J. Physiol. (Lond.)* **310**, 97–115.

Chapman, R. A., Coray, A., and McGuigan, J. A. S. (1983). Sodium/calcium exchange in mammalian ventricular muscle: A study done with sodium-sensitive microelectrodes. *J. Physiol. (Lond.)* **343**, 253–276.

Cohen, C. J., Fozzard, H. A., and Sheu, S-S. (1982). Increase in intracellular sodium ion activity during stimulation in mammalian cardiac muscle. *Circ. Res.* **50**, 651–662.

Cohen, I., Falk, R., and Kline, R. (1981). Membrane currents following activity in canine cardiac Purkinje fibers. *Biophys. J.* **33**, 281–288.

Coray, A., Fry, C. H., Hess, P., McGuigan, J. A. S., and Weingart, R. (1980). Resting Ca in sheep cardiac tissue and frog skeletal muscle measured with ion-selective microelectrodes. *J. Physiol. (Lond.)* **305**, 60P.

Ebashi, S., and Endo, M. (1968). Calcium ion and muscle contraction. *Prog. Biophys. Molec. Biol.* **18**, 123–184.

Eisner, D. A., Lederer, W. J., and Vaughan-Jones, R. D. (1981). The dependence of sodium pumping and tension on intracellular sodium activity in voltage-clamped sheep Purkinje fibres. *J. Physiol. (Lond.)* **317**, 163–187.

214   Harry A. Fozzard

Ellis, D. (1977). The effects of external cations and ouabain on the intracellular sodium activity of sheep heart Purkinje fibres. *Physiol. (Lond.)* **273**, 211–240.

Fabiato, A. (1981). Myoplasmic free calcium concentration reached during the twitch of an intact isolated cardiac cell and during calcium-induced release of calcium from the sarcoplasmic reticulum of a skinned cardiac cell from the adult rat or rabbit ventricle. *J. Gen. Physiol.* **78**, 457–497.

Fabiato, A. (1983). Calcium-induced release of calcium from the cardiac sarcoplasmic reticulum. *Am. J. Physiol. (Cell)* **14**, C1–C14.

Fabiato, A., and Fabiato, F. (1978). Effects of pH on the myofilaments and the sarcoplasmic reticulum of skinned cells from cardiac and skeletal muscles. *J. Physiol. (Lond.)* **276**, 233–255.

Fozzard, H. A., (1977). Heart: Excitation–contraction coupling. *Ann. Rev. Physiol.* **39**, 201–220.

Fozzard, H. A., and Hellam, D. C. (1968). Relationship between membrane voltage and tension in voltage-clamped cardiac Purkinje fibres. *Nature (Lond.)* **218**, 588–589.

Gadsby, D. C. (1980). Activation of electrogenic Na^+/K^+ exchange by intracellular K in canine cardiac Purkinje fibers. *Proc. Natl. Acad. Sci. (USA)* **77**, 4035–4039.

Gibbons, W. R., and Fozzard, H. A. (1971a). Voltage dependence and time dependence of contraction in sheep cardiac Purkinje fibers. *Circ. Res.* **28**, 446–460.

Gibbons, W. R., and Fozzard, H. A. (1971b). High potassium and low sodium contractures in sheep cardiac muscle. *J. Gen. Physiol.* **58**, 483–510.

Gibbons, W. R., and Fozzard, H. A. (1975a). Relationships between voltage and tension in sheep cardiac Purkinje fibre. *J. Gen. Physiol.* **65**, 345–365.

Gibbons, W. R., and Fozzard, H. A. (1975b). Slow inward current and contraction of sheep cardiac Purkinje fibers. *J. Gen. Physiol.* **65**, 367–384.

Glitsch, H, G., and Pusch, H. (1980). Correlation between changes in membrane potential and intracellular sodium activity during K activated response in sheep Purkinje fibres. *Pfluegers Arch.* **384**, 184–191.

Hajdu, S. (1953). Mechanism of staircase and contracture in ventricular muscle. *Am. J. Physiol.* **174**, 371–380.

Hale, C. C., Slaughter, R. S., Ahrens, D., and Reeves, J. P. (1984). Identification and partial purification of the cardiac sodium–calcium exchanger. *Biophys. J.* **45**, 81a (abstract).

Hodgkin, A. L., and Horowicz, P. (1960). Potassium contractures in single muscle fibres. *J. Physiol. (Lond.)* **153**, 386–403.

Kadoma, M., Froehlich, J., Reeves, J., and Sutko, J. (1982). Kinetics of sodium ion induced calcium ion release in calcium ion loaded cardiac sarcolemmal vesicles: Determination of initial velocities by stopped-flow spectrophotometry. *Biochemistry* **21**, 1914–1918.

Lado, M. G., Sheu, S-S., and Fozzard, H. A. (1982). Changes in intracellular Ca^{2+} activity with stimulation in sheep cardiac Purkinje strands. *Am. J. Physiol.* **243**, H133–H137.

Lado, M. G., Sheu, S-S., and Fozzard, H. A. (1984). Effects of tonicity on tension and intracellular sodium and calcium activities in sheep heart. *Circ. Res.* **54**, 576–585.

Langer, G. A. (1965). Calcium exchange in dog ventricular muscle: Relation to frequency of contraction and maintenance of contractility. *Circ. Res.* **17**, 78–90.

Langer, G. A. (1982). Sodium–calcium exchange in the heart. *Ann. Rev. Physiol.* **44**, 435–449.

Lee, C. O., and Dagostino, M. (1982). The effect of strophanthidin on intracellular Na ion activity and twitch tension of constantly driven canine cardiac Purkinje fibers. *Biophys. J.* **40**, 185–198.

Lee, C. O., and Fozzard, H. A. (1975). Activities of potassium and sodium in rabbit heart muscle. *J. Gen. Physiol.* **65**, 694–708.

Lee, C. O., Kang, D. H., Sokol, J. H., and Lee, K. S. (1980a). Relation between intracellular Na ion activity and tension of sheep cardiac Purkinje fibers exposed to dihydro-ouabain. *Biophys. J.* **29**, 315–330.

Lee, C. O., Uhm, D. Y., and Dresdner, K. (1980b). Sodium–calcium exchange in rabbit heart muscle cells: Direct measurement of sarcoplasmic Ca^{2+} activity. *Science (Wash. DC)* **209**, 699–701.

Lüttgau, H. C., and Niedergerke, R. (1958). The antagonism between Ca and Na ions on the frog's heart. *J. Physiol. (Lond.)* **143**, 486–502.

Marban, E., Rink, T. J., Tsien, R. W., and Tsien, R. Y. (1980). Free calcium in heart muscle at rest and during contraction measured with Ca-selective microelectrodes. *Nature (Lond.)* **286**, 845–850.

Morad, M., and Trautwein, W. (1968). Effect of the duration of the action potential on contraction in the mammalian cardiac muscle. *Pfluegers Arch.* **299**, 66–82.

Mullins, L. J. (1979). The generation of electric currents in cardiac fibers by Na/Ca exchange. *Am. J. Physiol. (Cell Physiol.)* **236**, C103–C110.

Mullins, L. J., and Brinley, F. J., Jr. (1975). Sensitivity of calcium efflux from squid axons to changes in membrane potential. *J. Gen. Physiol.* **65**, 135–152.

Niedergerke, R. (1956). The potassium chloride contracture of the heart and its modification by calcium. *J. Physiol. (Lond.)* **134**, 584–603.

Oehme, M., Kessler, M., and Simon, W. (1976). Neutral carrier Ca^{2+}-microelectrode. *Chimia* **30**, 204–206.

Philipson, K. D., and Nishimoto, A. Y. (1980). $Na^+ - Ca^{2+}$ exchange is affected by membrane potential in cardiac sarcolemmal vesicles. *J. Biol. Chem.* **255**, 6880–6882.

Philipson, K. D., and Nishimoto, A. Y. (1982). $Na^+ - Ca^{2+}$ exchange in inside-out cardiac sarcolemmal vesicles. *J. Biol. Chem.* **257**, 5111–5117.

Pitts, B. J. R. (1979). Stoichiometry of sodium–calcium exchange in cardiac sarcolemmal vesicles. *J. Biol. Chem.* **254**, 6232–6235.

Reeves, J. P., and Hale, C. C. (1984). The stoichiometry of the cardiac sodium–calcium exchange system. *J. Biol. Chem.* **259**, 7733–7739.

Reeves, J. P., and Sutko, J. L. (1979). Sodium–calcium ion exchange in cardiac membrane vesicles. *Proc. Natl. Acad. Sci. U.S.A.* **76**, 590–594.

Reeves, J. P., and Sutko, J. L. (1980). Sodium–calcium exchange activity generates a current in cardiac membrane vesicles. *Science (NY)* **208**, 1461–1463.

Reeves, J. P., and Sutko, J. L. (1983). Competitive interactions of sodium and calcium with the sodium–calcium exchange system of cardiac sarcolemmal vesicles. *J. Biol. Chem.* **258**, 3178–3182.

Reuter, H. (1973). Divalent cations as charge carriers in excitable membranes. *Prog. Biophys. Mol. Biol.* **26**, 1–43.

Reuter, H., and Seitz, N. (1968). The dependence of calcium efflux from cardiac muscle on temperature and external ion composition. *J. Physiol. (Lond.)* **195**, 451–470.

Sheu, S-S., and Fozzard, H. A. (1982). Transmembrane Na^+ and Ca^{2+} electrochemical gradients in cardiac muscle and their relationship to force development. *J. Gen. Physiol.* **80**, 325–351.

Sheu, S-S., Korth, M., Lathrup, D. A., and Fozzard, H. A. (1980). Intra- and extracellular K^+ and Na^+ activities and resting membrane potential in sheep cardiac Purkinje strands. *Circ. Res.* **47**, 692–700.

Steiner, R. A., Oehme, M., Ammann, D., and Simon, W. (1979). Neutral carrier sodium ion-selective microelectrode for intracellular studies. *Anal. Chem.* **51**, 351–353.

Vassalle, M. (1970). Electrogenic suppression of automaticity in sheep and dog Purkinje fibers. *Circ. Res.* **27**, 361–377.

Wasserstrom, J. A., Schwartz, D. J., and Fozzard, H. A. (1983). Relation between intracellular sodium and twitch tension in sheep cardiac Purkinje strands exposed to cardiac glycosides. *Circ. Res.* **52**, 697–705.

Wier, W. G. (1980). Calcium transients during excitation–contraction coupling in mammalian heart: Aequorin signals of canine Purkinje fibers. *Science (Wash. DC)* **207**, 1085–1087.

Wilbrandt, W., and Koller, H. (1948). Die Calciumwirkung am Froschherzen als Funktion des Ionengleichgewichts zwischen Zellmembran and Umgebung. *Helv. Physiol. Acta* **6**, 208–221.

Winegrad, S., McClellan, G., Tucker, M., and Lin, L-E. (1983). Cyclic AMP regulation of myosin isozymes in mammalian cardiac muscle. *J. Gen. Physiol.* **81**, 749–765.

8

The Regulation of Tension in Heart Muscle by Intracellular Sodium

W. J. Lederer, R. D. Vaughan-Jones, D. A. Eisner, S-S. Sheu, and M. B. Cannell

I. INTRODUCTION

Force developed by the heart during contraction depends on the release of calcium from intracellular stores, which is triggered by the cardiac action potential. The force of contraction can be modulated by varying either (1) the increase of intracellular calcium concentration ($[Ca^{2+}]_i$) during each contraction or (2) the sensitivity of the contractile proteins to $[Ca^{2+}]_i$. In this chapter we show how certain physiological and pharmacological maneuvers alter contractility. In particular, we will concentrate on the role of intracellular sodium (a^i_{Na}) in modulating the production of force by the heart. Intracellular sodium can have an effect on the development of tension because of the existence of a Na–Ca exchange mechanism in the surface membrane (Reuter and Seitz, 1968; Baker *et al.*, 1969; also, e.g., Glitsch *et al.*, 1970; Deitmer and Ellis, 1978a; Chapman and Tunstall, 1980, 1981). The Na–Ca exchanger allows a^i_{Na} to influence calcium influx and hence the intracellular calcium activity. Sarcoplasmic reticulum calcium uptake will depend on intracellular calcium activity and, therefore, calcium release from the sarcoplasmic reticulum will be linked to a^i_{Na} (Eisner *et el.*, 1983a, 1984). In this chapter we will present experimental evidence for such a link between changes of intracellular sodium ion activity and alterations of tension. The changes in a^i_{Na} may be produced by pharmacological interventions (e.g., Na-pump blockage or sodium-channel blockade—cf. Deitmer and Ellis, 1978b;

CARDIAC MUSCLE:
THE REGULATION OF EXCITATION AND CONTRACTION

Shue *et al.*, 1983; January and Fozzard, 1984) or physiological variations of cardiac function such as change in heart rate (Cohen *et al.*, 1982; see also Lado *et al.*, 1982; Lederer and Sheu, 1983).

We conclude that changes of a_{Na}^i are important in determining the tension generated by the heart and in bringing about changes in tension that follow physiological and pharmacological maneuvers. Intracellular sodium can play an important role even when the changes in intracellular sodium are very small, because there is a steep dependence of tension on sodium activity.

II. METHODS

A. General

Sheep cardiac Purkinje fibers used in these experiments were dissected from both left and right ventricles of the hearts obtained from sheep killed at a local slaughterhouse (cf. Eisner and Lederer, 1979a). They were stored in physiological saline (see below) at room temperature until needed. The two-microelectrode voltage-clamp method (Eisner and Lederer, 1979a,b), the construction and testing of recessed-tip electrodes (Thomas, 1978; Eisner *et al.*, 1981a) and liquid ion-exchanger electrodes (Thomas, 1978; Sheu and Fozzard, 1982; Eisner *et al.*, 1983d; Lederer *et al.*, 1984), and the details of fabricating the tension-transducer (Eisner and Lederer, 1979a) have been described previously.

B. Solutions

The standard superfusion solution contained (in mM) 145 NaCl, 2 CaCl$_2$, 1 MgCl$_2$, 10 glucose, and 10 Tris–HCl, pH 7.4 at 37°C. The concentration of potassium or rubidium chloride is indicated in the figure legends. Potassium and rubidium are essentially equal in their abilities to activate the Na pump (Eisner and Lederer, 1980; Eisner *et al.*, 1981a; Glitsch *et al.*, 1981).

C. Liquid Ion-Exchanger Cocktails

We obtained the liquid ion-exchanger cocktails containing the Na ionophore (ETH 227, cf. Steiner *et al.*, 1979) and the proton-ion-exchanger cocktail (containing 10 wt% tri-*n*-dodecylamine in *o*-nitrophenyl octyl ether with 0.7% sodium tetraphenylborate, cf. Ammann *et al.*, 1981) from Professor W. Simon (Swiss Federal Institute of Technology, Zurich, Switzerland). There compounds are now commercially available from Fluka Chemical Corp. (order No. 71176 for the Na cocktail and No. 82500 for the proton cocktail).

D.   Activity

We determined sodium-ion activity (as in many previous studies; cf. Eisner *et al.*, 1981a) by calibrating the sodium electrode in solutions of known sodium concentration and assuming an activity coefficient of 0.75 (Eisner *et al.*, 1981a) in both the intracellular compartments and the extracellular compartments. The pH electrodes were calibrated directly against established pH standards, and no compensation was made for possible interference from other ions in the intracellular environment.

III.   RESULTS AND DISCUSSION

A.   Twitch Tension

Changes in the duration of the action potential are known to accompany interventions that alter a_{Na}^i (cf. Lederer, 1976; Eisner *et al.*, 1982b). Because these variations in membrane potential may have direct effects on calcium transport (i.e., via calcium channels or a voltage-dependent Na–Ca exchange mechanism), it is important to control membrane potential when examining the relationship between sodium and tension. We therefore used the voltage-clamp technique to allow dissociation of the effects of potential on tension from those due to changes in a_{Na}^i.

When the sodium pump is inhibited, there is an increase in intracellular sodium activity from approximately 6 mM to between 15 to 35 mM (Ellis, 1977; Deitmer and Ellis, 1978b). The effects on a_{Na}^i and tension of applying the Na-pump inhibitor strophanthidin (10 μM) are shown in Fig. 1. This record shows the early portion of an experiment and indicates the time course of the elevation of intracellular sodium from the control level (about 6 mM) to about 12 mM. Twitch tension (resulting from each voltage-clamp depolarization) begins to rise as soon as an increase in a_{Na}^i becomes detectable. The details of the tension record are clearer in Fig. 2, which shows sample records (a), (b), and (c) from Fig. 1. In addition to the increase in twitch tension, a component of voltage-dependent tonic tension develops as a_{Na}^i increases (see Section III, C). Although not discussed further, aftercontractions and the arrhythmogenic transient inward current, I_{TI}, develop at higher levels of a_{Na}^i as is illustrated in Fig. 3 (see Lederer and Tsien, 1976; Eisner *et al.*, 1983d, 1984).

The dependence of twitch tension, tonic tension, aftercontraction, and I_{TI} amplitudes on sodium are shown graphically in Fig. 3. With the voltage protocol used in this experiment, there is little voltage-dependent tonic tension until a_{Na}^i has risen above 7 mM; however, twitch tension increases dramatically as soon as a_{Na}^i begins to increase.

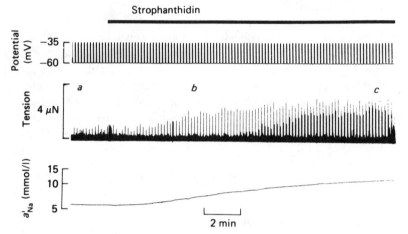

Fig. 1. Time course of the effects of Na–K pump inhibition on a_{Na}^i and tension. Strophanthidin (10 μM) was applied for the period shown above the record. The membrane potential was held at −60 mV and a 2-sec depolarizing pulse to −35 mV was applied at 0.1 Hz. The tension record has been filtered at 0.1 Hz (high-pass) to remove slow drifts in the base line tension. This means that only the twitch component of tension can be resolved accurately. These results, as well as those illustrated in the following figures, were obtained from sheep cardiac Purkinje fibers. [Taken from Eisner *et al.* (1984). Use with the permission of the *Journal of Physiology.*]

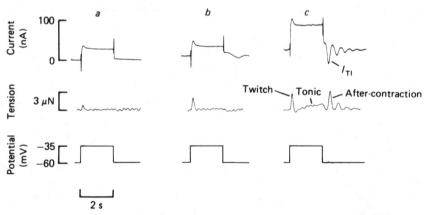

Fig. 2. Sample records of membrane current, tension, and membrane potential obtained when the sodium pump is inhibited by the application of strophanthidin (10 μM). Panels (a), (b), and (c) were taken from the record shown in Fig. 1 as indicated. Note the description of the labels identifying the different components of tension seen in panel (c). Twitch tension occurred with the depolarization and corresponds with the component of tension that would be noted with an action potential. The slow voltage-dependent tonic tension is observed to develop when intracellular sodium is elevated (see Figs. 6 and 7). Accompanying the development of the tonic tension is an oscillation of tension seen on repolarization, the aftercontraction. I_{TI}, the arrhythmogenic transient inward current, accompanies the aftercontraction. [Taken from Eisner *et al.* (1984). Used with the permission of the *Journal of Physiology.*]

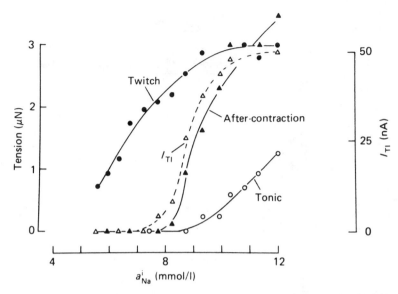

Fig. 3. Sodium dependence of twitch tension, tonic tension, the aftercontraction, and the arrhythmogenic transient inward current, I_{TI}. Data taken from the experiment shown in Fig. 1. (●) Twitch tension; (○) tonic tension; (▲) aftercontraction; (△) transient inward current, I_{TI}. Note that although twitch tension begins to rise as soon as a change of intracellular sodium is detectable, there is little effect on tonic tension, the aftercontraction, or I_{TI} until a^i_{Na} has risen, in this case, by approximately 50%. [Taken from Eisner *et al.* (1984). Used with the permission of the *Journal of Physiology.*]

The sodium dependence and voltage dependence of twitch tension are shown in greater detail in Fig. 4. In this experiment, the sodium pump is inhibited by removing the rubidium from the superfusion solution (which contained no potassium). The resulting increase in intracellular sodium and the concomitant development of twitch tension are shown in Fig. 4A. The voltage dependence of the tension and the time course of the twitches are shown in greater detail in Fig. 4B. A doubling of intracellular sodium is associated with approximately an eightfold increase in twitch tension when the membrane potential is depolarized to 0 mV. Figure 5 shows the dependence of twitch tension on sodium from a similar experiment. The main panel shows the results in linear coordinates, and the inset shows the same data plotted on logarithmic coordinates for a^i_{Na} between 5 and 10 m*M*. Because the data, when plotted in logarithmic coordinates, can be fitted by a straight line, it appears that over this range of a^i_{Na} the following relationship applies:

$$\text{Twitch tension} = b(a^i_{Na})^n$$

where n is the slope of the relationship and b is independent of a^i_{Na} but dependent on membrane potential. In seven fibers, the mean slope was found to be 3.2 ±

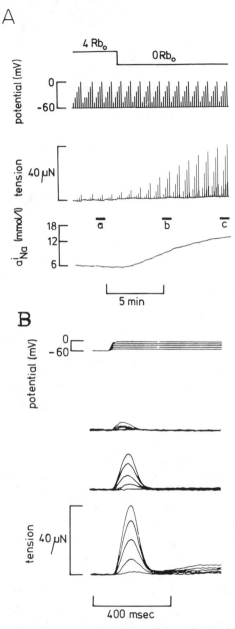

Fig. 4. The effects of membrane potential and intracellular sodium on the development of twitch tension. Panel (A) shows the time course of the change of intracellular sodium activity (a_{Na}^i) and tension when the sodium pump is inhibited. The Na pump was inhibited by removal of external rubidium from a superfusion solution containing no potassium. Panel (B) shows the sample tension records for five different depolarizing levels (-48, -36, -24, -12, and 0 mV) at three different levels of a_{Na}^i as indicated by the periods marked on Panel (A) by (a), (b), and (c). [Taken from Eisner *et al.* (1984). Used with the permission of the *Journal of Physiology*.]

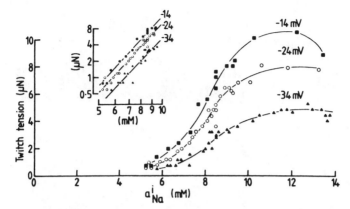

Fig. 5. The dependence of twitch tension on intracellular sodium activy (a_{Na}^i). Twitch tension evoked by depolarizations from -64 to -14 mV (■), to -24 mV (○), and to -34 mV (▲) are plotted as a function of a_{Na}^i. The plots are clearly nonlinear over most of the graph. The initial sodium dependence of twitch tension (5–10 mM) has been replotted in the inset, which shows that the logarithm of tension is a linear function of the logarithm of a_{Na}^i over this range of a_{Na}^i. The lines shown in the inset are based on the linear regression of the data and have the following slopes: 5.7 (-14 mV), 5.6 (-24 mV), and 5.2 (-34 mV). [Taken from Eisner *et al.* (1983e). Used with the permission of the *Journal of Physiology.*]

0.6 (S.E.M.). The exact value of the slope has no simple physical interpretation but will be a complicated function of (1) the properties of the Na–Ca exchange; (2) other calcium transport mechanisms across the surface membrane; (3) calcium sequestration and release by the sarcoplasmic reticulum; (4) calcium buffering by the mitochondria and intracellular proteins; and (5) the relationship between a_{Ca}^i and tension (see Cannell *et al.*, 1985). Thus, in contrast to some earlier reports showing a *linear* dependence of tension on a_{Na}^i (Lee *et al.*, 1980; Lee and Dagostino, 1982; Wasserstrom *et al.*, 1983), we find a steep and nonlinear relationship. The physiological significance of our observations is illustrated in Section III, G.

B. Tonic Tension

In Figs. 3, 4, 6, and 7 it is clear that as intracellular sodium rises, there is a considerable increase in voltage-dependent tonic tension. Figure 8A uses linear coordinates to show the dependence of tonic tension on intracellular sodium, whereas Fig. 8B shows the same data using logarithmic coordinates. The fact that, at any potential, the relationship can be fitted by a straight line (in logarithmic coordinates) indicates that over this range of intracellular sodium, the following empirical relationship holds:

$$\text{Tonic tension} = b(a_{Na}^i)^n$$

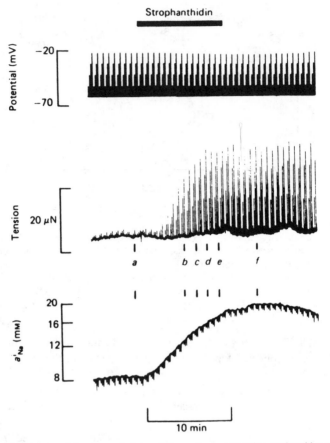

Fig. 6. Time course of the change in intracellular sodium and tension produced by exposure to strophanthidin (10 μM). Although this is a different experiment than is shown in Fig. 1, it resembles the latter in many ways. Note, however, that the sodium rises to a higher level and that this difference from preparation to preparation is typical. The detailed records at four pulse potentials are shown in Fig. 7. [Taken from Eisner *et al.* (1983e). Used with the permission of the *Journal of Physiology*.]

where n is the slope of the relationship (and is independent of membrane potential) and b is independent of a_{Na}^i but dependent on the voltage-clamp pulse potential. In five experiments the mean slope of this logarithmic plot was found to be 3.7 ± 0.7 (S.E.M.). Thus, like twitch tension, tonic tension is steeply dependent on a_{Na}^i (see also Eisner *et al.*, 1982a; Vaughan-Jones *et al.*, 1984).

C. Voltage Dependence of Tonic Tension

What causes the voltage-dependent tonic tension? Such tension may reflect the contribution of a voltage-dependent Na–Ca exchange mechanism to calcium

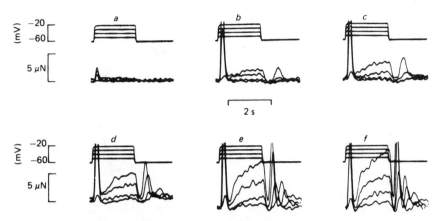

Fig. 7. Effects of intracellular sodium activity (a_{Na}^i) and membrane potential on tonic tension. Panels (a) through (f) were taken at different times from an experiment in which a sheep cardiac Purkinje fiber was exposed to strophanthidin (10 μM). The times at which the records were taken are indicated in Fig. 6. In each panel, records have been superimposed and show a 2-sec depolarizing pulse that was applied sequentially from the holding potential (-63 mV) to -53, -43, -33, and -23 mV. The twitch is off scale in several of the records. In each of the tension records shown, the larger the depolarizing pulse, the greater the tonic tension. Note also that after larger depolarizing pulses, there are larger aftercontractions. [Taken from Eisner *et al.* (1983e). Used with the permission of the *Journal of Physiology*.]

metabolism (Chapman and Tunstall, 1981). The Na–Ca exchange mechanism has been shown to be voltage dependent in a variety of tissues (see Eisner and Lederer, 1985, for review); however, to analyze our data in terms of this mechanism requires several assumptions: (1) There is a unique relationship between calcium and tension. (2) The Na–Ca exchange mechanism alone determines the level of intracellular calcium. (3) The Na–Ca exchange mechanism is at equilibrium at any test potential. However, as we will describe in greater detail later, it is unlikely that assumptions (1) and (2) are correct. Furthermore, assumption (3) is improbable because there are known leak conductances for calcium. For the Na–Ca exchanger to balance these leaks (a condition required by assumption (2)), it must extrude calcium from the cell and therefore cannot be at equilibrium. Thus while the Na–Ca exchange mechanism may explain the presence of voltage-dependent tonic tension, the slope of the relationship between log(tonic tension) and log(a_{Na}^i) is not interpretable in terms of the stoichiometry of the Na–Ca exchange (for more complete discussion, see Eisner *et al.*, 1983b; Eisner and Lederer, 1985). Supporting this point, Eisner *et al.* (1983b) showed that, in addition to the Na–Ca exchanger, other mechanisms can, in principle, adequately explain the voltage dependence and a_{Na}^i dependence of tonic tension. Nevertheless, because steady-state sources (other than the Na–Ca exchange mechanism) of activator calcium that depend on a_{Na}^i and membrane potential

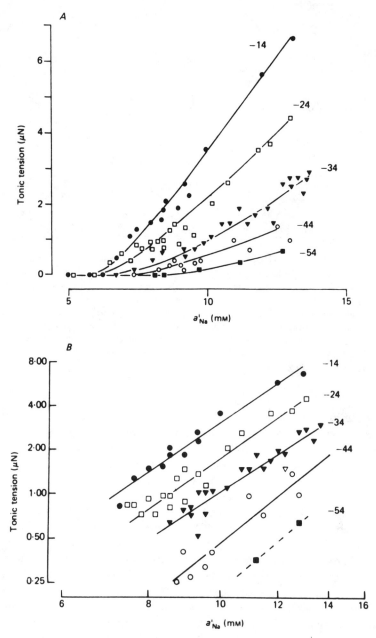

Fig. 8. The dependence of tonic tension on intracellular sodium activity (a^i_{Na}). Panel (A) shows data taken from an experiment that was different, but comparable, to that shown in Fig. 7. Tonic tension is plotted as a function of a^i_{Na} and indicates that there is marked nonlinearity of the relationship over the range of a^i_{Na} investigated (5–13 mM). Panel (B) shows that when the logarithm of tonic tension is plotted against the logarithm of a^i_{Na}, the data can be well fitted by a straight line over much of the range. Because the smaller values of tension are associated with greater fractional errors of measurement, they have not been plotted. [Taken from Eisner *et al.* (1983e). Used with the permission of the *Journal of Physiology*.]

remain poorly defined, a voltage-dependent Na–Ca exchange mechanism is the most plausible mechanism for producing the tonic tension that we have observed.

D. Sodium and Voltage Dependence of Twitch Tension

The effect of membrane potential and increasing a_{Na}^i on twitch tension can be seen in Figs. 1, 3, and 4. The fact that twitch tension is steeply dependent on both a_{Na}^i and membrane potential can be seen more clearly in Fig. 5. The similarity of the dependence of twitch tension on a_{Na}^i and voltage to that described earlier for tonic tension is made even more apparent by the inset in Fig. 5. Over the limited range of a_{Na}^i examined, we find that the relationship between $\log(a_{Na}^i)$ and log(twitch tension) is linear — as was shown for tonic tension; therefore, we can use the above empirical relationship (with different constants) also to describe the relationship between twitch tension and a_{Na}^i. It is notable, however, that the power function relationship between twitch tension and a_{Na}^i holds over a more limited range than that for tonic tension. This observation alone suggests that the processes responsible for determining twitch tension may be more complex than those for tonic tension.

A phasic rise in intracellular calcium initiates the twitch, and there are two possible sources for this calcium in cardiac muscle. Depolarization causes calcium release from the sarcoplasmic reticulum and an increased calcium influx from outside the cell; the level of tension development reflects modulation of both processes. We can explain a part of the a_{Na}^i dependence of twitch tension by assuming that a_{Na}^i will determine both the level of calcium loading of the sarcoplasmic reticulum immediately before the twitch (and therefore also the amount of calcium released) and calcium influx during the twitch. As described for tonic tension, the most plausible mechanism for linking a_{Na}^i to mean intracellular calcium is the Na–Ca exchanger. With this link between a_{Na}^i and calcium in mind, one might expect both twitch and tonic tension to display a similar dependence on a_{Na}^i. However, when one considers that the twitch reflects a transient increase in intracellular calcium, it is surprising that twitch tension and tonic tension should depend similarly on a_{Na}^i. This is because processes that determine tension production are likely to be further from equilibrium during the twitch than during tonic tension. Nevertheless, in order to describe how a nonmonotonic relationship between a_{Na}^i and twitch tension might come about, we must consider some additional factors that will affect tension production.

E. Influence of Intracellular pH on Twitch and Tonic Tension

The relationship between tension and a_{Na}^i described above is, in fact, the product of the relationship between a_{Na}^i and intracellular calcium and the rela-

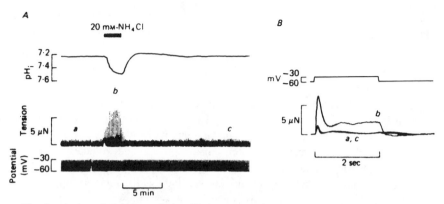

Fig. 9. Action of rapid intracellular pH change on twitch and tonic tension. (A) At the time indicated by the bar, 20 mM NH_4Cl was added to the modified Tyrode solution. In this experiment, the Tyrode solution contained 4 mM KCl and 10 mM Tris–HCl (as the extracellular pH buffer). Panel (A) shows the time course of the action of NH_4Cl on pH_i and tension. With the alkalinization of the intracellular compartment, there is an increase in tension. On removal of the NH_4Cl, there is a rapid acidification of the intracellular compartment such that pH_i is even less than in the control period. This "rebound" acidification of the intracellular compartment is associated with a reduction of twitch tension to a level below that of control. In the steady state, however, when pH_i has returned to control level, so have both twitch and tonic tension. The tension trace has been filtered (high-pass). (B) Specimen records (unfiltered) have been superimposed to facilitate comparison. [From Eisner *et al.* (1982b). Used with the permission of the *Journal of Physiology*.]

tionship between intracellular calcium and tension. One factor that is known to affect the relationship between intracellular calcium and tension is the intracellular pH (pH_i) (Fabiato and Fabiato, 1978; Allen and Orchard, 1983).

Figure 9 shows that a sudden change in intracellular pH (pH_i) can affect both twitch and tonic tension markedly. In the experiment shown, intracellular alkalinization is brought about by the application of extracellular NH_4Cl (20 mM). The uncharged NH_3 (in equilibrium with NH_4^+) crosses the cell membrane rapidly and, on entering the cell, acts as a H^+ sink leading to the rapid alkalinization of the cell. There is a dramatic and very large increase in both twitch and tonic tension produced by the alkalinization. On removal of the extracellular (NH_4Cl, there is a slight rebound intracellular acidification, and there is a reduction of tension. The rebound is due to the lipid-soluble NH_3 diffusing across the cell membrane leaving a proton behind. The increase in tension with increased intracellular alkalinization is expected on the basis of published data on the effect of pH on the pCa_i–tension relationship (Fabiato and Fabiato, 1978).

The observation that pH_i can affect tension production is relevant to the relationship between a_{Na}^i and tension, because interventions that produce an elevation in intracellular calcium also produce an intracellular acidification (Deitmer and Ellis, 1980; Vaughan-Jones *et al.*, 1983; Cannell *et al.*, 1984). While the mechanism of this effect is still unclear, it could come about by calcium

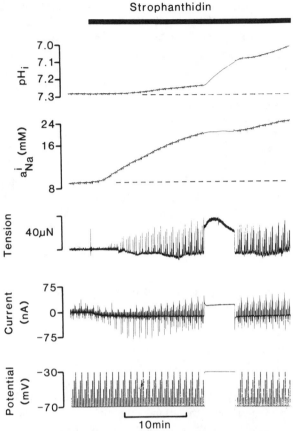

Fig. 10. Effect of depolarization on intracellular pH, intracellular sodium activity (a^i_{Na}), and tension. During the period indicated by the bar, strophanthidin (20 μM) was added to the superfusion solution. This blockade of the Na pump is associated with a large and rapid rise in a^i_{Na} and a slower and less dramatic acidification. From a holding potential of -70 mV, 5-sec depolarizing pulses were applied every 15 sec to -60, -50, -40, and -30 mV. Accompanying the increase in intracellular sodium are the gradual elevations of both twitch tension and tonic tension. A prolonged depolarization to -30 mV is accompanied also by a contracture. This contracture, lasting for the period of the depolarization, shows a significant relaxation that is accompanied not by a reduction of intracellular sodium, but by significant intracellular acidification. [Taken from Cannell *et al.* (1984). Used with the permission of the *Journal of Physiology.*]

either displacing protons from common buffers or accelerating metabolism, leading to an increase in the rate of proton production.

From the previous discussion, it would appear that changes in Ca$_i$ not only will affect tension directly but also will have an indirect effect on tension that is mediated by a change in pH$_i$. An example of this is shown in Fig. 10. This figure shows that during the rise in a^i_{Na}, the cell starts to acidify (as discussed above).

Of particular relevance to the question of the relationship between tension and a^i_{Na} is the relaxation of tonic tension during the long depolarizing pulse, *without any change in a^i_{Na} or membrane potential*. Concomitant with this relaxation there is a marked intracellular acidification. Thus, while the depolarization causes an increase in tension, mediated via an increase in Ca_i, this increase in Ca_i also produces an effect on pH_i that tends to reduce the tension developed. Analysis of this type of experiment shows that the a^i_{Na} dependence of tonic tension (on a logarithmic plot as shown in Fig. 8B) is shifted to the right (it takes a greater a^i_{Na} to produce a unit of tension) at more acidic pH_i, but there is no change in slope (Cannell, *et al.*, 1986).

Although pH_i can modify the relationship between a^i_{Na} and tension by affecting the relationship between calcium and tension (see discussion by Wier and Hess, 1984), an additional factor that must be considered is that at high levels of a^i_{Na}, oscillations of intracellular calcium can develop (Allen *et al.*, 1984). These oscillations may be responsible for the differences in response of twitch and tonic tension to increasing a^i_{Na} at high levels of a^i_{Na} (Cannell *et al.*, 1985).

F. Can Spatial Asynchrony of Calcium Release Explain a Reduction in Twitch Tension at High a^i_{Na}?

As a^i_{Na} becomes elevated, there is an initial steep rise of twitch tension (see Fig. 5). With higher a^i_{Na}, however, further increases of a^i_{Na} lead to either no increase of twitch tension or a decline (see Figs. 3, 5, and 8, this chapter, and Fig. 3 in Eisner and Lederer, 1979a). Although, in general, as a^i_{Na} rises, so does intracellular calcium activity (Sheu and Fozzard, 1982; Bers and Ellis, 1982), this increase in calcium activity does not necessarily lead to an increase in twitch tension. An explanation for this phenomenon is that at high levels of intracellular calcium, a calcium overload takes place (cf. Kass *et al.*, 1978; Vassalle and Lin, 1979; Vassalle, Chapter 9). In a calcium-overloaded state, the sarcoplasmic reticulum function seems to change, so that instead of releasing calcium only in response to depolarization, calcium release takes place spontaneously (Kass *et al.*, 1978; Lakatta and Lappé, 1981; Kass and Tsien, 1982; Allen *et al.*, 1984). This spontaneous release gives rise to spontaneous fluctuations of intracellular calcium (Orchard *et al.*, 1983; Wier *et al.*, 1983; Allen *et al.*, 1984), of calcium-dependent membrane current (Kass and Tsien, 1982; Matsuda *et al.*, 1982), and of tension (Lakatta and Lappé, 1981; Kass and Tsien, 1982). If the sarcoplasmic reticulum spontaneously releases calcium between beats, then the mean amount of calcium that can be released by depolarization will be reduced. This can be demonstrated by a simple model that shows that when asynchronous release of calcium develops (at a given level of mean intracellular calcium), there is a decline in twitch tension (Cannell *et al.*, 1985).

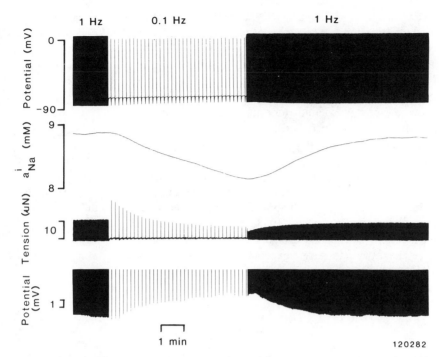

Fig. 11. Rate-dependent changes in tension are mediated in part by rate-dependent changes in intracellular sodium. In a Purkinje fiber bathed in Tris–HCl-buffered (10 mM), modified Tyrode solution containing 4 mM KCl and 2 mM CaCl$_2$, changing the action potential stimulation rate from 1 to 0.1 Hz and back to 1 Hz leads to reproducible changes in twitch tension. On slowing the rate of stimulation, there is a nearly immediate increase in twitch tension at unchanged a^i_{Na}. There is, however, a gradual reduction of twitch tension with the maintained lower rate, and this secondary reduction in tension is accompanied by a decrease in intracellular sodium. On reestablishing the original rate of 1.0 Hz, there is an immediate reduction in twitch tension. With the maintained higher rate, however, there is a gradual increase in twitch tension back to the control level as a^i_{Na} returns to its original value. [Taken from Lederer and Sheu (1983). Used with the permission of the *Journal of Physiology*.]

G. Rate-Dependent Changes of Tension: A Role for a^i_{Na}

For a^i_{Na} to be considered as a regulator of tension, it must be shown to play a role during physiological interventions. Figure 11 shows that changes in rate alter a^i_{Na} (see also Cohen *et al.*, 1982) thereby affecting tension (see also Koch-Weser and Blinks, 1965; Allen *et al.*, 1976). The immediate effect of reducing the stimulation rate from 1.0 to 0.1 Hz is to produce an increase in twitch tension. This initial action occurs without any change in a^i_{Na} and is probably due, at least in part, to the increased time available for the sarcoplasmic reticulum to take up calcium (Allen et al., 1976; Lederer and Sheu, 1983). More importantly, as a^i_{Na} falls, there is a reduction of twitch tension, but the rate of stimulation is constant. Furthermore, as a^i_{Na} rises when the rate of 1.0 Hz is resumed, there is an increase in twitch tension even though the rate of stimulation is constant. Presumably, more sodium enters at higher stimulation rates because the sodium current (I_{Na}) is activated more frequently. Note, however, that there is a trade-off between increased sodium entry due to the greater number of stimulated action potentials and the decreased mean electrochemical potential that occurs at a higher rate (see Eisner et al., 1981b, 1983b; Lederer and Sheu, 1983; January and Fozzard, 1984). In Fig. 11, at higher rates of stimulation, there is a net increase in sodium influx. As a^i_{Na} rises, the steady-state sodium efflux rises also, because the Na pump is activated by increasing a^i_{Na}, until Na efflux equals Na influx (see Eisner et al., 1983c). From experiments similar to those shown in Fig. 11 (Lederer and Sheu, 1983, 1986), it is clear that during physiological interventions, tension is extremely sensitive to changes in a^i_{Na}, just as it appears to be under the more severe experimental conditions illustrated in Fig. 1 through 10.

IV. CONCLUSIONS

Increasing a^i_{Na} in heart muscle increases twitch and tonic tension. These changes may result from the administration of a therapeutic agent (e.g., a cardiotonic steroid) or the imposition of a physiological maneuver (e.g., changing heart rate). Changes in a^i_{Na} appear to be effective in modifying tension because of the existence of a Na–Ca exchange mechanism that translates any change in a^i_{Na} into a change in a^i_{Ca}. The very steep dependence of tension on a^i_{Na} indicates how important this process must be in mediating therapeutic and physiological changes in tension. To complete our understanding of the relationship between a^i_{Na} and tension, however, we must have additional information on both intracellular pH and the presence or absence of nonuniformities in the spatial distribution of intracellular calcium. Finally, quantitative kinetic descriptions of the interdependence of a^i_{Na}, a^i_{Ca}, sarcolemmal Ca conductances, Na–Ca exchange, and the dynamic calcium buffers (e.g., the sarcoplasmic reticulum) would enable us to appreciate more fully the dependence of tension on a^i_{Na}.

ACKNOWLEDGMENTS

We thank the following for grant support: British Heart Foundation and the M.R.C. (D.A.E.); the M.R.C. and The Wellcome Trust (R.D.V-J.); the Maryland Heart Association (M.B.C.); the American Heart Association (S-S.S.); and the NIH (HL25675), the American Heart Association, and the

Maryland Heart Association (W.J.L.). This work was carried out during an Established Investigatorship supported by the American and the Maryland Heart Associations W.J.L.). We would like to acknowledge the excellent assistance of Mr. David Darragh, who has provided technical support while many of the experiments were carried out and has aided us in the preparation of the figures. We would like to acknowledge, also, Professor W. Simon (Swiss Federal Institute of Technology, Zurich, Switzerland) for his kind gifts of liquid ion-exchanger cocktails.

REFERENCES

Allen, D. G., and Orchard, C. H. (1983). The effects of changes of pH on intracellular calcium transients in mammalian cardiac muscle. *J. Physiol.* **335**, 555–567.

Allen, D. G., Jewell, B. R., and Wood, E. H. (1976). Studies on the contractility of mammalian myocardium at low rates of stimulation. *J. Physiol.* **254**, 1–17.

Allen, D. G., Eisner, D. A., and Orchard, D. H. (1984). Characterization of oscillation of intracellular calcium concentration in ferret ventricular muscle. *J. Physiol.* **352**, 113–128.

Ammann, D., Lanter, F., Steiner, R., Schulthess, P., Shijo, Y., and Simon, W. (1981). Neutral carrier based hydrogen ion selective microelectrode for intra- and extracellular studies. *Anal. Chem.* **53**, 2267–2269.

Baker, P. F., Blaustein, M. P., Hodgkin, A. L., and Steinhardt, R. A. (1969). The influence of calcium on sodium efflux in squid axons. *J. Physiol.* **200**, 431–458.

Bers, D. N., and Ellis, D. (1982). Intracellular calcium and sodium activity in sheep heart Purkinje fibres. Effects of changes of external sodium and intracellular pH. *Pflügers Arch.* **393**, 171–178.

Cannell, M. B., Lederer, W. J., and Vaughan-Jones, R. D. (1984). The effect of membrane potential on intracellular pH in sheep cardiac Purkinje fibres. *J. Physiol.* **349**, 45P.

Cannell, M. B., Vaughan-Jones, R. D., and Lederer, W. J. (1985). Ryanodine block of calcium oscillations in heart muscle affects the sodium–tension relationship. *Fed. Proc.* **44**, 2964–2969.

Cannell, M. B., Lederer, W. J., and Vaughan-Jones, R. D. (1986). In preparation.

Chapman, R. A., and Tunstall, J. (1980). The interaction of sodium and calcium ions at the cell membrane and the control of contractile strength in frog atrial muscle. *J. Physiol.* **305**, 109–123.

Chapman, R. A., and Tunstall, J. (1981). The tension–depolarization relationship of frog atrial trabeculae as determined by potassium contractures. *J. Physiol.* **310**, 97–115.

Cohen, C. J., Fozzard, H. A., and Sheu, S-S. (1982). Increase in intracellular sodium ion acitivty during stimulation in mammalian cardiac muscle. *Circ. Res.* **50**, 651–662.

Deitmer, J. W., and Ellis, D. (1978a). Changes in the intracellular sodium activity of sheep heart Purkinje fibres produced by calcium and other divalent cations. *J. Physiol.* **277**, 437–453.

Deitmer, J. W., and Ellis, D. (1978b). The intracellular sodium activity of cardiac Purkinje fibres during inhibition and re-activation of the Na/K pump. *J. Physiol.* **284**, 241–259.

Deitmer, J. W., and Ellis, D. (1980). Interactions between the regulation of the intracellular pH and sodium activity of sheep cardiac Purkinje fibres. *J. Physiol.* **304**, 471–488.

Eisner, D. A., and Lederer, W. J. (1979a). Inotropic and arrhythmogenic effects of potassium depleted solutions on mammalian cardiac muscle. *J. Physiol.* **294**, 255–277.

Eisner, D. A., and Lederer, W. J. (1979b). The role of the sodium pump in the effects of potassium depleted solutions on mammalian cardiac muscle. *J. Physiol.* **294**, 475–494.

Eisner, D. A., and Lederer, W. J. (1980). Characterization of the electrogenic sodium pump in cardiac Purkinje fibres. *J. Physiol.* **303**, 441–474.

Eisner, D. A., and Lederer, W. J. (1985). Na–Ca exchange: Stoichiometry and electrogenicity. *Am. J. Physiol.* **248**, C189–C202.

Eisner, D. A., Lederer, W. J., and Vaughan-Jones, R. D. (1981a). The dependence of sodium pumping and tension on intracellular sodium activity in voltage-clamped sheep Purkinje fibres. *J. Physiol.* **317**, 163–187.

Eisner, D. A., Lederer, W. J., and Vaughan-Jones, R. D. (1981b). The effects of rubidium ions and membrane potential on the intracellular sodium activity of voltage-clamped sheep cardiac Purkinje fibres. *J. Physiol.* **317**, 189–205.

Eisner, D. A., Lederer, W. J., and Vaughan-Jones, R. D. (1982a). The relationship between intracellular Na activity and tonic tension in sheep cardiac Purkinje fibres. *J. Physiol.* **326**, 67–68P.

Eisner, D. A., Lederer, W. J., and Giles, W. (1982b). Pacemaker activity in cardiac Purkinje fibers. *In* "Cellular Pacemakers" Vol. 1 (D. Carpenter, ed.), pp. 67–89. John Wiley and Sons, Inc., New York.

Eisner, D. A., Lederer, W. J., and Vaughan-Jones, R. D. (1983a). The control of tonic tension by membrane potential and intracellular sodium activity in the sheep cardiac Purkinje fibre. *J. Physiol.* **335**, 723–743.

Eisner, D. A., Lederer, W. J., and Vaughan-Jones, R. D. (1983b). Effects of sodium pump inhibition on contraction in sheep cardiac Purkinje fibers. *Curr. Top. Membr. Transp.* **19**, 885–890.

Eisner, D. A., Vaughan-Jones, R. D., and Lederer, W. J. (1983c). Comments on "Active transport and inotropic state in guinea pig left atrium." *Circ. Res.* **63**, 834–835.

Eisner, D. A., Lederer, W. J., and Sheu, S-S. (1983d). The role of intracellular sodium activity in the antiarrhythmic action of local anesthetics in sheep cardiac Purkinje fibres. *J. Physiol.* **340**, 239–257.

Eisner, D. A., Lederer, W. J., and Vaughan-Jones, R. D. (1983e). The relationship between twitch tension and intracellular Na activity in sheep cardiac Purkinje fibres. *J. Physiol.* **341**, 28–29P.

Eisner, D. A. Lederer, W. J., and Vaughan-Jones, R. D. (1984). The quantitative relationship between twitch tension and intracellular Na activity in sheep cardiac Purkinje fibres. *J. Physiol.* **355**, 251–266.

Ellis, D. (1977). The effects of external cations and ouabain on the intracellular sodium activity of sheep heart Purkinje fibres. *J. Physiol.* **273**, 211–240.

Fabiato, A., and Fabiato, F. (1978). Effects of pH on the myofilaments and the sarcoplasmic reticulum of skinned cells from cardiac and skeletal muscles. *J. Physiol.* **276**, 233–255.

Glitsch, H. G., Reuter, H., and Scholz, H. (1970). The effect of the internal sodium concentration on calcium fluxes in isolated guinea-pig auricles. *J. Physiol.* **204**, 25–43.

Glitsch, H. G., Kampmann, W., and Pusch, H. (1981). Activation of active Na transport in sheep Purkinje fibres by external K or Rb ions. *Pflügers Arch.* **391**, 28–34.

January, C. T., and Fozzard, H. A. (1984). The effects of membrane potential, extracellular potassium, and tetrodotoxin on the intracellular sodium ion activity of sheep cardiac muscle. *Circ. Res.* **54**, 652–665.

Kass, R. S., and Tsien, R. W. (1982). Fluctuations in membrane current driven by intracellular calcium in cardiac Purkinje fibers. *Biophys. J.* **38**, 259–269.

Kass, R. S., Lederer, W. J., Tsien, R. W., and Weingart, R. (1978). Role of calcium ions in transient inward currents and aftercontractions induced by strophanthidin in cardiac Purkinje fibres. *J. Physiol.* **281**, 187–208.

Koch-Weser, J., and Blinks, J. R. (1965). The influence of the interval between beats on myocardial contractility. *Pharm. Rev.* **15**, 601–652.

Lado, M. G., Sheu, S-S., and Fozzard, H. A. (1982). Changes in intracellular Ca^{2+} activity with stimulation in sheep cardiac Purkinje strands. *Am. J. Physiol.* **243**, H133–H137.

Lakatta, E. G., and Lappé, E. M. (1981). Diastolic scattered light fluctuation, resting force and twitch force in mammalian cardiac muscle. *J. Physiol.* **315**, 369–394.

Lederer, W. J. (1976). "Ionic basis of arrhythmogenic effects of cardiotonic steroids in cardiac Purkinje fibers." Ph.D. Dissertation, Yale University. University Microfilms No. 76-13681, Ann Arbor, Michigan.

Lederer, W. J., and Sheu, S-S. (1983). Heart rate-dependent changes in intracellular sodium activity and twitch tension in sheep cardiac Purkinje fibres. *J. Physiol.* **345**, 44P.

Lederer, W. J., and Sheu, S-S. (1986). In preparation.

Lederer, W. J., and Tsien, R. W. (1976). Transient inward current underlying arrhythmogenic effects of cardiotonic steroids in Purkinje fibres. *J. Physiol.* **253**, 73–100.

Lederer, W. J., Sheu, S-S., Vaughan-Jones, R. D., and Eisner, D. A. (1984). The effects of Na–Ca exchange on membrane current in sheep cardiac Purkinje fibers. *In* "Electrogenic Transport: Fundamental Principles and Physiological Implications" (M. P. Blaustein and M. Lieberman, eds.), pp. 373–380. Raven Press, New York.

Lee, C. O., and Dagostino, M. (1982). Effect of strophanthidin on intracellular Na ion activity and twitch tension of constantly driven canine cardiac Purkinje fibers. *Biophys. J.* **40**, 185–198.

Lee, C. O., Kang, D. H., Sokol, J. H., and Lee, K. S. (1980). Relation between intracellular Na ion activity and tension of sheep cardiac Purkinje fibers exposed to dihydro-ouabain. *Biophys. J.* **29**, 315–330.

Matsuda, H., Noma, A., Kurachi, Y., and Irisawa, H. (1982). Transient depolarization and spontaneous fluctuations in isolated single cells from guinea pig ventricles: Calcium-mediated membrane potential fluctuations. *Circ. Res.* **51**, 142–151.

Orchard, C. H., Eisner, D. A., and Allen, D. G. (1983). Oscillations of intracellular Ca^{2+} in mammalian cardiac muscle. *Nature* **304**, 735–738.

Reuter, H., and Seitz, N. (1968). The dependence of calcium efflux from cardiac muscle on temperature and external ion composition. *J. Physiol.* **195**, 451–470.

Sheu, S-S., and Fozzard, H. A. (1982). Transmembrane Na^{2+} and Ca^{2+} electrochemical gradients in cardiac muscle and their relationship to force development. *J. Gen. Physiol.* **80**, 325–351.

Sheu, S-S., Hamlyn, J. M., and Lederer, W. J. (1983). Low-dose cardiotonic steroids, intracellular sodium and tension in heart. *Circulation* **68**, Suppl. III, 250a.

Steiner, R. A., Oehme, M., Ammann, D., and Simon, W. (1979). Neutral carrier sodium ion-selective microelectrode for intracellular studies. *Anal. Chem.* **51**, 351–353.

Thomas, R. D. (1978). "Ion-Sensitive Intracellular Microelectrodes". Academic Press, New York and London.

Vassalle, M., and Lin, C. I. (1979). Effect of calcium on strophanthidin-induced electrical and mechanical toxicity in cardiac Purkinje fibers. *Am. J. Physiol.* **236**, H689–H697.

Vaughan-Jones, R. D., Lederer, W. J., and Eisner, D. A. (1983). Ca^{2+} ions can affect intracellular pH in mammalian cardiac muscle. *Nature* **301**, 522–524.

Vaughan-Jones, R. D., Eisner, D. A., and Lederer, W. J. (1984). The effect of intracellular Na on contraction and intracellular pH in mammalian cardiac muscle. *Adv. Myocard.* **5**, 313–330.

Wasserstrom, J. A., Schwartz, D. J., and Fozzard, H. A. (1983). Relation between intracellular sodium and twitch tension in sheep cardiac Purkinje strands exposed to cardiac glycosides. *Circ. Res.* **52**, 697–705.

Wier, W. G., and Hess, P. (1984). Excitation–contraction coupling in cardiac Purkinje fibers: Effects of cardiotonic steroids on the intracellular $[Ca^{2+}]$ transient, membrane potential and contraction. *J. Gen. Physiol.* **83**, 395–415.

Wier, W. G., Kort, A. A., Stern, M. D., Lakatta, E. G., and Marban, E. (1983). Cellular calcium fluctuations in mammalian heart: Direct evidence from noise analysis of aequorin signals in Purkinje fibers. *Proc. Natl. Acad. Sci. U.S.A.* **80**, 7361–7371.

9

Cardiac Glycosides: Regulation of Force and Rhythm

Mario Vassalle

I. INTRODUCTION

The usefulness of cardiac glycosides in clinical practice is probably matched by our degree of uncertainty about the mechanism of their therapeutic actions. This does not mean that the effects of cardiac glycosides have not been studied sufficiently. On the contrary, the literature is as extensive as the interpretation of some of the results is varied. Cardiac glycosides sustain our interest not only because of their widespread clinical use but also because they provide a tool to study various aspects of cellular functions such as the development of contractile force or arrhythmias. In this chapter, I consider first the effects of cardiac glycosides on contractile force and then the effects on rhythm. I use the term cardiac glycosides (or digitalis) even though some of the agents studied are aglicones. A partial justification for this simplification is that the active part of cardiac glycosides resides in the aglicone, even if the sugar moiety modifies their action in several respects.

II. CARDIAC GLYCOSIDES AND THE REGULATION OF CONTRACTILE FORCE

Cardiac glycosides are used clinically to increase myocardial contractile force in cardiac failure. The positive inotropic effect of cardiac glycosides is not limited, however, to the correction of the mechanical deficit associated with

237

cardiac failure: cardiac glycosides increase force in the nonfailing heart, too (Smith and Braunwald, 1980). Still, the inotropic action in normal and failing tissues does not need to be identical, at least quantitatively. The inotropic effect is relatively larger when contractile force is depressed before administration of digitalis (Cattell and Gold, 1938). This may be of some relevance in comparing concentrations of cardiac glycosides used clinically and those used in isolated tissues, because in cardiac failure, a small concentration of digitalis could induce a larger percentage increase in force than in a nondepressed tissue.

A. The Changes in Force Caused by Cardiac Glycosides

An analysis of cardiac glycoside actions is complicated because the actions themselves are complex. Different cardiac glycosides act differently in the various cardiac tissues and by modifying one function may affect other functions. The same tissue can react differently depending on several variables, including, for example, age and sex (Surawicz and Mortelmans, 1969). Moreover, cardiac glycosides act not only on cardiac fibers but also on cardiac nerves, on the arterial and venous circulations, and on autonomic reflex activity (Hoffman and Bigger, 1980; Smith and Braunwald, 1980). Thus, *in vivo,* the direct positive inotropic effects are modified by indirect effects such as changes in rate, fiber length, autonomic reflexes, etc.

The study of tissues perfused *in vitro* has established beyond doubt that cardiac glycosides increase contractile force through a direct effect (Cattell and Gold, 1938); however, experiments *in vitro* show also that depending on the tissue, ionic composition of perfusing solution, duration of exposure, and cardiac glycoside and its concentration, the effects on force are not limited to the development of positive inotropy.

Low concentrations (10^{-9} to 10^{-8} M) of cardiac glycosides have been reported to have a slight positive, a slight negative, or no inotropic effect (Noble, 1980; Grupp *et al.,* 1982). If there is a decrease in force, it may be persistent or replaced eventually by an increase in force (Hart *et al.,* 1983).

Only rarely do high concentrations ($\geq 10^{-7}$ M) cause an initial, negative inotropic effect (Lee and Dagostino, 1982). Usually, the force increases monotonically to a steady state (e.g., see Lin and Vassalle, 1978, 1983b; Lee *et al.,* 1980); however, during exposure to high concentrations, the contractile force eventually decreases, whereas the resting force can increase (e.g., see Lin and Vassalle, 1983b). Although the positive inotropy is the therapeutic effect, the other force changes need to be accounted for, also because their mechanisms may be either similar or dissimilar (qualitatively or quantitatively) to the therapeutic one.

1. Mechanism of the Increase in Force at High Concentrations

The positive inotropic effect of cardiac glycosides is likely to involve an increase in calcium released on excitation. How this might be accomplished at different concentrations is disputed (Lee and Klaus, 1971; Langer, 1977; Akera and Brody, 1977; Schwartz *et al.*, 1975; Okita, 1977; Noble, 1980). I consider the effects of high concentrations ($\geq 10^{-7}$ M) first because, in this connection, several important findings concur. One undisputed action is that high concentrations ($\geq 10^{-7}$ M) block active transport of Na^+ and K^+ across the cell membrane (Schatzmann, 1953) by inhibiting the Na^+, K^+-activated adenosine triphosphatase (Skou, 1957). Because cardiac glycosides impair transport of both Na^+ and K^+ (the sodium pump), $[Na^+]_i$ increases and $[K^+]_i$ decreases (Lee and Klaus, 1971; Schwartz *et al.*, 1975; Akera and Brody, 1977).

a. The Sodium Pump and Contractile Force. Digitalis-induced inhibition of the sodium pump raises the question of how altered pump function can modify contractile force.

In the absence of cardiac glycosides, activity of the sodium pump responds to changes in intracellular sodium concentration to maintain ionic homeostasis. Thus, such pump activity should moderate (rather than induce) changes in contractile force.

In the presence of high concentrations of cardiac glycosides, inhibition of the sodium pump is the primary event that results in an increased intracellular sodium activity (a_{Na}^i). Cardiac glycosides at concentrations of 10^{-7} M or higher have been reported to increase a_{Na}^i consistently (Ellis, 1977; Deitmer and Ellis, 1978b; Lee *et al.*, 1980; Lee and Dagostino, 1982; Sheu and Fozzard, 1982; Wasserstrom *et al.*, 1983; Vassalle and Lee, 1984). Such an increase begins at a threshold concentration of 10^{-7} M for dihydroouabain (Lee *et al.*, 1980) and at 5 $\times$ 10^{-8} M for strophanthidin (Lee and Dagostino, 1982).

The increase in a_{Na}^i alters the sodium gradient across the cell membrane and therefore Na–Ca exchange (Mullins, 1979; Chapman, 1983): intracellular calcium activity (a_{Ca}^i) increases also (Lee and Dagostino, 1982). It is interesting that at 10^{-7} M (or less) strophanthidin, a_{Ca}^i does not increase but the force does. With high concentrations of cardiac glycosides (when the sodium pump is certainly inhibited), a_{Na}^i correlates generally with an increase in force (Fig. 1 and Lee *et al.*, 1980; Lee and Dagostino, 1982; Wasserstrom *et al.*, 1983). The increase in force is large (100–400%) and depends on the tissue as well as the concentration and duration of exposure to the cardiac glycoside (e.g., Wasserstrom *et al.*, 1983; Lin and Vassalle, 1983b).

b. Role of Internal Sodium in the Inotropy of High Concentrations. That an increase in a_{Na}^i augments contractile force is supported by the correlation be-

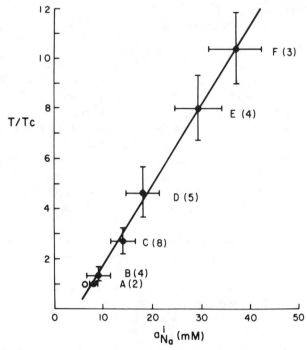

Fig. 1. Relation between tension and intracellular sodium activity at different dihydroouabain concentrations in sheep Purkinje fibers. The ordinate shows relative tension (ratio of tension during dihydroouabain exposure to control tension). The abscissa shows sodium activity (a_{Na}^i) in mM. The concentrations of dihydroouabain were: 5×10^{-8} M (A); 10^{-7} M (B); 5×10^{-7} M (C); 10^{-6} M (D); 5×10^{-6} M (E); and 10^{-5} M (F). The numbers in parentheses indicate the number of experiments. The open circle shows the mean control a_{Na}^i. [Reproduced from Lee *et al.* (1980) with permission.]

tween these two parameters (see above). Reciprocally, in Purkinje fibers, the administration of local anesthetics or tetrodotoxin (TTX) decreases markedly both contractile force (Vassalle and Bhattacharyya, 1980; Bhattacharyya and Vassalle, 1981b) and a_{Na}^i (Deitmer and Ellis, 1980; Vassalle and Lee, 1984). Strophanthidin has little effect on force when a_{Na}^i has been reduced by TTX (Vassalle and Lee, 1984).

One reason why the action of digitalis depends on a_{Na}^i may be its increased binding when intracellular sodium is higher (Temma and Akera, 1982). Thus, a fast rate of discharge and substances that increase sodium influx (monensin, grayanotoxin I, and batrachotoxin) enhance the binding of ouabain to sarcolemmal Na^+–K^+ ATPase, probably because the enhanced Na influx increases turnover of the sodium pump. In turn, this hastens the rate of development of the inotropic effect (Temma and Akera, 1982). It is of interest that guinea pig hearts exposed to ouabain in the absence of calcium can later develop a positive inotropic effect when Ca is restored, but this does not happen if both Na and Ca are absent from the perfusing fluid (Akera *et al.*, 1979). This suggests that sodium is required for the interaction of ouabain with its receptor. Still, the question remains whether the increase in force is related predominantly to increased binding or to the increased intracellular sodium (see below). In Purkinje fibers exposed to a sodium-free solution, the force does not increase and arrhythmias do not develop in the presence of strophanthidin, even though the fibers accelerate when reexposed to Tyrode solution without strophanthidin (Lin and Vassalle, 1979).

In support of a role for sodium in digitalis inotropy is the finding that strophanthidin produces a greater percentage increase in tension when added to a solution that is low in calcium or high in sodium instead of a standard Tyrode solution (Vassalle *et al.*, 1984). Low-calcium (Ellis, 1977; Deitmer and Ellis, 1978a; Lee and Vassalle, 1983) or high-sodium solutions (Abete *et al.*, 1985; Lee, *et al.*, 1985) increase a^i_{Na}. In Purkinje fibers, the force is increased also by lowering $[Na]_o$ in the absence of strophanthidin (Li and Vassalle, 1984) because a^i_{Na} decreases but less than does $[Na]_o$ (Abete *et al.*, 1985). In fact, the inotropic action is conditioned by the level of a^i_{Na} prior to strophanthidin administration (Abete and Vassalle, 1985b; Lee *et al.*, 1985).

These findings introduce the concept that the regulation of force is related not only to a^i_{Na} but also to the sodium gradient across the cell membrane. If the a^o_{Na} decreases *more* than a^i_{Na}, calcium will accumulate, and the force will increase. Instead, if a^i_{Na} decreases and the sodium gradient increases (e.g., by administration of TTX), the force decreases.

An analysis of experimental results obtained with different procedures (i.e., strophanthidin, TTX, different $[K]_o$) has led to a quantitative evaluation of the role of sodium in the development of tension. It has been concluded that the changes in force are usually proportional to a^i_{Na} raised approximately to the sixth power (Im and Lee, 1984); therefore, relatively little change in a^i_{Na} may be expected to modify the contractile force substantially.

While a direct relationship between a^i_{Na} and force is prerequisite for a role of the increased a^i_{Na} in digitalis inotropy, it should not be taken as an unequivocal proof of the exclusive role of a^i_{Na}. Thus, a higher $[Na]_o$ increases a^i_{Na} and force linearly. Adding tetrodotoxin decreases force more than a^i_{Na}: the relation remains linear but its slope changes. Thus there is a direct relation between a^i_{Na} and force both in the absence and presence of TTX, but the slope of the relation is conditioned by factors other than a^i_{Na} (Abete and Vassalle, 1985b). Similarly, digitalis could modify the slope of the relation by bringing into play factors other than the inhibition of the sodium pump.

c.   Role of Intracellular Calcium in the Inotropy of High Concentrations. The importance of calcium in digitalis inotropy is shown by the following experiments. In the presence of TTX, strophanthidin has little effect on force (as

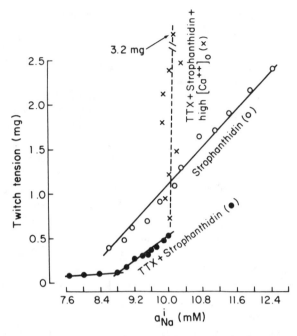

Fig. 2. Relationships between twitch tension and intracellular sodium activity (a^i_{Na}) in dog Purkinje fibers. The ordinate shows twitch tension in mg. The abscissa shows a^i_{Na} in mM. The open circles show the relationship obtained in the presence of strophanthidin (5×10^{-7} M) and in the absence of TTX. The first open circle shows control a^i_{Na} and tension. The solid circles show the relationship in the presence of strophanthidin of TTX. The X's show the relationship during exposure to high [ca]$_o$ in the presence of TTX and strophanthidin. All curves were obtained from the same fiber [Reproduced from Vassalle and Lee (1984) with permission.]

mentioned above) but increases a^i_{Na} gradually (Vassalle and Lee, 1984). In the presence of TTX, norepinephrine and high [Ca]$_o$ increase contractile force more than does strophanthidin (Bhattacharyya and Vassalle, 1981b) but *decrease* a^i_{Na} (Lee and Vassalle, 1983). In the presence of TTX and strophanthidin, the addition of Ca or norepinephrine increases force much more than in the absence of strophanthidin (Bhattacharyya and Vassalle, 1981b). Potentiation of the inotropic effect of strophanthidin by high [Ca]$_o$ (Fig. 2) or norepinephrine is not associated with an increase in a^i_{Na}; therefore, the increase in a^i_{Na} by strophanthidin must require sufficient stores of calcium for the development of positive inotropy. Also, the inotropic effect of strophanthidin is least in a low-Na–Ca solution (Vassalle *et al.*, 1984) because a^i_{Na} decreases to a low level, and strophanthidin increases it more slowly, as in the presence of TTX (Abete *et al.*, 1985).

2. The Changes in Force with Low Concentrations of Cardiac Glycosides

The therapeutic plasma concentrations of cardiac glycosides in patients are approximately 10^{-9} to 10^{-8} M, depending on the cardiac glycoside (Smith and Braunwald, 1980; Bernabei et al., 1980). Thus, it becomes important to establish whether these low concentrations act as the high concentrations do or in some different manner. This is where discrepancies begin. First, one difference between low and high concentrations is that low concentrations may stimulate the sodium pump, thereby decreasing intracellular sodium and increasing intracellular potassium concentrations (Lee and Klaus, 1971; Noble, 1980) as well as reducing a^i_{Na} (Deitmer and Ellis, 1978b). This would indicate still that Na^+-K^+ ATPase is the receptor for cardiac glycosides: the difference would be that low concentrations stimulate and high concentrations inhibit the sodium pump. The problem is that stimulation of the sodium pump and sodium depletion should lead to a *decrease* in force. If such a decline (see above) were the only effect of low concentrations of cardiac glycosides, the therapeutic action of these low doses in cardiac failure would be difficult to understand. In the heart *in situ*, low concentrations of digitalis augment contractile force (measured as dP/dt) by some 40% (Smith and Braunwald, 1980). This introduces the necessity of another mechanism (possibly an increase in exchangeable calcium) to increase force *in spite* of the decrease in a^i_{Na}. This additional mechanism may or may not be related to binding of cardiac glycosides to the Na^+-K^+ ATPase.

In an interesting approach, Godfraind et al. (1982) have studied the actions of ouabain on systolic tension and sodium pump activity in the absence and presence of dihydroouabain in an attempt to distinguish the increase in force caused by sodium-pump inhibition from that caused by the postulated additional mechanism. Dihydroouabain competes with ouabain for both high- and low-affinity binding sites (the latter being involved in sodium-pump inhibition). Ouabain had a similar effect on sodium-pump activity in the absence and presence of 10^{-7} M dihydroouabain, but at the smallest concentration, the inotropic effect produced by the mechanism unrelated to sodium-pump inhibition was abolished, presumably because of binding of dihydroouabain to the high-affinity sites (Fig. 3). Only at higher concentrations did ouabain overcome the dihydroouabain antagonism. What is less clear is (1) whether ouabain alone, at the lowest concentration, should have stimulated uptake of potassium, (2) why dihydroouabain does not stimulate the pump at low doses (Lee et al., 1980) even though it, too, binds to high-affinity sites, and (3) why the mechanism unrelated to sodium-pump inhibition should contribute more to the increase in force at higher concentrations (when pump inhibition is more marked and should therefore contribute more to the inotropic effect).

At higher concentrations, the mechanism that is unrelated to pump inhibition

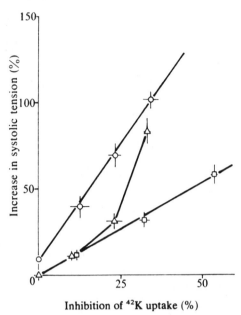

Inhibition of ^{42}K uptake (%)

Fig. 3. Relationship between the increase in tension in guinea pig atria and the inhibition of ^{42}K uptake. The ordinate is the percentage increase in systolic tension. The abscissa shows the percentage inhibition of ^{42}K uptake. The circles were obtained in the presence of 10^{-8}, 10^{-7}, 3×10^{-7}, and 6×10^{-7} M ouabain. The squares were obtained in the presence of 10^{-6}, 3×10^{-6}, and 10^{-5} M dihydroouabain. The triangles show the relation after a 30-min preincubation with 10^{-7} M di-hydroouabain and then exposure to the concentrations of ouabain indicated by the corresponding circles. Preincubation with dihydroouabain abolished the positive inotropic effect of the lowest concentration of ouabain but had a gradually smaller inhibitory effect as the concentration of ouabain was increased. [Reproduced from Godfraind *et al.* (1982) with permission.]

and that operates at lower concentrations should make little (if any) contribution to the total inotropic effect because the force correlates with a^i_{Na} (but see Abete and Vassalle, 1985b). Still, the mechanism related to sodium pump inhibition at high concentrations is not necessarily the most important mechanism for positive inotropy in patients. It would be significant only if the increase in force at low concentrations were caused exclusively by a milder inhibition of the sodium pump and a consequent increase (however small) of a^i_{Na}. Otherwise, the large increase in tension caused by a substantial inhibition of the sodium pump may not come into play unless electrical signs of digitalis toxicity develop. Even then, pump inhibition may involve predominantly the more sensitive Purkinje fibers (Polimeni and Vassalle, 1971).

It is assumed generally that the effectiveness of low concentrations of digitalis is similar *in vivo* and *in vitro*. Yet *in vivo* conditions differ in several respects from those *in vitro,* and these differences are likely to affect the action of digitalis. For example, digitalis may modify the release and reuptake of catecholamines and, therefore, reflex or direct sympathetic activity (Hoffman and Bigger, 1980; Smith and Braunwald, 1980). In addition inotropic and arrhythmogenic actions of digitalis may be modified by circulating catecholamines (Vassalle and Bhattacharyya, 1981). Different cardiac glycosides may act predominantly on sympathetic or vagal nerves (Cook *et al.*, 1982). Furthermore, results from different tissues are often quoted in support of one or the other conclusion, even though there are remarkable differences in sensitivity among different tissues (e.g., Purkinje fibers and ventricular muscle fibers, Vassalle *et al.*, 1962) and in like tissues from various organisms within one species. Finally, disease may alter sensitivity to digitalis. For example, smaller concentrations of cardiac glycosides may induce arrhythmias in infarcted hearts (Brennan and Bonn, 1980). These differences are emphasized because not only therapeutic (digoxin, 1-2 $\times$ 10^{-9} M) but also toxic (2-4 $\times$ 10^{-9} M) concentrations are lower *in vivo* (Table 16-7 in Smith and Braunwald, 1980; Bernabei *et al.*, 1980). The latter concentrations may not have even a therapeutic effect *in vitro* (let alone a toxic effect; Grupp *et al.*, 1982). Moreover, if comparisons of effective concentrations *in vitro* and *in vivo* are to be valid, the ratio between digitalis bound to the receptor and that in the extracellular fluid should be the same in both conditions.

The shift of both therapeutic and toxic concentrations to lower values *in vivo* seems to indicate that (for reasons that are unclear) the *in vivo* and *in vitro* relationships between concentration of cardiac glycoside and force differ. If so, then a direct comparison of effective concentrations in the two situations becomes uncertain. For example, the inotropic effect of low concentrations of strophanthidin *in vitro* is potentiated by low concentrations of norepinephrine (Vassalle *et al.*, 1984; Abete and Vassalle, 1985a): this catecholamine factor would be operating presumably *in vivo*.

Mechanism(s) Underlying the Therapeutic Effect of Low Concentrations. The definition of therapeutic effect is most clearly understood when the strengthening of contractile force leads to the restoration of a normal cardiac output and to the abolition of cardiac failure. If there is no failure, therapeutic effects can be approximated only by an increase in force that occurs in the absence of signs of toxicity; nevertheless, it is difficult to determine the minimum concentration that would have abolished cardiac failure.

Among the mechanisms that are possibly responsible for the positive inotropic effect of low concentrations of cardiac glycosides (when found) is inhibition of the sodium pump. In support of this, dihydroouabain ($\geq 10^{-7}$ M) increases force only when it increases a_{Na}^i (Lee *et al.*, 1980). It is true that dihydroouabain does not stimulate the sodium pump at low concentrations, but strophanthidin (which does) increases force only when it increases a_{Na}^i, also (Lee and Dagostino,

1982). Similar conclusions were reached by Wasserstrom et al. (1983). In the rat, 10^{-7} M ouabain, a concentration that is relatively low (for the rat), increases myocardial force and a^i_{Na} simultaneously, but does not inhibit the Na^+-K^+ ATPase. Nevertheless, the increase in a^i_{Na} was taken as evidence of inhibition of the sodium pump, even though the same concentration of ouabain did not inhibit the Na^+-K^+ ATPase *isolated* from that tissue (Grupp et al., 1985). These and other results (Schwartz et al., 1975; Akera and Brody, 1977) support the idea that low concentrations and high concentrations act similarly, the difference being merely quantitative.

Inhibition of the sodium pump by digitalis has been measured after the isolation of the Na^+-K^+ ATPase, and this procedure is open to several objections (Noble, 1980). For this reason, attempts have been made to study activity of the pump indirectly in intact tissues. In one approach, low concentrations of cardiac glycosides ($\leq 10^{-7}$ M) were found to have a positive inotropic effect when Na-pump activity was stimulated, as suggested by a negative shift of the reversal potential for the pacemaker current. In some fibers, stimulation of the pump resulted in a decreased contractile force (Hart et al., 1983).

In another approach (Bernabei and Vassalle, 1984), Purkinje fibers were exposed to zero $[K^+]_o$ to increase cellular Na^+. The return to normal potassium solution caused a hyperpolarization, apparently in response to electrogenic sodium extrusion, because the hyperpolarization was reduced by tetrodotoxin and by substituting lithium for sodium. In the presence of 5×10^{-8} M strophanthidin, the force increased by some 90%, but the hyperpolarization was affected only slightly. With increasing concentrations ($>10^{-7}$ M), tension increased up to 340%, and the hyperpolarization was abolished. Metabolic inhibitors decreased force and reduced the hyperpolarization. Strophanthidin (0.5-5×10^{-7} M) increased force even in the presence of metabolic inhibitors (see, also, Bhattacharyya and Vassalle, 1981a), although there was no hyperpolarization. The conclusion was that low concentrations of strophanthidin can increase force without an apparent inhibition of the sodium pump.

If pump activity is not suppressed (or is even stimulated) by low concentrations, then other possible mechanisms have to be considered. These mechanisms may involve a change in calcium movements across the sarcolemma, because cardiac glycosides have little effect on internal structures of the cell (Hoffman and Bigger, 1980; Smith and Braunwald, 1980). The major difference would be that at a low concentration of digitalis, calcium entering the fiber might somehow increase without accumulating, whereas at higher concentrations, calcium would accumulate intracellularly because of the increased sodium.

One obvious mechanism is an increase in the slow inward current. On this point, however, there is no agreement: some investigators did not find such an increase (McDonald et al., 1975; Greenspan and Morad, 1975) and others did (Weingart et al., 1978; Marban and Tsien, 1982). Such an increase may not be a direct effect of cardiac glycosides but could result from a rise in cellular calcium (Marban and Tsien, 1982). This hypothesis requires identification of the cause of the increased intracellular calcium.

Another mechanism has been proposed by Schwartz and collaborators (Gervais et al., 1977), who suggested that cardiac glycosides might bind to the $Na^+ - K^+$ ATPase and thereby modify its configuration. As a result, more Ca^{2+} could be mobilized from the sarcolemma, and this extra calcium would be available to increase force. As pointed out by Noble (1980), this mechanism would account for the simultaneous mobilization of calcium and the stimulation of Na^+-pump activity (actually a disinhibition caused by removal of calcium). Whether force would increase or decrease would depend on the net balance of these two factors.

By these mechanisms, the positive inotropy of low concentrations would be related to an increased availability of calcium independent of sodium-pump inhibition. The calcium released on excitation would increase because of the increased calcium influx. The calcium in the SR might increase in relation of the increased calcium influx, but there would be no progressive accumulation of calcium in the cell as in the toxic stage (see Lee and Klaus, 1971).

3. Calcium Overload and the Late Decline in Force

As mentioned above, cardiac glycosides increase and then decrease contractile force. The decline in force needs explanation also. The increase and decrease are related in that the higher the concentration of strophanthidin, the faster and greater (within limits) the positive inotropic effect and the sooner the onset of the decline in contractile force (Lin and Vassalle, 1983b). If the increase in contractile force is a therapeutic effect, the decline has to be a manifestation of toxicity. Accordingly, in cardiac muscle the resting force may also increase, and, in Purkinje fibers, oscillatory potentials (see below) appear when the contractile force begins to decline (Ishikawa and Vassalle, 1982).

The first question is whether the decline in contractile force represents an exaggeration of events that lead initially to the therapeutic effect or results from a different mechanism. Such a decline occurs with concentrations of strophanthidin (Lin and Vassalle, 1983b) that inhibit the sodium pump and increase a^i_{Na}, eventually to the point that intracellular calcium rises beyond an optimal level for maintained inotropy (calcium overload).

The reasons for proposing that the decline in contractile force results from calcium overload are several. First, decreasing $[Ca]_o$ decreases contractile force in the absence of strophanthidin, but increases contractile force during the declining phase of inotropy induced by strophanthidin (Fig. 4). Reciprocally, augmenting $[Ca]_o$ increases contractile force in the absence, but decreases it during administration, of strophanthidin (Vassalle and Lin, 1979). Also, strophanthidin does not increase (or even decreases) contractile force in the presence of caffeine

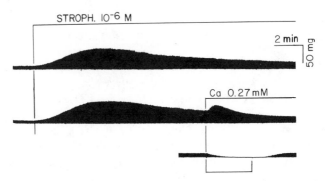

Fig. 4. Low [ca]$_o$ decreases force in Tyrode solution but transiently increases it during the declining phase of strophanthidin inotropy in dog Purkinje fibers. The top trace shows the increase and decrease in force by strophanthidin (10^{-6} M). The middle trace shows the transient increase in force when [Ca]$_o$ was lowered from 2.7 to 0.27 mM during declining phase of strophanthidin inotropy. The bottom trace shows decrease in force when [Ca]$_o$ was reduced in the absence of strophanthidin. In the upper two panels, strophanthidin superfusion was begun at the vertical line. [Reproduced from Vassalle and Lin (1979) with permission.]

(which also causes calcium overload, Paspa and Vassalle, 1984; Di Gennaro *et al.*, 1984), but the positive inotropic effect can be restored if either caffeine or [Ca]$_o$ is lowered (Lin and Vassalle, 1983a). In Purkinje fibers, a solution containing low Na and low Ca in a suitable proportion causes an initial transient increase in force followed by a return of force to a value similar to that present in Tyrode solution (Li and Vassalle, 1983). The initial increase results apparently from an increase in cellular calcium in response to the diminished Na gradient. In the presence of a low concentration of strophanthidin, a low-Na–Ca solution increases contractile force initially even more than does Tyrode solution; in the presence of a high concentration of strophanthidin, the low-Na–Ca solution decreases force. If only [Na]$_o$ is decreased, the force increases in Tyrode and low-strophanthidin solutions (Fig. 5A) and decreases in the presence of high strophanthidin (Fig. 5B). Opposite results are obtained with low [Ca]$_o$ alone (Figs. 5C and 5D). That these results are related to calcium overload is shown by the fact that low [Na]$_o$ increases contractile force in normal [Ca]$_o$ and decreases it in high (10.8 mM) [Ca]$_o$ (Li and Vassalle, 1984).

High [K]$_o$ decreases a^i_{Na} (Ellis, 1977), decreases force in Purkinje fibers, and apparently reduces cellular calcium because it causes relaxation of strophanthidin-induced contracture in ventricular muscle fibers (Lin and Vassalle, 1980). By reducing cellular calcium, high [K]$_o$ may abolish the fall in force (see Fig. 5B) induced by calcium overload. When high strophanthidin is given in the presence of high [K]$_o$, the force increases, but no calcium overload develops, as evidenced by the fact that decreasing [Na]$_o$ increases contractile force (in contrast to the finding illustrated in Fig. 5B), and a low-Na–Ca solution causes an initial increase in force (instead of a decrease as at normal [K]$_o$; Li and Vassalle,

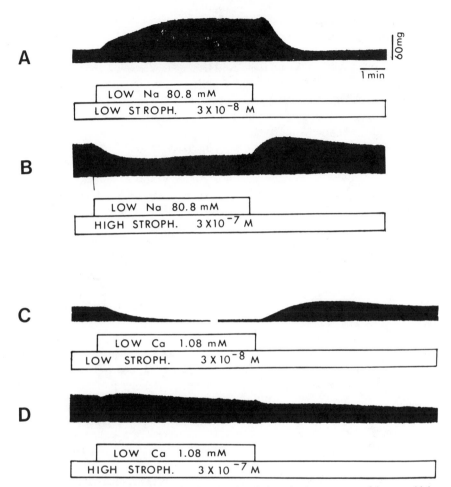

Fig. 5. Effects of low-sodium or low-calcium solutions in the presence of low- or high-strophanthidin concentrations. Traces (A) and (B) were recorded before, during, and after exposure of dog Purkinje fibers to a low-Na solution (80.8 m*M*) in the presence of 3×10^{-8} and $3 \times 10^{-7} M$ strophanthidin solutions, respectively. Traces (C) and (D) were recorded before, during, and after exposure to a low-Ca solution (1.08 m*M*) in the presence of low- and high-strophanthidin solutions, respectively. [Reproduced from Li and Vassalle (1984) with permission.]

1984). In Purkinje fibers (in the absence of strophanthidin), increasing $[Ca]_o$ to approximately 8 m*M* increases force, but at higher $[Ca]_o$, tension becomes less (Vassalle and Lin, 1979). The relationship between calcium and force is modified by low $[Na]_o$ (and more so by low $[Na]_o$ plus strophanthidin) in such a way that force becomes greater at low $[Ca]_o$ and lesser at higher $[Ca]_o$. The transient recovery of force in calcium-overloaded Purkinje fibers upon exposure to lower

$[Ca]_o$ (see Fig. 4) is exaggerated if $[Na]_o$ has been decreased, and even more so if strophanthidin has also been present (Li and Vassalle, 1984). In a low-Na solution, strophanthidin reduces force, but this effect is reversed by decreasing $[Ca]_o$ (Metha and Vassalle, 1981). High $[K]_o$ (Lin and Vassalle, 1980) and local anesthetics (Bhattacharyya and Vassalle, 1981c) decrease force in Tyrode solution, but increase it during the stage of declining strophanthidin inotropy. Thus, when force declines, it is clear that fibers exposed to high concentrations of strophanthidin are undergoing calcium overload. Such a decline is even greater when other conditions are also increasing the calcium load.

Because calcium overload may be brought about by several interventions, this factor could determine whether the same concentration of cardiac steroids is therapeutic or toxic, that is, whether the positive inotropic effect becomes a negative inotropic effect.

The Possible Cause of the Fall in Force during Calcium Overload. The mechanism by which calcium overload decreases contractile force is not clear, but accumulating evidence suggests that calcium overload can affect contractile force as well as other cell functions (Nayler and Grinwald, 1981; Dhalla *et al.*, 1982). One possible mechanism is a reduced availability of high-energy phosphates (Dhalla *et al.*, 1982) that could result from increased uptake of calcium by the mitochondria at the expense of ATP production (Lehninger, 1974). High-energy phosphates are reduced during the toxic stage of cardiac glycoside administration (Wollenberger, 1949, 1951; Furchgott and De Gubareff, 1958). Dinitrophenol also decreases force and high-energy phosphates in ventricular muscle: under these conditions, cardiac glycosides fail to increase force and decrease stores of high-energy phosphates further (Wollenberger and Karsh, 1952). Similarly, inhibitors of oxidative phosphorylation reduce the inotropic effect of strophanthidin and accelerate the onset of the decline in force (Lin and Vassalle, 1983b). That the decline in contractile force may involve a deficit in the production of high energy phosphates is supported by the fact that such a decline during the exposure to strophanthidin or high $[Ca]_o$ can be reversed by providing suitable substrates (Ishikawa and Vassalle, 1985). The fact that the force increases rapidly when $[K]_o$ is raised in the presence of calcium overload (Lin and Vassalle, 1983b) suggests that the excessive increase in calcium is related to an excessive increase in a^i_{Na}. In fact, it has been shown (Abete and Vassalle, 1985c) that $10^{-6}\,M$ strophanthidin increases both a^i_{Na} and force, but when a^i_{Na} increases to about 11 mM, contractile force begins to decrease (whereas a^i_{Na} continues to increase). In higher $[K]_o$, strophanthidin increases a^i_{Na} less and the force does not show a late decline. However, the late decline is present even in high $[K]_o$, if a^i_{Na} is increased prior to strophanthidin administration by increasing $[Na]_o$ (Abete and Vassalle, 1985c). Under such circumstances, the late decline in force would result from an exaggeration of the effects of inhibition of the sodium pump.

III. CARDIAC GLYCOSIDES AND THE REGULATION OF RHYTHM

A major indication for administering cardiac glycosides is the reduction of ventricular rate in the presence of atrial flutter or fibrillation. This action may occur indirectly, however, through a change in the function of parasympathetic and sympathetic nerves (Hoffman and Bigger, 1980; Smith and Braunwald, 1980). Moreover, if cardiac function improves because of the removal of failure, some irregularities in rhythm might be eliminated. On the other hand, toxic concentrations of cardiac glycosides are known to cause a variety of cardiac arrhythmias. This analysis of changes in rhythm is confined primarily to those occurring in ventricular Purkinje fibers, as this is the tissue in which the most recent advances in the understanding of digitalis toxicity have been made.

The fact that digitalis modifies cardiac rhythm in both the therapeutic and toxic stages elicits the question of whether these changes are caused by different mechanisms.

A. Site of Origin of Ventricular Extrasystoles and Influence of Rate

In 1958, Dudel and Trautwein showed that cardiac glycosides increase the rate of discharge of Purkinje fibers. In a comparative study (Vassalle *et al.*, 1962), Purkinje and ventricular muscle fibers from the same animals were superfused simultaneously with equal concentrations of ouabain. Purkinje fibers showed shortening of the action potential, a decrease in the amplitude and rate of rise of the upstroke, and a progressive increase in the slope of diastolic depolarization, whereas fibers from ventricular muscle showed comparatively normal action potentials. Some Purkinje fibers became quiescent and inexcitable, but in the majority, the enhanced diastolic depolarization resulted in multiple extrasystoles and then a rapid spontaneous rhythm. The ventricular muscle fibers depolarized much more slowly until they became inexcitable, but no diastolic depolarization was ever observed. Moreover, inexcitability occurred sooner if the muscle fibers were driven (rather than left quiescent) or were driven at a faster rate. Thus, Purkinje fibers were shown to be more sensitive to ouabain than ventricular muscle fibers, and only in the former were spontaneous rhythms brought about by a steepened diastolic depolarization. And the onset of toxicity was shown to be related to the driving rate.

1. The Relationship between Rate and Arrhythmias

The relationship between rate and arrhythmias was studied also *in vivo* (Vassalle *et al.*, 1963). During the infusion of ouabain, the sinus rhythm slowed, as expected. During successive vagal stimulations, ventricular standstill become shorter and the rate of the escape idioventricular rhythm became faster. At a later stage, a fast idioventricular rhythm occurred immediately after the beginning of vagal stimulation and eventually became intermingled with the sinus rhythm in the absence of vagal stimulation. In many experiments, a progressive slowing preceded acceleration of the idioventricular rhythm, and occasionally there was no escape during one minute of vagal stimulation. Another type of arrhythmia was the appearance of extrasystoles that showed a constant or variable coupling with the sinus beats. The extrasystoles disappeared when the sinus node was suppressed by vagal stimulation, but, interestingly, upon graded vagal stimulation that slowed the sinus node, the extrasystoles became trigemini (instead of bigemini), and the coupling interval became prolonged. Further slowing of the sinus rate by graded vagal stimulation led to disappearance of the extrasystoles. When the rate was increased by driving the heart, the number of extrasystoles increased. Also, the sinus rate increased spontaneously after vagal stimulation (postvagal tachycardia, Vassalle, 1978), and, in the presence of ouabain, this acceleration induced extrasystoles (which were abolished if vagal stimulation was applied once more). The extrasystoles could sometimes sustain themselves, in which case they could not be suppressed by vagal stimulation; however, if vagal stimulation suppressed the initiating sinus beat, no runs of extrasystoles appeared.

The initial slowing of the idioventricular rhythm was attributed tentatively to an initial stimulation of active transport by ouabain, although other possibilities could not be excluded. The acceleration of the ventribular rhythm was attributed to an enhanced diastolic depolarization. Vassalle *et al.* (1963) concluded that the mechanism of the extrasystoles was "still a matter of speculation and an adequate explanation cannot be formulated on the basis of available evidence." In retrospect, these extrasystoles showed the characteristics of rhythms induced by oscillatory potentials (see below).

To study the response of idioventricular pacemakers to cardiac glycosides in the absence of sinus node influences, ouabain was administered in animals with complete AV block (Greenspan *et al.,* 1962). The idioventricular rate decreased initially, but was followed by the relatively rapid onset of a fast rhythm (see Fig. 8-8 in Vassalle and Musso, 1976b). Thus, the sinus node influence is not essential for either the slowing or acceleration of the idioventricular rhythm.

2. Mechanism of Ventricular Asystole and Its Modification by Cardiac Glycosides

Initially, the slowing of the idioventricular rhythm might appear to be a therapeutic effect similar to slowing of the sinus node rate, but on occasion, ventricular standstill persisted through the 60 sec of vagal stimulation. Thus, the action could hardly be considered therapeutic. In addition, it occurred after prolonged treatment with ouabain, which had induced ventricular tachycardia in other animals. Even in the same animal, the prolonged ventricular standstill could be followed by tachyarrhythmias during postvagal tachycardia. These findings suggest that digitalis may either increase or suppress automatic discharge. We shall see that the suppression may result from a slow repolarization during diastole.

The more common finding in the presence of digitalis is a progressive shortening of ventricular standstill. This requires a brief consideration of the mechanism of ventricular arrest upon vagal stimulation in the absence of ouabain (Vassalle, 1970, 1977, 1982). The intrinsic rate of ventricular Purkinje fibers (30–40 beats/min) is slower than that of the sinus node (70–80 beats/min). Because the sinus node discharges Purkinje fibers at its own rate, the Purkinje fibers are overdriven, that is, driven at a rate faster than their own intrinsic rate. This overdrive leads to a suppression of spontaneous activity (overdrive suppression), which becomes apparent when the sinus node activity is interrupted abruptly by vagal stimulation. When Purkinje fibers are driven at a rate faster than their own, intracellular sodium is increased and sodium-pump activity is stimulated. If the extrusion of sodium is electrogenic, the outward current thus created maintains diastolic depolarization negative to the threshold potential. During standstill, the decreased influx and increased efflux of sodium leads to a decrease in intracellular sodium and a decline in the activity of the sodium pump and the outward current associated with it. As a result, diastolic depolarization attains threshold, and activity is resumed. Changes in the distribution of other ions occur with overdrive (Vassalle, 1977, 1982), but if electrogenic sodium extrusion is the major mechanism, concentrations of digitalis that inhibit the sodium pump should decrease and eventually abolish overdrive suppression. The progressive shortening of ventricular standstill by cardiac glycosides can be explained by this mechanism because strophanthidin abolishes overdrive hyperpolarization (Carpentier and Vassalle, 1971) as do metabolic inhibitors (dinitrophenol, Vassalle, 1970; 2-deoxy-D-glucose, Carpentier and Vassalle, 1971; antimycin and iodoacetic acid, Bhattacharyya and Vassalle, 1980).

B. Cardiac Glycosides and Diastolic Depolarization in Purkinje Fibers

The onset of repetitive extrasystoles with a faster rate of firing (Vassalle *et al.*, 1963) indicates that cardiac glycosides must cause other changes in addition to those that shorten ventricular arrest. This is likely because overdrive in the presence of cardiac glycosides accelerates (rather than suppresses) idioventricular rhythm (Wittenberg *et al.*, 1970, 1972). The same rate-dependent phenomena are likely to account for the observation that in dogs recovering from acetyl-strophanthidin-induced tachycardia, a single premature beat induced ventricular extrasystoles. When the repetitive responses disappeared, an increase of the atrial pacing rate made the extrasystoles reappear (Hagemeijer and Lown, 1970). Thus, the repetitive ventricular responses are facilitated by shorter cycle lengths.

The relation between fast rates and arrhythmias could be related presumably to enhanced binding of cardiac glycosides (Temma and Akera, 1982). Although this factor should play a role in digitalis toxicity of fibers driven at different rates, it is less likely to play a major role in the changes that occur within a few beats or even a single extrasystole. Instead, it appears that digitalis, by increasing cellular calcium, makes the fibers respond to a rate increase by steepening diastolic depolarization.

In the toxic stage, digitalis inhibits the sodium pump and increases a_{Na}^i and a_{Ca}^i (Lee et al., 1980; Lee and Dagostino, 1982). If the rate of discharge increases in the absence of digitalis, a_{Na}^i (Cohen et al., 1982) and a_{Ca}^i (Lado et al., 1982) increase also; therefore, in the presence of digitalis, these changes should be greater. Such ionic changes are likely to be more pronounced in Purkinje fibers because active transport is more severely depressed by digitalis in this tissue than in ventricular muscle fibers (Polimeni and Vassalle, 1971): this is likely to contribute to the higher sensitivity of Purkinje fibers. Because of their inhibition of the sodium pump, cardiac glycosides abolish the outward current generated by electrogenic sodium extrusion (Gadsby and Cranefield, 1979) and enhance simultaneously the ionic changes associated with overdrive. In fact, in the absence of strophanthidin overdrive causes an increase in a_{Na}^i and cessation of overdrive is associated with a temporary undershoot of a_{Na}^i. In the presence of strophanthidin (10^{-7} M), a_{Na}^i increases more during overdrive and remains higher than control after overdrive (Abete and Vassalle, 1986).

In this context, we must now focus on the increase in cellular calcium and its effect on diastolic depolarization. High $[Ca]_o$ increases the slope of diastolic depolarization, and, after a fast drive, the enhanced diastolic depolarization attains a larger peak and then decays again (Temte and Davis, 1967). Although not recognized as such, the peaking and decaying of diastolic depolarization was caused by an oscillatory potential superimposed on diastolic depolarization. In 1973, several papers described the oscillatory potential and its behavior in the presence of cardiac glycosides: Davis (1973) showed that in Purkinje fibers exposed to ouabain, the slope of diastolic depolarization increased when the driving rate was increased. Moreover, a fast drive could be followed by spontaneous beats, especially if a premature beat was introduced at the end of the drive. Ferrier et al. (1973) reported that the steepening of diastolic depolarization was caused by superimposed oscillatory potentials. These oscillatory potentials are rate dependent in that the amplitude of the oscillatory potential increases and its cycle length decreases (within limits) when the preceding drive is faster. If the preparation is quiescent, upon initiation of the drive, the oscillatory potentials increase in magnitude with each successive action potential. They can also attain threshold and cause repetitive activity. It was stressed by Ferrier *et al.* (1973) that the oscillatory potentials are different from the normal process of diastolic depolarization and that diastolic depolarization would be depressed by digitalis. The induction of oscillatory potentials by cardiac glycosides was reported also by Rosen *et al.* (1973) and by Hogan *et al.* (1973). Their results showed that although cardiac glycosides reduced the influence of overdrive suppression, they led to the development of a depolarizing event (the oscillatory potential) that steepened diastolic depolarization and could cause repetitive activity.

1. Ionic Events Underlying the Oscillatory Potential

The oscillatory potentials are increased by high $[Ca]_o$ and are decreased by low $[Ca]_o$, manganese, and verapamil (Ferrier and Moe, 1973). These findings point clearly to a role of calcium in the induction of the oscillatory potentials. At first, it was believed that the current responsible for the oscillatory potential was carried by calcium (Ferrier and Moe, 1973; Lederer and Tsien, 1976), but it soon became apparent that the oscillatory potential disappears when $[Na]_o$ is reduced (Lin and Vassalle, 1976, 1978). Because low $[Na]_o$ increases calcium overload, the finding indicated that Na^+ was the charge carrier. Voltage-clamp experiments (Kass *et al.*, 1978a,b) showed that the oscillatory current induced by cardiac steroids was dependent on an increase of $[Ca]_i$ (calcium overload) and was carried mostly (but not exclusively) by sodium ions (Kass *et al.*, 1978b). On repolarization, an oscillatory release of calcium from the sarcoplasmic reticulum would increase a nonspecific membrane conductance and thus allow the flow of an inward current with a reversal potential of approximately -5 mV. The oscillatory current was shown to be different from the slow inward current and to be increased by conditions that increase cellular calcium and decreased by those that decrease $[Ca]_i$. The oscillatory current was superimposed on an unaltered pacemaker current (Lederer and Tsien, 1976) and was not affected by tetrodotoxin (Kass *et al.*, 1978b).

A similar current occurs in the absence of $[K]_o$, a condition that also leads to inhibition of the sodium pump (Eisner and Lederer, 1979a,b). In addition, the oscillatory current is often superimposed on a tail of inward current (the creep current) that may also be present during the administration of cardiac glycosides (Eisner and Lederer, 1979b). The oscillatory current can be found also in fibers superfused with Tyrode solution in the *absence* of pump inhibition (Vassalle and Mugelli, 1981; Lipsius and Gibbons, 1982). To appear, this oscillatory current requires a prior depolarization to approximately -20 mV or more positive values for a duration of approximately 1 sec or more, and then repolarization to -40 mV or more negative values. It becomes smaller at more negative potentials and

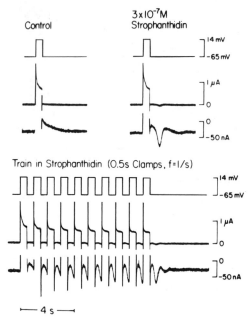

Fig. 6. Effect of a train of voltage clamps on the rate of development of oscillatory current in the presence of strophanthidin in sheep Purkinje fibers. The traces were recorded in the absence (control) and presence ($3 \times 10^{-7} M$) of strophanthidin. In the control (upper left traces), a 0.5-sec step to $+14$ mV was applied from a holding potential of -65 mV. The traces show the voltage (top), current (middle), and current at higher gain (bottom). The same clamp pulse applied in the presence of strophanthidin was followed by a large oscillatory current. When a train of 10 clamps was applied (botton part of the figure), the oscillatory current developed at a faster rate after each successive pulse and peaked sooner after the last. [Reproduced from Vassalle and Mugelli (1981) with permission.]

can be shown to be separable from all other known currents. The oscillatory current is exaggerated by conditions that increase calcium load of the cell such as high $[Ca]_o$, low $[K]_o$, repetitive activity, norepinephrine, and strophanthidin (Vassalle and Mugelli, 1981). Its enhancement with repetitive activity (Fig. 6) provides the basis for the growth of the oscillatory potential (Ferrier *et al.*, 1973) with successive action potentials.

2. Events Responsible for the Oscillatory Current

The event that triggers release of calcium from the sarcoplasmic reticulum is not clear. It has been demonstrated that the oscillatory current can be triggered not only after a depolarizing voltage clamp but also during a depolarizing test pulse applied after a conditioning one (Lin *et al.*, 1983). The two preconditions for induction of oscillatory current upon depolarization are that the sheep Purkinje fiber be loaded with calcium and that the depolarizing pulse induce a calcium influx to trigger release of calcium from the sarcoplasmic reticulum. If the oscillatory current is activated and a depolarizing clamp applied at its peak, the current disappears but does not reverse direction at less negative potentials. Furthermore, measurements of membrane resistance during the oscillatory current show that the membrane resistance does not decrease (instead it increases). On the basis of these findings, it has been proposed that the oscillatory current results from an electrogenic sodium–calcium exchange (Lin *et al.*, 1983, 1986; see also Noble, Chapter 6).

When no reversal potential was found in other tissues, investigators proposed that the oscillatory current was caused by an electrogenic sodium–calcium exchange (Karagueuzian and Katzung, 1982; Clusin *et al.*, 1983; Brown *et al.*, 1984; Arlock and Katzung, 1985; Henning and Meinertz, 1985). The hypothesis that Na–Ca exchange is the mechanism for the oscillatory current is supported by the fact that adriamycin, an inhibitor of Na–Ca exchange in canine sarcolemmal vesicles (Caroni *et al.*, 1981), reduces the oscillatory potentials induced by ouabain in canine Purkinje fibers (Binah *et al.*, 1983).

The Role of Sarcoplasmic Reticulum. The sarcoplasmic reticulum is a likely site for the cyclic release of calcium because the oscillatory current is often associated with an aftercontraction (Kass *et al.*, 1978a,b). Supporting this concept is the finding that caffeine abolishes the oscillatory current in fibers exposed to zero $[K]_o$ (Eisner and Lederer, 1982) as well as in fibers superfused with Tyrode solution (Vassalle and Di Gennaro, 1983). Caffeine abolishes the oscillatory current and at the same time enhances or induces a tail of inward current that becomes more evident under conditions of calcium overload (high $[Ca]_o$, strophanthidin, low $[Na]_o$) (Vassalle and Di Gennaro, 1984). The tail current shares many of the characteristics of the oscillatory current (i.e., follows a depolarizing clamp, can be triggered twice on repolarization, becomes greater the larger or longer the preceding depolarizing clamp, etc.). The major difference is that caffeine abolishes one current (the oscillatory current) but increases the other (the tail of inward current). The reason for this is unclear, but it may be related to the fact that when uptake of calcium into the SR is impaired, electrogenic extrusion of calcium through the sarcolemma has to increase.

If the oscillatory potential is responsible for digitalis arrhythmias, caffeine should abolish them. In fact, caffeine (10 m*M*) not only abolishes ventricular tachyarrhythmias in the isolated guinea pig heart but also induces contracture (Di Gennaro *et al.*, 1983). In Purkinje fibers superfused *in vitro*, caffeine is quick to abolish oscillatory potentials resulting from calcium overload and causes slowing of repolarization (the tail). The latter effect may lead to repetitive activity at a depolarized level followed by quiescence (Di Gennaro and Vassalle, 1985). Oscillatory potentials induced in guinea pig ventricular muscle by digitalis are also abolished by caffeine (Matsuda et al., 1982; Di Gennaro et al., 1984).

3. The Initiation of Spontaneous Activity in Quiescent Fibers

Because the oscillatory potential follows the action potential, it cannot be responsible for the induction of spontaneous activity by strophanthidin in Purkinje fibers rendered quiescent by a 5.4 mM K solution (Vassalle and Musso, 1976a). The initiation of activity is brought about by a gradual decrease in resting potential that begins to oscillate in the threshold region and initiates the first action potential. It is significant that the action potential is not followed by an oscillatory potential. The gradual decline in resting potential could be related to inhibition of electrogenic extrusion of sodium. Alternatively, it could be caused by a decrease in membrane conductance (Kassebaum, 1963). In fibers that are active spontaneously or driven at a very slow rate, strophanthidin increases the slope of diastolic depolarization and the rate of discharge without the appearance of an oscillatory potential. On the other hand, it is clear that the oscillatory potential is present at faster driving rates (Vassalle and Musso, 1976a).

In a different approach (Ishikawa and Vassalle, 1982), Purkinje fibers were driven in the absence or presence of strophanthidin, and the drive was interrupted periodically (the pause), a procedure reminiscent of the periodical suppression of sinus node drive *in vivo*. In the presence of strophanthidin and during the successive pauses, the slope of the diastolic depolarization increased, and the fibers began their spontaneous discharging sooner and at faster rate. This occurred while the force was increasing toward its maximum value. When the force reached its peak or had started to decline, there appeared oscillatory potentials that could attain threshold and initiate a fast discharge. These results suggest that during vagal stimulation *in vivo*, digitalis shortens ventricular standstill and accelerates idioventricular rhythms by increasing the rate of diastolic depolarization; it causes fast rhythms by the development of oscillatory potentials. These two phenomena occur at different stages of digitalis action. That the early steepening of diastolic depolarization is not caused by a shallow and prolonged oscillatory potential is shown by the use of cesium. Cesium abolishes diastolic depolarization (Ishikawa and Vassalle, 1982) but not the oscillatory current (Mugelli, 1982) and prevents the early acceleration of activity but not the development of oscillatory potentials. In the presence of cesium, the oscillatory potential may be followed by a repolarization during the pause (instead of a depolarization). This repolarization is likely to be caused by the decay of the inward tail current. In the absence of cesium, the effects of decay of the inward tail current may be masked by decay of the pacemaker current (Ishikawa and Vassalle, 1982). These experiments may explain the apparent paradox that cardiac glycosides depress the pacemaker potential (Ferrier et al., 1973). In actuality, the pacemaker current is not affected by strophanthidin (Lederer and Tsien, 1976).

C. The Elimination of Cardiac Glycoside Arrhythmias

Because the oscillatory potentials can initiate fast rhythms, an appropriate treatment of digitalis-induced tachyarrhythmias (in addition to discontinuing digitalis or removing it from its binding sites by means of specific antibodies; see Smith and Braunwald, 1980) would be the administration of slow channel blockers that reduce calcium overload by decreasing influx of calcium. Although these drugs do indeed reduce the oscillatory potentials (Ferrier and Moe, 1973), several drugs with different mechanisms of action have been reported to eliminate both the oscillatory potentials and aftercontractions. Thus, quinidine (McCall, 1976), procainamide, and lignocain (McCall, 1978) have been shown to reduce passive sodium influx in cultured heart cells. Quinidine, procainamide, lidocaine, and diphenylhydantoin abolished the aftercontraction and oscillatory potential in cultured cardiac cells (Goshima, 1976, 1977), as diphenylhydantoin and quinidine reduced ouabain-induced oscillatory potentials in Purkinje fibers (Rosen et al., 1976). That the effects noted are not exclusively related to a reduction of sodium influx has been shown in cultured heart cells (Goshima and Wakabayashi, 1983). Quinidine and procainamide prevented the onset of arrhythmias and reduced not only the increase in ^{24}Na content but also the rate of ^{45}Ca uptake in both beating and quiescent cells. The increased rate of Ca uptake is related at least in part to the increased Na content. Interestingly, but not unexpectedly, ouabain inhibited ^{24}Na release, but neither quinidine nor procainamide affected release of sodium, Na–Ca exchange, or the $Na^+–K^+$ ATPase in either the absence or presence of ouabain (Goshima and Wakabayashi, 1983).

Thus, drugs that diminish sodium influx are also effective against digitalis arrhythmias because they decrease the intracellular sodium concentration, the very factor that initiates the calcium overload. Tetrodotoxin was the first agent demonstrated to reduce or abolish the oscillatory potential (Vassalle, 1975; Vassalle and Scida, 1979). Local anesthetics have also been shown to diminish calcium overload and the oscillatory potential in Purkinje fibers (Bhattacharyya and Vassalle, 1981c). An increased potassium concentration is also very effective in abolishing digitalis arrhythmias. High $[K]_o$ acts in several ways: it increases potassium conductance and reduces digitalis binding (see Lin and Vasalle, 1980), but its most important effect is to decrease the oscillatory potential (Lin and Vassalle, 1980), probably by diminishing intracellular sodium (as a result of stimulating the Na pump; see Ellis, 1977) and therefore calcium through Na–Ca exchange.

IV. CONCLUSIONS

The mechanism of action of cardiac glycosides remains of undiminished interest, as it bears on some basic processes that regulate cardiac contraction and arrhythmogenesis. A few facts seem to be generally established: that the inhibition of the sodium pump occurs at higher concentrations, that such inhibition leads to accumulation of intracellular sodium, and that this, in turn, increases cellular calcium. That inhibition of the sodium pump leads to an increase in force is unquestionable, as can be demonstrated easily by manipulating a^i_{Na} by various means. Such inhibition may be responsible for the largest increase in force, as the correlation between a^i_{Na} and contractile force at high glycoside concentrations would suggest. This in itself may not mean too much, because in patients given concentrations in the therapeutic range, an increase in contractile force of only 40% may be sufficient to relieve cardiac failure. But it is in these lower ranges of concentrations that disagreement on mechanisms is most significant because, *in vitro*, low concentrations have a small positive, a small negative, or no inotropic effect at all. In addition, these low concentrations may increase slightly, decrease slightly, or not change a^i_{Na}. Clearly, there are two major possibilities: that even at low concentrations the sodium pump is inhibited (although relatively little) or that another action (perhaps even related to the binding of digitalis to the $Na^+–K^+$ ATPase) involves primarily greater release of calcium upon excitation. Such enhanced release would increase contractile force, sometimes in spite of greater Na-pump activity. Evaluation of this problem is difficult because both therapeutic and toxic concentrations are smaller *in vivo* than *in vitro*, making uncertain the extrapolation of *in vitro* results to *in vivo* studies. Another difficulty is that the same concentration of digitalis may have a different action (and even act through a different mechanism) depending on variables such as cardiac glycoside used, rate of discharge, $[K]_o$, tissue studied, presence of catecholamines, calcium load, presence of disease, etc. On the one hand, these factors complicate analysis of the effects of small concentrations; on the other, they favor the chance of disparate results. Such discrepancies preclude resolution of the issue at present—firm conclusions can be drawn only when additional evidence accounts satisfactorily for the differing results.

As for the toxic actions of cardiac glycosides, an excessive amount of digitalis leads to calcium overload through inhibition of the sodium pump and because of rising intracellular sodium, reduction of calcium efflux through Na–Ca exchange. In turn, this brings about a decline in contractile force and changes in the process of impulse formation. It is then that mechanical and electrical toxicity share a common mechanism in the increased cellular calcium.

ACKNOWLEDGMENTS

Original work in this chapter was supported by grants from the NIH Heart, Lung, and Blood Institute and the New York Heart Association.

REFERENCES

Abete, P., and Vassalle, M. (1985a). The role of intracellular sodium activity in the inotropy potentiation among high $[Ca]_o$, norepinephrine and strophanthidin. *Arch. Internat. Pharmacodyn.* **278,** 87–96.

Abete, P., and Vassalle, M. (1985b). A role of calcium in strophanthidin inotropy. *Physiologist* **28,** 364.

Abete, P., and Vassalle, M. (1985c). Intracellular sodium activity and strophanthidin inotropy under conditions that vary cellular sodium. *Circulation* **72,** 379.

Abete, P., and Vassalle, M. (1986) Strophanthidin inotropy, overdrive and intracellular sodium activity. *Proc. XXX. Intern. Congr. Physiol. Sci.* (In press.)

Abete, P., Lee, C. O., Pecker, M., Sonn, J. K., and Vassalle, M. (1985). Strophanthidin inotropy: Role of intracellular Na ion activity and Na–Ca exchange. *Fed. Proc.* **44,** 1579.

Akera, T., and Brody, T. M. (1977). The role of Na^+-K^+ ATPase in the inotropic action of digitalis. *Pharmacol. Rev.* **29,** 187–220.

Akera, T., Hirai, M., and Oka, T. (1979). Sodium ions and development of the inotropic action of ouabain in guinea pig heart. *European J. Pharmacol.* **60,** 189–198.

Arlock, P., and Katzung, B. G. (1985). Effects of sodium substitutes on transient inward current and tension in guinea-pig and ferret papillary muscle. *J. Physiol. (London)* **360,** 105–120.

Bernabei, R., and Vassalle, M. (1984). The inotropic effects of strophanthidin in Purkinje fibers and the sodium pump. *Circulation* **69,** 618–631.

Bernabei, R., Perna, G. P., Carosella, L., Di Nardo, P., Cocchi, A., Weisz, A. M., and Carbonin, P. U. (1980). Digoxin serum concentration measurement in patients with suspected digitalis-induced arrhythmias. *J. Cardiovas. Pharmacol.* **2,** 319–329.

Bhattacharyya, M., and Vassalle, M. (1980). Metabolism dependence of overdrive induced hyperpolarization. *Arch. Internat. Pharmacodyn. Therap.* **246,** 28–37.

Bhattacharyya, M. L., and Vassalle, M. (1981a). The effect of metabolic inhibitors on strophanthidin induced arrhythmias and contracture in cardiac Purkinje fibers. *J. Pharmacol. Exp. Ther.* **219,** 75–84.

Bhattacharyya, M. L., and Vassalle, M. (1981b). Role of calcium and sodium in strophanthidin inotropy in cardiac Purkinje fibers. *Am. J. Physiol.* **240,** H561–H570.

Bhattacharyya, M. L., and Vassalle, M. (1981c). The effect of local anaesthetics on strophanthidin toxicity in canine cardiac Purkinje fibers. *J. Physiol. (London)* **312,** 125–142.

Binah, O., Cohen, I. S., and Rosen, M. (1983). The effects of adriamycin on normal and oubain-toxic canine Purkinje and ventricular muscle fibers. *Circ. Res.* **53,** 655–662.

Brennan, J. F., and Bonn, J. R. (1980). Effects of oubain on the electrophysiological properties of subendocardial Purkinje fibers surviving in regions of acute myocardial infarction. *Am. Heart J.* **100**, 201–212.

Brown, H. F., Kimura, J., Noble, D., Noble, S. J., and Taupignon, A. (1984). The slow inward current, I_{si}, in the rabbit sino-atrial node investigated by voltage-clamp and computer simulation. *Proc. R. Soc. B.* **222**, 305–328.

Caroni, P., Villani, F., and Carafoli, E. (1981). The cardiotoxic antibiotic doxorubicin inhibits the Na^+/Ca^{2+} exchange of dog heart sarcolemmal vesicles. *FEBS Lett.* **30**, 184–186.

Carpentier, R., and Vassalle, M. (1971). Enhancement and inhibition of a frequency-activated electrogenic sodium-pump in cardiac Purkinje fibers. *In* "Research in Physiology, a Liber Memorialis in Honor of Prof. C. McC. Brooks" (F. F. Kao, K. Koizumi, and M. Vassalle, eds.), pp. 81–96. A. Gaggi Publisher, Bologna.

Cattell, M., and Gold, H. (1938). The influence of digitalis glycosides on the force of contraction of mammalian cardiac muscle. *J. Pharmacol. Exp. Therap.* **62**, 116–125.

Chapman, R. A. (1983). Control of cardiac contractility at the cellular level. *Am. J. Physiol.* **245**, H535–H552.

Clusin, W. T., Fischmeister, R., and DeHaan, R. (1983). Caffeine-induced current in embryonic heart cells: Time course and voltage dependence. *Am. J. Physiol.* **245**, H523–H532.

Cohen, C. J., Fozzard, H. A., and Sheu, S-S. (1982). Increase in intracellular sodium ion activity during stimulation in mammalian cardiac muscle. *Circ. Res.* **65**, 651–662.

Cook, L. S., Caldwell, R. W., Nash, C. B., Doherty, J. E., and Straub, K. D. (1982). Adrenergic and cholinergic mechanisms in digitalis inotropy. *J. Pharmacol. Exp. Therap.* **223**, 761–765.

Davis, L. D. (1973). Effect of changes in cycle length on diastolic depolarization produced by ouabain in canine Purkinje fibers. *Circ. Res.* **32**, 206–214.

Deitmer, J., and Ellis, D. (1978a). Changes in the intracellular sodium activity of sheep heart Purkinje fibres produced by calcium and other divalent cations. *J. Physiol. (London)* **277**, 437–453.

Deitmer, J. W., and Ellis, D. (1978b). The intracellular sodium activity of cardiac Purkinje fibers during inhibition and re-activation of the Na–K pump. *J. Physiol. (London)* **284**, 241–259.

Deitmer, J. W., and Ellis, D. (1980). The intracellular sodium activity of sheep heart Purkinje fibers: Effects of local anesthetics and tetrodotoxin. *J. Physiol. (London)* **300**, 269–282.

Dhalla, N. S., Pierce, G. N., Panagia, V., Singal, P. K., and Beamish, R. E. (1982). Calcium movements in relation to heart function. *Basic Res. Cardiol.* **77**, 117–139.

Di Gennaro, M., and Vassalle, M. (1985). Relationship between caffeine effects and calcium in canine cardiac Purkinje fibers. *Am. J. Physiol.* **249**, H520–H533.

Di Gennaro, M., Valle, R., Pahor, M., and Carbonin, P. (1983). Abolition of digitalis tachyarrhythmias by caffeine. *Am. J. Physiol.* **244**, H215–H222.

Di Gennaro, M., Carbonin, P., and Vassalle, M. (1984). On the mechanism by which caffeine abolishes the fast rhythms induced by cardiotonic steroids. *J. Mol. Cell. Cardiol.* **16**, 851–862.

Dudel, J., and Trautwein, W. (1958). Elektrophysiologische Messungen zur Strophanthinwirkung am Herzmuskel. *Naunyn Schmiedeberg's Arch. exp. Pathol.* **232**, 393–407.

Eisner, D. A., and Lederer, W. J. (1979a). Inotropic and arrhythmogenic effects of potassium-depleted solutions on mammalian cardiac muscle. *J. Physiol. (London)* **294**, 255–277.

Eisner, D. A., and Lederer, W. J. (1979b). The role of the sodium pump in the effects of potassium-depleted solutions on mammalian cardiac muscle. *J. Physiol. (London)* **294**, 279–301.

Eisner, D. A., and Lederer, W. J. (1982). Effects of caffeine on the inward current in cardiac Purkinje fibers. *J. Physiol. (London)* **322**, 48P–49P.

Ellis, D. (1977). The effect of external cations and ouabain on the intracellular sodium activity of sheep heart Purkinje fibers. *J. Physiol. (London)* **273**, 211–240.

Ferrier, G. R., and Moe, G. K. (1973). Effect of calcium on acetylstrophanthidin-induced transient depolarizations in canine Purkinje tissue. *Circ. Res.* **33**, 508–515.

Ferrier, G. R., Saunders, J. H., and Mendez, C. (1973). A cellular mechanism for the generation of ventricular arrhythmias by acetylstrophanthidin. *Circ. Res.* **32,** 600–609.

Furchgott, R. F., and De Gubareff, T. (1958). The high energy phosphate content of cardiac muscle under various experimental conditions which alter contractile strength. *J. Pharmacol. Exp. Therap.* **124,** 203–218.

Gabsby, D. C., and Cranefield, P. F. (1979). Direct measurement of changes in sodium pump current in canine cardiac Purkinje fibers. *Proc. Natl. Acad. Sci. USA* **76,** 1783–1787.

Gervais, A., Lane, L. K., Anner, B. M., Lindenmayer, G. E., and Schwartz, A. (1977). A possible molecular mechanism of the action of digitalis: Ouabain action on calcium binding to sites associated with a purified sodium–potassium-activated adenosine triphosphatase from kidney. *Circ. Res.* **40,** 8–14.

Godfraind, T., Ghysel-Burton, J., and De Pover, A. (1982). Dihydroouabain is an antagonist of ouabain inotropic action. *Nature (London)* **299,** 824–826.

Goshima, K. (1976). Arrhythmic movements of myocardial cells in culture and their improvement with antiarrhythmic drug. *J. Mol. Cell. Cardiol.* **8,** 217–238.

Goshima, K. (1977). Ouabain-induced arrhythmias of single isolated myocardial cells and cell clusters cultured *in vitro* and their improvement by quinidine. *J. Mol. Cell. Cardiol.* **9,** 7–23.

Goshima, K., and Wakabayashi, S. (1983). Inhibition of ouabain-induced increase in Na content of cultured myocardial cells by quinidine and procainamide. *J. Pharmacol. Exp. Therap.* **224,** 239–246.

Greenspan, A. M., and Morad, M. (1975). Electromechanical studies on the inotropic effects of acetylstrophanthidin in ventricular muscle. *J. Physiol. (London)* **253,** 357–384.

Greenspan, K., Vassalle, M., and Hoffman, R. F. (1962). Ouabain toxicity in complete heart block. *Fed. Proc.* **21,** 134 (Abstract).

Grupp, G., Grupp, I. L., Ghysel-Burton, J., Godfraind, T., and Schwartz, A. (1982). Effect of very low concentrations of ouabain on contractile force of isolated guinea pig, rabbit and cat atria and right ventricular papillary muscles: An interinstitutional study. *J. Pharmacol. Exp. Ther.* **220,** 141–151.

Grupp, I., Im, W-B. Lee, C. O., Lee, S-W., Pecker, M. S., and Schwartz, A. (1985). Relation of sodium pump inhibition to positive inotropy at low concentrations of ouabain in rat heart muscle. *J. Physiol. (London).* **360,** 149–160.

Hagemeijer, F., and Lown, M. (1970). Effect of heart rate on electrically induced repetitive ventricular responses in the digitalized dog. *Circ. Res.* **27,** 333–344.

Hart, G., Noble, D., and Shimoni, Y. (1983). The effects of low concentration of cardiotonic steroids on membrane currents and tension in sheep Purkinje fibers. *J. Physiol. (London)* **334,** 103–131.

Henning, B., and Meinertz, T. (1985). Voltage dependance of the transient inward current. *Circulation* **72,** 111–380.

Hoffman, B. F., and Bigger, J. T., Jr. (1980). Digitalis and allied cardiac glycosides. *In* "The Pharmacological Basis of Therapeutics" (A. Goodman, L. S. Goodman, and A. Gilman, eds.), pp. 729–760. MacMillan Publishing Co., New York.

Hogan, P. M., Wittenberg, S. M., and Klocke, F. J. (1973). Relationship of stimulation frequency to automaticity in the canine Purkinje fiber during ouabain administration. *Circ. Res.* **32,** 377–384.

Im, W-B., and Lee, C. O. (1984). Quantitative relation of twitch and tonic tensions to intracellular sodium ion activity during positive and negative inotropy in canine cardiac Purkinje fibers. *Am. J. Physiol. (Cell. Physiol.)* **247,** C478–C487.

Ishikawa, S., and Vassalle, M. (1982). Different forms of spontaneous discharge induced by strophanthidin in cardiac Purkinje fibers. *Am. J. Physiol.* **243,** H767–H778.

Ishikawa, S., and Vassalle, M. (1985). Reversal of strophanthidin negative inotropy by metabolic substrates in cardiac Purkinje fibres. *Cardiovasc. Res.* **19,** 537–551.

Karagueuzian, H. S., and Katzung, B. G. (1982). Voltage clamp studies of transient inward current and mechanical oscillations induced by ouabain in ferret papillary muscle. *J. Physiol. (London)* **327**, 255–271.

Kass, R. S., Lederer, W. J., Tsien, R. W., and Weingart, R. (1978a). Role of calcium ions in transient inward currents and aftercontractions induced by strophanthidin in cardiac Purkinje fibres. *J. Physiol. (London)* **281**, 187–208.

Kass, R. S., Tsien, R. W., and Weingart, R. (1978b). Ionic basis of transient inward current induced by strophanthidin in cardiac Purkinje fibres. *J. Physiol. (London)* **281**, 209–226.

Kassebaum, D. G. (1963). Electrophysiological effects of strophanthidin in the heart. *J. Pharmacol. Exp. Therap.* **140**, 329–338.

Lado, M. G., Sheu, S-S., and Fozzard, H. A. (1982). Changes in intracellular Ca^{2+} activity with stimulation in sheep cardiac Purkinje strands. *Am. J. Physiol.* **243**, H133–H137.

Langer, G. A. (1977). Relationship between myocardial contractility and the effects of digitalis on ionic exchange. *Fed. Proc.* **36**, 2231–2234.

Lederer, W. J., and Tsien, R. W. (1976). Transient inward current underlying arrhythmogenic effects of cardiac steroids in Purkinje fibres. *J. Physiol. (London)* **263**, 73–100.

Lee, C. O., and Dagostino, M. (1982). Effect of strophanthidin on intracellular Na ion activity and twitch tension of constantly driven canine cardiac Purkinje fibers. *Biophys. J.* **40**, 185–198.

Lee, C. O., and Vassalle, M. (1983). Modulation of intracellular Na^+ activity and cardiac force by norepinephrine and Ca^{2+}. *Am. J. Physiol.* **244**, C110–C114.

Lee, C. O., Kang, D. H., Sokol, J. H., and Lee, K. S. (1980). Relation between intracellular Na ion activity and tension of sheep cardiac Purkinje fibers exposed to dihydro-ouabain. *Biophys. J.* **29**, 315–330.

Lee, C. O., Abete, P., Pecker, M., Sonn, J. K., and Vassalle, M. (1985). Strophanthidin inotropy: Role of intracellular sodium activity and sodium-calcium exchange. *J. Mol. Cell. Cardiol.* **17**, 1043–1053.

Lee, K. S., and Klaus, W. (1971). The subcellular basis for the mechanism of inotropic action of cardiac glycosides. *Pharmacol. Rev.* **23**, 193–261.

Lehninger, A. L. (1974). Ca^{2+} transport by mitochondria and its possible role in the cardiac contraction–relaxation cycle. *Circ. Res.* **34/35** (Suppl. III), 83–88.

Li, T., and Vassalle, M. (1983). Sodium–calcium exchange in Purkinje fibers: Electrical and mechanical effects. *Basic Res. Cardiol.* **78**, 396–414.

Li, T., and Vassalle, M. (1984). The negative inotropic effect of calcium overload in cardiac Purkinje fibers. *J. Mol. Cell. Cardiol.* **16**, 65–77.

Lin, C-I., and Vassalle, M. (1976). Role of sodium in strophanthidin toxicity in cardiac Purkinje fibers. *Physiologist* **19**, 271.

Lin, C-I., and Vassalle, M. (1978). Role of sodium in strophanthidin toxicity of Purkinje fibers. *Am. J. Physiol.* **234**, H477–H486.

Lin, C-I., and Vassalle, M. (1979). Sodium lack prevents strophanthidin toxicity in Purkinje fibers. *Cardiology* **64**, 110–121.

Lin, C-I., and Vassalle, M. (1980). The antiarrhythmic effect of potassium and sodium in strophanthidin toxicity. *Eur. J. Pharmacol.* **62**, 1–15.

Lin, C-I., and Vassalle, M. (1983a). Role of calcium in the inotropic effects of caffeine in cardiac Purkinje fibers. *Int. J. Cardiol.* **3**, 421–434.

Lin, C-I., and Vassalle, M. (1983b). Calcium overload and strophanthidin induced mechanical toxicity in cardiac Purkinje fibers. *Can. J. Physiol. Pharmacol.* **61**, 1329–1339.

Lin, C-I., Kotake, H., and Vassalle, M. (1983). On the mechanism underlying the oscillatory current in cardiac Purkinje fibers. *Physiologist* **26**, A-90.

Lin, C.-I, Kotake H., and Vassalle M. (1986). On the mechanism underlying the oscillatory current in cardiac Purkinje fibers. *J. Cardiovasc. Pharmacol.* (In press.)

Lipsius, S. L., and Gibbons, R. W. (1982). Membrane currents, contractions, and aftercontractions in cardiac Purkinje fibers. *Am. J. Physiol.* **243**, H77–H86.

McCall, D. (1976). Effect of quinidine on cation exchange in cultured cells. *J. Pharmacol. Exp. Therap.* **197**, 605–614.

McCall, D. (1978). Responses of cultured heart cells to procainamide and lignocaine. *Cardiovasc. Res.* **12**, 529–536.

McDonald, T. F., Nawrath, H., and Trautwein, W. (1975). Membrane currents and tension in cat ventricular muscle treated with cardiac glycosides. *Circ. Res.* **37**, 674–682.

Marban, E., and Tsien, R. W. (1982). Enhancements of calcium current during digitalis inotropy in mammalian heart: Positive feed-back regulation by intracellular calcium. *J. Physiol. (London)* **329**, 589–614.

Matsuda, H., Akinori, K., Yoshihisa, K., and Irisawa, H. (1982). Transient depolarizations and spontaneous voltage fluctuations in isolated single cells from guinea pig ventricles: Calcium-mediated potential fluctuations. *Circ. Res.* **51**, 142–151.

Metha, N. L., and Vassalle, M. (1981). The dependence of strophanthidin inotropy on sodium concentration and calcium overload. *Circulation* **64**, IV-273.

Mugelli, A. (1982). Separation of the oscillatory current from other currents in cardiac Purkinje fibers. *Cardiovasc. Res.* **16**, 637–645.

Mullins, L. J. (1979). The generation of electric currents in cardiac fibers by Na/Ca exchange. *Am. J. Physiol.* **136**, C103–C110.

Nayler, W. G., and Grinwald, P. (1981). Calcium entry blockers and myocardial function. *Fed. Proc.* **40**, 2855–2861.

Noble, D. (1980). Mechanism of action of therapeutic levels of cardiac glycosides. *Cardiovasc. Res.* **14**, 495–514.

Okita, G. T. (1977). Dissociation of Na^+, K^+-ATPase inhibition from digitalis inotropy. *Fed. Proc.* **36**, 2225–2230.

Paspa, P., and Vassalle, M. (1984). Mechanism of caffeine-induced arrhythmias in canine cardiac Purkinje fibers. *Am. J. Cardiol.* **53**, 313–319.

Polimeni, P. I., and Vassalle, M. (1971). On the mechanism of ouabain toxicity in Purkinje and ventricular muscle fibers at rest and during activity. *Am. J. Cardiol.* **27**, 622–629.

Rosen, M. R., Gelband, H., Merker, C., and Hoffman, B. F. (1973). Mechanisms of digitalis toxicity. Effect of ouabain on phase four of canine Purkinje fiber transmembrane potentials. *Circulation* **47**, 681–689.

Rosen, M. R., Danilo, P., Jr., Alonso, M. B., and Pippenger, C. E. (1976). Effects of therapeutic concentrations of diphenylhydantoin on transmembrane potentials of normal and depressed Purkinje fibers. *J. Pharmacol. Exp. Therap.* **197**, 597–604.

Schatzmann, H. J. (1953). Herzglykoside als Hemmstoffe für den aktiven Kalium- und Natriumtransport durch die Erythrocytenmembran. *Helv. Physiol. Pharmacol. Acta* **11**, 346–354.

Schwartz, A., Lindenmayer, G. E., and Allen, J. C. (1975). The sodium–potassium adenosine triphosphatase: Pharmacological, physiological and biochemical aspects. *Pharmacol. Rev.* **27**, 1–134.

Sheu, S. S., and Fozzard, H. A. (1982). Transmembrane Na^+ and Ca^{2+} electrochemical gradients in cardiac muscle and their relationship to force development. *J. Gen. Physiol.* **80**, 325–351.

Skou, J. C. (1957). The influence of some cations on an adenosine triphosphatase from peripheral nerves. *Biochim. Biophys. Acta* **23**, 394–401.

Smith, T. W., and Braunwald, E. (1980). The management of heart failure. *In* "Heart Disease. A Textbook of Cardiovascular Medicine" (E. Braunwald, ed.), pp. 510–570. W. B. Saunders Co., Philadelphia.

Surawicz, B., and Mortelmans, S. (1969). Factors affecting individual tolerance to digitalis. *In* "Digitalis" (C. Fisch and B. Surawicz, eds.), pp. 127–147. Grune & Stratton, New York.

Temma, K., and Akera, T. (1982). Enhancement of cardiac actions of ouabain and its binding to Na^+, K^+-adenosine triphosphatase by increased sodium influx in isolated guinea pig heart. *J. Pharmacol. Exper. Ther.* **223,** 490–496.

Temte, J. V., and Davis, L. D. (1967). Effect of calcium concentration on the transmembrane potentials of Purkinje fibers. *Circ. Res.* **20,** 32–44.

Vassalle, M. (1970). Electrogenic suppression of automaticity in sheep and dog Purkinje fibers. *Circ. Res.* **27,** 361–377.

Vasslle, M. (1975). Toxic mechanisms of strophanthidin in cardiac Purkinje fibers. *Physiologist* **18,** 429.

Vassalle, M. (1977). The relationship among cardiac pacemakers. Overdrive suppression. *Circ. Res.* **41,** 269–277.

Vassalle, M. (1978). The acceleratory action of the vagus on the sinus node. *In* "The Sinus Node: Structure, Function, and Clinical Relevance" (F. I. M. Bonke, ed.), pp. 279–289. Martinus Nijhoff, The Hague.

Vassalle, M. (1982). The role of the electrogenic sodium pump in controlling excitability in nerve and cardiac fibers. *In* "Current Topics in Membrane and Transport" Vol. 16 (C. L. Slayman, ed.), pp. 467–483. Academic Press, New York.

Vassalle, M., and Bhattacharyya, M. (1980). Local anesthetics and the role of sodium in the force development by canine ventricular muscle and Purkinje fibers. *Circ. Res.* **47,** 666–674.

Vassalle, M., and Bhattacharyya, M. (1981). Interactions of norepinephrine and strophanthidin in cardiac Purkinje fibers. *Int. J. Cardiol.* **1,** 179–194.

Vassalle, M., and Di Gennaro, M. (1983). Caffeine eliminates the oscillatory current in cardiac Purkinje fibers. *Eur. J. Pharmacol.* **94,** 361–362.

Vassalle, M., and Di Gennaro, M. (1984). Caffeine actions on currents induced by calcium overload in Purkinje fibers. *Fed. Proc.* **43,** 2055.

Vassalle, M., and Lee, C. O. (1984). The relationship among intracellular sodium activity, calcium, and strophanthidin inotropy in canine cardiac Purkinje fibers. *J. Gen. Physiol.* **83,** 287–307.

Vassalle, M., and Lin, C-I. (1979). Effect of calcium on strophanthidin-induced electrical and mechanical toxicity in cardiac Purkinje fibers. *Am. J. Physiol.* **236,** H689–H697.

Vassalle, M., and Mugelli, A. (1981). An oscillatory current in sheep cardiac Purkinje fibers. *Circ. Res.* **48,** 618–631.

Vassalle, M., and Musso, E. (1976a). On the mechanisms underlying digitalis toxicity in cardiac Purkinje fibers. *In* "Recent Advances in Studies on Cardiac Structure and Metabolism. The Sarcolemma" Vol. 9 (P. E. Roy and N. S. Dhalla, eds.), pp. 355–375. University Park, Baltimore.

Vassalle, M., and Musso, E. (1976b). Therapeutic and toxic actions of digitalis. *In* "Cardiac Physiology for the Clinician" (M. Vassalle, ed.), pp. 203–239. Academic Press, New York.

Vassalle, M., and Scida, E. E. (1979). The role of sodium in spontaneous discharge in the absence and presence of strophanthidin. *Fed. Proc.* **38,** 880.

Vassalle, M., Karis, J., and Hoffman, B. F. (1962). Toxic effects of ouabain on Purkinje fibers and ventricular muscle fibers. *Am. J. Physiol.* **203,** 433–439.

Vassalle, M., Greenspan, K., and Hoffman, B. F. (1963). An analysis of arrhythmias induced by ouabain in intact dogs. *Circ. Res.* **13,** 132–148.

Vassalle, M., Bernabei, R., Carbonin, P., and Li, T. (1984). The inotropic action of strophanthidin at different sodium and calcium concentrations. *Physiologist* **27,** 235.

Wasserstrom, J. A., Schwartz, D. J., and Fozzard, H. A. (1983). Relation between intracellular sodium and twitch tension in sheep cardiac Purkinje strands exposed to cardiac glycosides. *Circ. Res.* **52,** 697–705.

Weingart, R., Kass, R. S., and Tsien, R. W. (1978). Is digitalis inotropy associated with enhanced slow inward calcium current? *Nature (London)* **273**, 389–392.

Wittenberg, S. M., Streuli, F., and Klocke, F. H. (1970). Acceleration of ventricular pacemakers by transient increases in heart rate in dogs during ouabain administration. *Circ. Res.* **26**, 705–716.

Wittenberg, S. M., Gandel, P., Hogan, P. M., Kreuzer, W., and Klocke, F. J. (1972). Relationship of heart rate to ventricular automaticity in dogs during ouabain administration. *Circ. Res.* **30**, 167–170.

Wollenberger, A. (1949). The energy metabolism of the failing heart and the metabolic action of cardiac glycosides. *Pharmacol. Rev.* **1**, 311–352.

Wollenberger, A. (1951). Metabolic action of cardiac glycosides. II. Effect of ouabain and digoxin on the energy-rich phosphate content of the heart. *J. Pharmacol. Exp. Therap.* **103**, 123–135.

Wollenberger, A., and Karsh, M. L. (1952). Effect of a cardiac glycoside on the contraction and the energy-rich phosphate content of the heart poisoned with dinitrophenol. *J. Pharmacol. Exp. Therap.* **105**, 477–485.

10

Calcium at the Sarcolemma: Its Role in Control of Myocardial Contraction

G. A. Langer

I. INTRODUCTION

The most widely accepted, current models for excitation–contraction coupling in mammalian heart muscle include two critical calcium (Ca) components. Largely on the basis of the elegant studies of Fabiato (1983), it is assumed that one component of coupling Ca is derived from the sarcoplasmic reticulum (SR) via the process of Ca-induced Ca release (CICR). The fraction of Ca from the SR varies among mammalian species with adult rat ventricular muscle the most dependent and adult rabbit ventricle the least dependent on SR Ca (Fabiato and Fabiato, 1978). The other component, that which serves to induce the release of SR Ca as well as to supply the myofilaments, comes directly from influx across the sarcolemma. Heart muscle, in contrast to skeletal muscle, ceases to contract if transsarcolemmal influx of Ca is interrupted, despite adequate stores of Ca in the SR.

At present two systems are recognized as responsible for the transsarcolemmal influx of Ca: the Ca channel and the Na–Ca exchanger (Langer *et al.*, 1982). [The latter operates also to produce a net efflux of Ca, dependent on transmembrane potential (Mullins, 1979).] The amount of Ca that enters the cell via these systems is a major determinant of the concentration of Ca at the myofilaments during systole and, therefore, a major determinant of the level of contractile force. The source of Ca for these systems has been a subject of investigation by our laboratory at UCLA over the past 10 years.

269

CARDIAC MUSCLE:
THE REGULATION OF EXCITATION AND CONTRACTION

II. EXTRACELLULAR CALCIUM

The primary source of Ca that enters the cell across the sarcolemma is the extracellular space. Recent studies using Ca-sensitive microelectrodes in the interstitial space (Bers, 1983) and Ca-sensitive dyes limited in their distribution to the extracellular space (Hilgemann and Langer, 1984) demonstrate clearly the extracellular depletion of Ca that follows excitation. These studies indicate a depletion of approximately 20 μmol Ca/kg wet weight ventricle at $[Ca]_o = 1.0$–2.0 mM. Because of the orientation of the microelectrode and because the dyes sample a mean value for the extracellular space, it is likely that both techniques underestimate the magnitude of the depletion but certainly not enough to make the value comparable to those obtained in guinea pig ventricle by Pytkowski *et al.* (1983). This group reports an uptake of cellular Ca greater than 200 μmol/kg wet weight per excitation or more than 10-fold the values measured in rabbit ventricle with microelectrode or dye. Fabiato (1983) has calculated from his studies in skinned fibers that 50% of maximum tension is achieved at a pCa $= 5.57$ $(2.7 \times 10^{-6} M)$, which, with the buffer capacity of the cell, would require 114 μmol/liter cell water. If we assume 1 : 1 distribution of cell to extracellular water, the calculated value is 57 μmol/kg weight. This value is much less than that reported by Pytkowski *et al.* but approximately threefold more than the amount reported by Bers (1983) and Hilgemann and Langer (1984). If the latter amount is more nearly correct (and Fabiato's assumption of buffering capacity applies to the intact cell), it is clear that amplification of transsarcolemmal flux, through CICR, is required to achieve 50% maximal force activation. This 50% force activation is approximately the level achieved in rabbit ventricle with 2 mM $[Ca]_o$ (Bers *et al.*, 1981).

Although the ratio of transsarcolemmal Ca influx to Ca released from the SR remains undetermined, it seems that the Ca that enters the cell across the sarcolemma is not derived directly from Ca that is free in solution. When Ca is removed from the perfusate in a vascularly perfused segment of rabbit ventricle, force declines 4–5 times more slowly than it is regained upon replacement of Ca in the perfusate (Philipson and Langer, 1979). The simplest explanation for the asymmetry of loss and return of force is that a component of Ca destined to enter the cell is *bound* at a cellular site that is in rapid equilibrium with Ca in the extracellular space. A site with a certain affinity for Ca would be expected to *wash off* more slowly than it would *wash on*. It seemed to us that the most likely site for a rapidly exchangeable component of Ca was the sarcolemma. We undertook, therefore, a series of studies designed to examine the hypothesis that Ca-binding sites within the sarcolemma are involved in supplying the Ca that enters the cell upon excitation.

III. SARCOLEMMAL CALCIUM BINDING

A. Binding Versus $[Ca]_o$

Bers and Langer (1979) examined Ca bound to sarcolemmal vesicles (isolated from neonatal rat hearts) as a function of $[Ca]_o$. The K_m for the low-affinity sites, which accounted for 80% of the total sites, was 1.2 mM. A similar study of sarcolemma derived from rabbit heart (Philipson *et al.*, 1980a) showed a pre-dominance of low-affinity sites with a $K_m = 2.7$ mM. In the rabbit ventricle, a plot of Ca bound to the sarcolemma vs. $[Ca]_o$ is superimposable on a plot of maximum rate of force developed (dF/dt_{max}) vs. $[Ca]_o$ over a range of $[Ca]_o$ from 0.5 to 9.0 mM (Philipson *et al.*, 1980a). These experiments can be in-terpreted as consistent with the proposal that Ca bound to sarcolemmal sites plays a major role in determining development of peak active force.

The total number of sarcolemmal Ca-binding sites derived from Scatchard analysis was greater than 2000 μmol/kg wet weight rabbit ventricle. According to the superimposable plots of $[Ca]_o$ vs. binding and dF/dt (see above), the amount of Ca bound when force development is 50% maximal is approximately 800 μmol/kg wet weight. This is some 14 times the amount of Ca required to enter the cytoplasm of the cell to produce 50% activation of force (57 μmol/kg wet weight—see above). The estimated influx of Ca from microelectrode and Ca-sensitive dyes is even less (approximately 20 μmol/kg wet weight). The point to be emphasized is that the quantity of Ca bound at sarcolemmal sites of relatively low affinity ($K_m = 1.2$–2.7 mM) is very large in comparison to the amounts required for activation during a contraction cycle. Less than 10% of this Ca would be used during a single activation to produce 50% maximal force development if *all* of the Ca went directly to the myofilaments. Much less would be required if the bound Ca supplied only that Ca necessary to induce release from the SR. These relative values imply that a great deal more Ca is bound to the sarcolemma than enters the cell and that the transsarcolemmal systems (Ca channel and Na–Ca exchanger) move only a small fraction with each beat. On the other hand, it should be noted that larger amounts of Ca could move from sarcolemmal sites and return within the bounds of a contraction cycle and not be measured with techniques currently available.

B. Competitive Cations and Ca Binding

Fifteen years ago we first used the trivalent cation lanthanum (La) as a specific uncoupler of excitation from contraction in cardiac muscle (Sanborn and Langer, 1970). Low concentrations of La (5–40 μM) produced a rapid decline of active force and an abrupt release of tissue-bound Ca in rabbit ventricle. After perfusion with La, action potentials demonstrated essentially normal regenerative depolarization. It was concluded from this study that ''contractile dependent Ca was derived primarily from 'superficially' located (cellular) sites.''

La has proved to be a useful probe for surface-bound Ca. There is abundant evidence that the ion does not penetrate beyond the sarcolemma of intact cells and that it *displaces* Ca specifically from sarcolemmal sites. Definitive proof of its specificity for surface-bound Ca comes from a recent study using monolayers of myocardial cells in tissue culture and sarcolemmal membrane derived from these cells (Langer and Nudd, 1983). Cultured cells are grown in monolayer on plastic disks that contain a scintillant compound. The disks are fitted into a flow cell, which is then inserted into the well of a specially designed scintillation spectrometer. ^{45}Ca is then perfused through the flow cell. As ^{45}Ca is taken up by cells in contact with the perfusate, β emissions activate the scintillant to produce photons, which are in turn recorded by the spectrometer. The system allows on-line measurement of ^{45}Ca uptake or washout from the cells over a period of hours. In addition to measuring ^{45}Ca exchange in whole cells, the system can measure ^{45}Ca binding kinetics in sheets of sarcolemmal membrane derived from these cells by gas dissection (Langer and Nudd, 1983). Cellular monolayers on the scintillation disk are exposed to a tangentially oriented, high-velocity stream of nitrogen gas. It appears that the upper surface of the cells is sheared open, the cellular material blown out, and the sarcolemma left fenestrated and flat and, in some areas, wrinkled or rolled. ^{45}Ca exchange of the membranes on the scintillator disks is measured in exactly the same manner as in the whole cells.

In cultured cells perfused in HEPES-buffered medium, 80–90% exchangeable Ca was rapidly exchangeable ($t_{1/2} < 1$ min) and accounted for 40–50% of total cellular Ca (Langer *et al.*, 1979). Addition of La to the whole cell produced an immediate displacement of > 80% of the rapidly exchangeable fraction or 3.32 mmol Ca/kg dry weight whole cells. After ^{45}Ca labeling of gas-dissected membranes, La was again used to displace the bound Ca from this preparation from which 99% of the cellular content had been removed (Langer and Nudd, 1983). To compare the quantity of Ca displaced from the membranes with that displaced from the whole cells, a membrane protein : dry cell weight ratio was applied (19.1 $\pm$ 1.8 μg protein/mg dry cell weight). Displacement of La from the membranes was 3.21 mmol/kg dry weight or 97% of the value from whole cells. Thus La is clearly a specific probe for Ca bound to sarcolemma. Its uncoupling of excitation from contraction might, therefore, be associated with displacement of Ca from sarcolemmal sites.

Further evidence of the participation of these sarcolemmal sites is derived from correlation of the ability of other cations to displace Ca with their ability to uncouple excitation from contraction (Langer and Nudd, 1983). Cadmium (Cd), at equimolar concentration, is nearly as effective as La in displacing Ca from whole cells and membranes and nearly as effective as an EC uncoupler. Manganese (Mn) exhibits intermediate potency in displacing Ca and uncoupling, and magnesium (Mg) is weakest in both displacing Ca and uncoupling. Effectiveness of the divalent cations as displacers and uncouplers is related to their unhydrated or crystal radii. Cd has a radius (0.97 Å) closest to that of Ca (0.99 Å), the radius of Mn is intermediate (0.80 Å), and that of Mg is the farthest removed (0.65 Å). This offers further evidence that specific sarcolemmal Ca-binding sites play a significant role in the control of myocardial force development.

The sequence for displacement of sarcolemma-bound Ca by multivalent cations is identical to that of inside-out vesicles made from red blood cells (Cohen and Solomon, 1976). This suggests that the membrane sites responsible for Ca binding may be common to a variety of tissues. In this respect, the displacement sequence is also identical to the sequence for cationic effects on the temperature of phospholipid phase transitions (Rainier et al., 1979) and the sequence of cation-enhanced fusion of phospholipid vesicles (Liao and Prestegard, 1980). These last two relationships suggest that phospholipid molecules within the sarcolemma may be primarily responsible for Ca binding. The following section examines this possibility.

IV. ROLE OF PHOSPHOLIPID IN Ca BINDING

We had proposed originally that anionic components of the glycocalyx, such as sialic acid, could account for a significant fraction of Ca binding at the cellular surface (Langer et al., 1976). A later study, in which sarcolemmal vesicles were subjected to lipid extraction and then reconstituted from the extracted material, showed, however, that at physiological $[Ca]_o$ more than 80% of the Ca was bound to bilayer phospholipids (PL) (Philipson et al., 1980b). In quantitative terms, the PL of the bilayer are, therefore, of much greater importance in terms of Ca binding than are the anionic components of the glycocalyx.

It would be expected that the PL with a net anionic charge would be those most likely to contribute to the binding of Ca. Of the PL naturally present in the sarcolemma, phosphatidylserine (PS) and phosphatidylinositol (PI) carry a net negative charge (Philipson et al., 1980b; Tibbits et al., 1981). Other PL present in greater concentration, such as phosphatidylethanolamine (PE), at pH > 7 (in the physiological range) undergo neutralization of the $-NH_3^+$ group to $-NH_2$ and release $-PO_4^-$ or $-COO^-$ from PO_4NH_3 and $COONH_3$ salts in the molecule. Ca can then react with the ionized PO_4^- or COO^- groups (Seimiya and Ohki, 1973). Thus those zwitterionic PL with NH_3^+ groups may also be candidates for Ca binding at physiological pH.

A. Polymyxin B

The contribution of negatively charged PL to Ca binding was tested with the cationic probe polymyxin B (PXB). PXB is an amphiphilic peptidolipid with hydrophilic diaminobutyric acid groups that carry a net positive charge. These groups lie in a heptapeptide ring that is connected through three more amino acids to a fatty acid (Storm et al., 1977). Thus, PXB has a highly charged cationic head group and a lipophilic tail. The tail inserts into the lipid bilayer and the cationic head group interacts with the hydrophilic negatively charged ends of the PL. In support of this proposed mechanism, PXB has been demonstrated to bind only to artificial membranes that contain negatively charged phospholipids or to phosphatidylethanolamine at pH > 7.2 (Feingold et al., 1974; Iwai et al., 1975; Teuber and Miller, 1977).

We have studied the effect of PXB on Ca binding to whole cultured cardiac cells (Burt et al., 1983) and to gas-dissected membranes from these cells (Burt and Langer, 1983). In the presence of 1.0 mM [Ca]$_o$, 0.1 mM PXB displaced 42% of total La-displaceable Ca from the membranes. Increasing concentrations of PXB displaced greater amounts of Ca. Pretreatment of the membranes with neuraminidase (to remove sialic acid) and protease (to remove Ca-binding protein components) led to a decrease in La-displaceable Ca but to an increase in the fraction displaced by PXB. Treating the membranes with phospholipase D (PLD) increased their phosphatidate content and, therefore, the level of anionic PL sites (see below). Such treatment increased La-displaceable Ca, and all of the increment was displaced by 0.1 mM PXB. Thus, there is strong evidence that a major fraction of sarcolemmal Ca binding is attributable to anionic PL sites.

In whole cells, 0.1 mM PXB displaced 1.4 mmol Ca/kg dry weight or 24% of total displaceable Ca. It inhibited also the rate of Ca uptake after displacement. This is consistent with the proposal that bound Ca feeds the systems responsible for transsarcolemmal influx of the ion.

B. Phospholipase

Gas-dissected membranes were used initially to measure the effect of phospholipases on Ca binding (Langer and Nudd, 1983). Phospholipase A$_2$ (PLA$_2$) cleaves the acyl group from the C2 position of phospholipids, producing lysophosphoglyceride and a fatty acid. The enzyme produced a significant increase in Ca binding that was eliminated completely by an albumin wash. The albumin binds and removes the fatty acid product. Thus the fatty acid product and not lysophosphoglyceride was responsible for the enhanced binding. This was to be expected because no change in net anionic charge would be produced by lysophosphoglyceride.

Phospholipase C (PLC) derived from *Bacillus cereus* has its major effect on neutral phosphatidylcholine and a negligible effect on anionic PL. It cleaves the entire phosphorylated base from the C3 position. PLC decreased Ca binding by a small but not statistically significant amount. This would be expected if Ca binding were associated predominantly with anionic or zwitterionic PL. If significant amounts were bound to PE (see previous page), a greater decrease in binding could have been expected with the PLC derived from *B. cereus*.

Treatment with phospholipase D (PLD) increased La-displaceable Ca binding, however, by nearly 60%. PLD cleaves the nitrogenous base from the PL, producing phosphatidic acid, and thereby increases the net anionic charge on the membrane. These findings were extended to whole cultured cells (Burt *et al.*, 1984) in which PLD treatment resulted in a 39% increase in Ca uptake. Seventy-eight percent of this increase remained La-displaceable and could, therefore, be localized to the sarcolemma. Moreover, PLD increased PXB-displaceable Ca by 85%, a clear indication that a major fraction was localized to anionic components of PL.

These effects of PLD on Ca binding make pertinent the recent study of Philipson and Nishimoto (1984). They found that treatment of canine cardiac sarcolemmal vesicles with PLD increased Na–Ca exchange activity by up to 400%. The effect was specific for Na–Ca exchange. Other sarcolemmal transport enzymes, such as Na–K ATPase, and ATP-dependent Ca transport were slightly inhibited. There is, at present, no proof that the augmented Ca binding induced by PLD is related directly to the striking augmentation of Na–Ca exchange. It is tempting, however, to propose such a cause and effect.

Finally, it has been demonstrated (Burt *et al.*, 1984) that treating ventricular strips from neonatal rat heart with PLD produces a significant increase (1.7- to 2.5-fold) in contractile force; therefore, the results of the experimental series with PLD indicate that Ca bound to anionic sites of sarcolemmal PL plays a major role in the control of transsarcolemmal flux and force development in the heart.

V. RELATIONSHIP OF Ca BINDING TO PRIMARY ALTERATION IN TRANSSARCOLEMMAL FLUX

To date, only one study has provided any information in this area. Burt and Langer (1982) studied the effect of Na–K pump inhibition by ouabain ($10^{-3} M$) and perfusion with a solution of low potassium concentration (0.5 mM). Both of these interventions produce increases in [Na]$_i$ and net uptake of Ca via the Na–Ca exchange system, and both produced significant increases in La-displaceable

Ca from cultured myocardial cells. Thus an increase in the amount of Ca bound to sarcolemmal sites might be correlated with an effect on the Na–Ca exchanger. This could indicate feedback between Na–Ca exchange activity and sites on or within the membrane that stores Ca.

VI. PRESENT CONCEPTS

The work that I have summarized and studies in progress have led us to certain concepts with respect to Ca at the sarcolemma: (1) Ca in the interstitial space is in rapid equilibrium with that bound within the sarcolemmal–glycocalyx complex of the cell. (2) At $[Ca]_o$ of 1.0–1.5 mM, 80–85% of this Ca is bound to phospholipids in the sarcolemmal bilayer. (3) The total Ca-binding capacity of the membrane is large—approximately 2000 μmol/kg wet weight tissue. At 1.5 mM $[Ca]_o$, 700–800 μmol Ca/kg wet weight is bound. (4) Phospholipids of net anionic charge and those of zwitterionic form are likely to play a predominant role in the binding. (5) Augmentation of net anionic charge, e.g., formation of phosphatidate by phospholipase D treatment, augments Ca binding and is positively inotropic. Conversely, insertion of a cationic amphiphile, e.g., poly-myxin B, into the membrane displaces Ca and is negatively inotropic. (6) The Ca that enters the cell via channel or Na–Ca exchanger is derived from the sarcolem-mal binding sites. (7) The amount of Ca derived from the binding sites is, by itself, insufficient to activate the myofibrils fully, and an intracellular amplifica-tion of Ca concentration is required, i.e., Ca-induced Ca release. It remains possible, however, that transsarcolemmal Ca influx is underestimated by present techniques. If so, a larger fraction of myofilament activation would occur from direct entry of Ca.

VII. CONCLUSIONS

Figure 1 is a schematic representation of current concepts of Ca movement in the mamalian myocardial cell and serves as a guide for future investigation of the EC coupling process. Sarcolemmal Ca binding is considered to be in rapid equilibrium with Ca in the interstitium. Most of the Ca is, as emphasized, thought to be bound to PL. A question that remains is: "To which PL is the Ca bound?" If the molecule or molecules can be identified, then possible rela-tionships between the bound Ca and the transsarcolemmal systems depicted in Fig. 1 (channel, Na–Ca exchanger, and Ca pump) might be modeled realistically and tested experimentally.

CALCIUM MOVEMENT

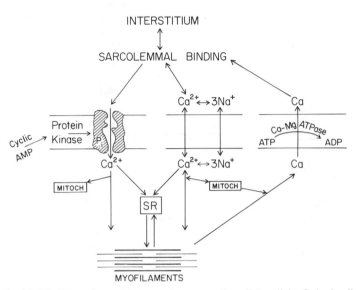

Fig. 1. Model of Ca exchange for mammalian myocardium. Extracellular Ca is visualized to be in rapid equilibrium with sarcolemmal binding sites, predominantly phospholipid in nature. The relation between the binding sites and the three transsarcolemmal systems (the channel controlled by phosphorylation, the bidirectional Na–Ca exchanger, and the sarcolemmal Ca pump) is not yet defined. It seems possible, however, that there is an interaction between bound Ca and these systems (see text for discussion). Ca that enters via the channel and/or exchanger may activate the myofilaments directly but is more likely to serve primarily as a trigger for SR Ca release. Mitochondria contribute little to beat-to-beat Ca fluxes, but serve as a large intracellular buffer under conditions of high cellular Ca load. The contribution of the sarcolemmal Ca pump (in comparison to that of the SR) to controlling the level of cytosolic Ca is not known. [Reproduced from Dintenfass, *et al.* (1983) with permission of Plenum Press, New York.]

Another significant problem concerns the amounts of Ca that move through each transsarcolemmal system during the contraction cycle. Do both channel and exchanger move Ca inward with each excitation, or is the exchanger operative only in the Ca-efflux mode? What role does the sarcolemmal Ca pump play in relation to the SR in removal of Ca from the sarcoplasm? What are the relative amounts of Ca derived from the SR through CICR and directly through sarcolemmal influx for activation of the myofilaments, and how do these amounts vary among species? Does the distribution of Ca within the cell differ with the system (channel or exchanger) responsible for influx of Ca? These are a few of the questions that require answers before a fully developed model of cardiac EC coupling can be realized.

UPDATE

Since this chapter was submitted for publication (June, 1984) further significant information relative to the role of sarcolemmal Ca has been obtained:

1. We used the divalent cation dimethonium (ethane-bis-trimethylammonium) as a probe for Ca in the diffuse double layer (Fintel, *et al.*, 1985). The diffuse double layer refers to the space directly adjacent to the sarcolemma where the ionic composition of the media is a direct function of the membrane surface potential. Dimethonium is a large organic cation that effectively screens negative surface charge with consequent removal of cation from the diffuse double layer, but does not adsorb to or displace cation from the membrane (McLaughlin, *et al.*, 1983). Concentrations of dimethonium sufficient to displace significant Ca^{2+} from the double layer had virtually no effect on force development of rabbit ventricle. Contractile function appears, therefore, to be supported mainly by Ca that is independent of the diffuse double layer. The results indicate that the Ca that is significant is the Ca *actually bound* to sarcolemmal constituents.

2. As noted, insertion of a cationic amphiphile, PXB, into the sarcolemma displaces Ca and is negatively inotropic. Insertion of an anionic amphiphile, dodecylsulfate (DDS), produces a specific increase in sarcolemmal bound Ca (Langer and Rich, 1986). The effect of DDS on force development in diverse tissues is informative. DDS produces a 60% increase in active force in ventricular tissue from adult rabbit and neonatal rat but virtually no increase in adult rat ventricle. However perfusion of rat ventricle with $10^{-6} M$ ryanodine markedly increased the relative response of adult rat ventricle to DDS but had little effect on the response of a rabbit or neonatal rat ventricle. It is generally accepted that ryanodine removes the contribution of the sarcoplasmic reticulum (SR) from the excitation–contraction process. The study confirms the importance of sarcolemmal-bound Ca in force control and is consistent with the concept that SR Ca plays a dominant role in force control in adult rat and a significantly lesser role in neonatal rat and adult rabbit ventricle.

3. pH Variation was used to alter the ionization of the putative sarcolemmal Ca binding sites (Langer, 1985). Increase of pH from 5.5 to 8.5 markedly increased Ca binding to whole myocardial cells and to isolated sarcolemma. Contraction amplitude increased in proportion to binding. The relation between sarcolemmal binding or contraction amplitude to pH was closely fit by a form of the Henderson–Hasselbach relation with pK of the ionized sites between 6.60 and 7.15. This pK is 3 orders of magnitude higher than that expected for phosphate or carboxyl Ca-binding sites on sarcolemmal phospholipid. This suggested another group of sites (as suggested by Seimya and Ohki, 1973; see previous discussion), e.g., amino groups, with higher pK value are neutralized ($NH_3^+ \rightarrow NH_2 + H^+$) as pH is increased from 5.5 to 8.5. They would, then, no longer shield, intra- or intermolecularly, the negatively charged phospholipid acidic groups that would then be

available to bind Ca. The pH study suggested a two-site model for control of sarcolemmal Ca-binding:

$$Ca\ bound = \frac{1}{antilog[pK - pH] + 1} \times \frac{Ca_{sat} \cdot [Ca]_0}{K_d + [Ca]_0}$$

The first factor predicts the ionization of the access sites with relatively high pK (possibly amino groups). The second factor is the Michaelis–Menten relation that predicts the actual Ca binding to the more acidic sites (carboxyl or phosphate) with their dissociation constant (K_d) for Ca^{2+}. Current work indicates that the relationship is highly predictive of ventricular force development at any pH between 6.0 and 8.0 and for a range of $[Ca]_0$ from 0.25 to 4.0 mM.

ACKNOWLEDGMENTS

This study was supported in part by a grant from USPHS(HL 28539-2) and the Castera Endowment.

REFERENCES

Bers, D. M. (1983). Early transient depletion of extracellular Ca during individual cardiac muscle contraction. Am. J. Physiol. **244**, H462–H468.

Bers, D. M., and Langer, G. A. (1979). Uncoupling cation effects on cardiac contractility and sarcolemmal Ca^{2+} binding. Am. J. Physiol. **237**, H333–H341.

Bers, D. M., Philipson, K. D., and Langer, G. A. (1981). Cardiac contractility and sarcolemmal calcium binding in several different cardiac muscle preparations. Am J. Physiol. **240**, H576–H583.

Burt, J. M., and Langer, G. A. (1982). Ca^{++} distribution after Na^{+} pump inhibition in cultured neonatal rat myocardial cells. Circ. Res. **51**, 543–550.

Burt, J. M., and Langer, G. A. (1983). Ca^{2+} displacement by Polymyxin B from sarcolemma isolated by "gas dissection" from cultured neonatal rat myocardial cells. Biochim. Biophys. Acta **729**, 44–52.

Burt, J. M., Duenas, C. J., and Langer, G. A. (1983). Influence of Polymyxin B, a probe for anionic phospholipids, on calcium binding and calcium and potassium fluxes of cultured cardiac cells. Circ. Res. **53**, 679–687.

Burt, J. M., Rich, T. L., and Langer, G. A. (1984). Phospholipase D increases cell surface Ca-binding and positive inotropy in rat heart. Am. J. Physiol. **247**, H880–H885.

Cohen, C. M., and Solomon, A. K. (1976). Ca binding to human cell membrane: Characterization of membrane preparations and binding sites. J. Membrane Biol. **29**, 345–372.

Dintenfass, L., Julian, D. G., and Seaman, G. V. F., eds. (1983). "Heart Perfusion, Energetics and Ischemia." Plenum, New York.

Fabiato, A. (1983). Calcium-induced release of calcium from the cardiac sarcoplasmic reticulum. Am. J. Physiol. **245**, C1–C14.

Fabiato, A., and Fabiato, F. (1978). Calcium-induced release of calcium from the sarcoplasmic reticulum of skinned cells from adult human, dog, cat, rabbit, rat, and frog hearts and from fetal and new-born rat ventricles. *Ann. N. Y. Acad. Sci.* **307**, 491–522.

Feingold, D. S., HsuChen, C. C., and Sud, I. J. (1974). Basis for the selectivity of action of the polymyxin antibiotics on cell membranes. *Ann. N. Y. Acad. Sci.* **235**, 480–492.

Fintel, M., Langer, G. A., Rohloff, J. C., and Jung, M. E. (1985). Contribution of myocardial diffuse double-layer calcium to contractile junction. *Am J. Physiol.* **249**, H989–H994.

Hilgemann, D. W., and Langer, G. A. (1984). Transsarcolemmal calcium movements in arterially perfused rabbit ventricle measured with extracellular calcium sensitive dyes. *Circ. Res.* **54**, 461–467.

Iwai, M., Inoue, K., and Nojima, S. (1975). Effect of Polymyxin B on liposomal membranes derived from *E. coli* lipids. *Biochim. Biophys. Acta* **375**, 130–137.

Langer, G. A. (1985). The effect of pH on cellular and membrane calcium binding and contraction of myocardium. A possible rule for sarcolemmal phospholipid in EC coupling. *Circ. Res.* **571**, 374–382.

Langer, G. A., and Nudd, L. M. (1983). Effects of cations, phospholipases, and neuraminidase on calcium binding to "gas-dissected" membranes from cultured cardiac cells. *Circ. Res.* **53**, 482–490.

Langer, G. A., and Rich, T. L. (1986). Augmentation of sarcolemmal calcium by anionic amphiphile. Contractile response of three ventricular tissues. *Am J. Physiol.* **19**, H247–H254.

Langer, G. A., Frank, J. S., Nudd, L. M., and Seraydarian, K. (1976). Sialic acid: Effect of removal on calcium exchangeability of cultured heart cells. *Science* **193**, 1013–1015.

Langer, G. A., Frank, J. S., and Nudd, L. M. (1979). Correlation of calcium exchange, structure, and function in myocardial tissue culture. *Am. J. Physiol.* **237**, H239–H246.

Langer, G. A., Frank, J. S., and Philipson, K. D. (1982). Ultrastructure and calcium exchange of the sarcolemma, sarcoplasmic reticulum and mitochondria of the myocardium. *Pharmacol. Ther.* **16**, 331–376.

Liao, M. J., and Prestegard, J. H. (1980). Ion specificity in fusion of phosphatidic acid–phosphatidylcholine mixed lipid vesicles. *Biochim. Biophys. Acta* **601**, 453–461.

McLaughlin, A., Eng, W., Vaio, G., Wilson, T., and McLaughlin, S. (1983). Dimethonium, a divalent cation that exerts only a screening effect on the electrostatic potential adjacent to negatively charged phospholipid bilayer membranes. *J. Membr. Biol.* **76**, 183–193.

Mullins, L. J. (1979). The generation of electric currents in cardiac fibers by Na/Ca exchange. *Am. J. Physiol.* **236**, C103–C110.

Philipson, K. D., and Langer, G. A. (1979). Sarcolemmal-bound calcium and contractility in the mammalian myocardium. *J. Mol. Cell. Cardiol.* **11**, 857–875.

Philipson, K. D., and Nishimoto, A. Y. (1984). Stimulation of $Na^+–Ca^{2+}$ exchange in cardiac sarcolemmal vesicles by phospholipase D. *J. Biol. Chem.* **259**, 16–19.

Philipson, K. D., Bers, D. M., Nishimoto, A. Y., and Langer, G. A. (1980a). Binding of Ca^{2+} and Na^+ to sarcolemmal membranes: Relation to control of myocardial contractility. *Am. J. Physiol.* **238**, H373–H378.

Philipson, K. D., Bers, D. M., and Nishimoto, A. Y. (1980b). The role of phospholipids in the Ca^{2+} binding of isolated sarcolemma. *J. Mol. Cell Cardiol.* **12**, 1159–1173.

Pytkowski, B., Lewartowski, B., Prokopczuk, A., Solanowski, K., and Lewandowska, K. (1983). Excitation- and rest-dependent shifts of Ca in guinea-pig ventricular myocardium. *Pflügers Arch.* **398**, 103–112.

Rainier, S., Mahendrok, J. K., Ramirez, F., Ponayiotis, V. I., Marecek, J. F., and Wagner, R. (1979). Phase transition characteristics of diphosphatidylglycerol (cardiolipin) and stereoisometric phosphatidylacylglycerol bilayers. Mono- and divalent metal ion effects. *Biochim. Biophys. Acta* **558**, 187–198.

Sanborn, W. G., and Langer, G. A. (1970). Specific uncoupling of excitation and contraction in mammalian cardiac tissue by lanthanum. *J. Gen. Physiol.* **56**, 191–217.

Seimiya, T., and Ohki, S. (1973). Ionic structure of phospholipid membranes and binding of calcium ions. *Biochim. Biophys. Acta* **298**, 546–561.

Storm, D. R., Rosenthal, K. S., and Swanson, P. F. (1977). Polymyxin and related peptide antibiotics. *Ann. Rev. Biochem.* **46**, 723–763.

Teuber, M., and Miller, R. (1977). Selective binding of Polymyxin B to negatively charged lipid monolayers. *Biochim. Biophys. Acta* **467**, 280–289.

Tibbits, G. F., Sasaki, M., Ikeda, M., Shimada, K., Tsuruhara, T., and Nagatomo, T. (1981). Characterization of rat myocardial sarcolemma. *J. Mol. Cell. Cardiol.* **13**, 1051–1061.

11

Release of Calcium from the Sarcoplasmic Reticulum

Alexandre Fabiato

I. INTRODUCTION

The physiological mechanism that releases calcium from the sarcoplasmic reticulum is not known for either cardiac or skeletal muscle (Fabiato, 1983). For cardiac muscle it is not even universally agreed that calcium is released from the sarcoplasmic reticulum during excitation–contraction coupling. Accordingly, the first section of this chapter reviews the arguments of whether a release of calcium from the sarcoplasmic reticulum participates in cardiac excitation–contraction coupling. Thereafter, alternative hypotheses for the mechanism of the release of calcium from the cardiac sarcoplasmic reticulum are discussed. These hypotheses suggest respectively that the release of calcium is induced by calcium, depolarization, sodium, change of pH, movement of transverse tubular or sarcolemmal charged particles, or inositol (1,4,5)-trisphosphate. Because none of these hypotheses is yet supported by compelling evidence, the chapter has no conclusions.

II. EVIDENCE FOR AND AGAINST A RELEASE OF CALCIUM FROM THE SARCOPLASMIC RETICULUM DURING CARDIAC EXCITATION–CONTRACTION COUPLING

Analyses of the force–frequency relationships (Antoni *et al.*, 1969; Koch-Weser and Blinks, 1963; Kruta and Bravený, 1968; Wohlfart and Noble, 1982;

283

Wood *et al.*, 1969); voltage-clamp studies of the relationships between calcium current and contraction (Beeler and Reuter, 1970; Morad and Goldman, 1973; Winegrad, 1979), aequorin bioluminescence recordings of changes in intracellular free calcium concentration (Wier, 1980; Wier and Isenberg, 1982), and studies of the effects of pharmacological and ionic interventions in intact cardiac muscle (Chapman, 1983) suggest that a release of calcium from an internal store participates in cardiac excitation–contraction coupling. The evidence is, however, indirect, and alternative hypotheses explain the results in intact cardiac muscle by either calcium stored in structures other than the sarcoplasmic reticulum or a direct activation of the myofilaments by transsarcolemmal influx of calcium without the help of any release of calcium from an internal store.

Among the hypotheses placing the calcium store in organelles other than the sarcoplasmic reticulum, the mitochondria have been proposed as a possible storage site (Affolter *et al.*, 1976). This seems very unlikely because the mitochondria have much too low an affinity for calcium and rate of calcium binding to participate in the beat-to-beat regulation of cytosolic calcium (Fabiato and Fabiato, 1979; Somlyo *et al.*, 1981). Another hypothesis locates the store in potential-dependent binding sites at the inner face of the sarcolemma (Lüllmann *et al.*, 1983), although this hypothesis is not supported by any direct evidence.

The hypotheses negating the need of a calcium store because the transsarcolemmal influx of calcium would be sufficient to activate the myofilaments directly (Langer, 1976; Mensing and Hilgemann, 1981; Lewartowski *et al.*, 1982) are based on the assumption that the changes of intracellular free calcium concentration resulting from the transsarcolemmal influx of calcium can be inferred from the change of total influx of calcium. This is, in fact, not possible on the basis of currently available information (Fabiato, 1983). Even if the transsarcolemmal influx of calcium could be found sufficient to permit direct activation of the myofilaments in some cardiac tissues, at some developmental stages, or under certain experimental conditions, this would still not prove that such a direct activation indeed takes place. Some of the calcium that has crossed the sarcolemma could be accumulated in the sarcoplasmic reticulum, and an about equal amount could be released from the sarcoplasmic reticulum (Fabiato, 1983).

Thus, the experiments in intact cardiac muscle provide no compelling argument against the participation of a release of calcium from the sarcoplasmic reticulum in cardiac excitation–contraction coupling. Direct evidence of an intracellular calcium store in the adult mammalian or avian cardiac cell and that the storage site is the sarcoplasmic reticulum (Fabiato, 1982, 1983) has been provided by experiments with single cardiac cells from which the sarcolemma had been removed by microdissection (skinned cardiac cells). Unfortunately, the procedures for obtaining these preparations may result in unphysiological modifications. This argument may be used to question the physiological role of a calcium release from the sarcoplasmic reticulum and, even more so, the specific hypotheses for the mechanism of this release that are discussed in the subsequent sections of this chapter.

III. HYPOTHESIS OF CALCIUM-INDUCED RELEASE OF CALCIUM FROM THE SARCOPLASMIC RETICULUM

The hypothesis of calcium-induced release of calcium from the cardiac sarcoplasmic reticulum is that the increase of free calcium at the outer surface of the sarcoplasmic reticulum, which results from the transsarcolemmal influx, induces a release of calcium from the sarcoplasmic reticulum, which, in turn, activates the myofilaments (Fabiato, 1983). The calcium-induced release of calcium can be triggered by an increase of free calcium concentration much lower than that needed to activate the myofilaments directly in the skinned cells from each of the adult mammalian and avian cardiac tissues studied, provided that the rate of increase is sufficiently high (Fabiato, 1982, 1983).

The amount of calcium released increases when the free calcium concentration used as a trigger rises to an optimum level, above which any further increase inhibits the process. Such an inhibition occurs at the level of free calcium concentration outside the sarcoplasmic reticulum that is reached at the peak of the release of calcium (Fabiato, 1983). This negative feedback helps to explain why calcium-induced release of calcium is graded rather than all or none as previously assumed (Costantin and Taylor, 1973).

The activation and inactivation of calcium-induced release of calcium are not only calcium dependent but also time dependent. Thus, a fast increase of free calcium at the outer surface of the sarcoplasmic reticulum triggers a release of calcium, whereas a slow increase to the same final level loads the sarcoplasmic reticulum with an amount of calcium that will be available for release during the subsequent contractions. The transsarcolemmal calcium current presents both a fast and a slow component (McDonald, 1982; Tsien, 1983), which may, therefore, serve respectively to trigger the release of calcium from the sarcoplasmic reticulum and to load the sarcoplasmic reticulum with calcium (Fig. 1). The transsarcolemmal influx of calcium is not, however, limited necessarily to calcium channels; it might occur also through sodium–calcium exchange.

After a release of calcium has been triggered by an increase of free calcium in the solution bathing a skinned cardiac cell, the release recurs cyclically through a different mechanism corresponding to a calcium overload of the sarcoplasmic reticulum (Fabiato, 1983), unless the concentration of free calcium at the outer surface of the sarcoplasmic reticulum is decreased approximately as much as it has been increased. Thus, if calcium-induced release of calcium from the sar-

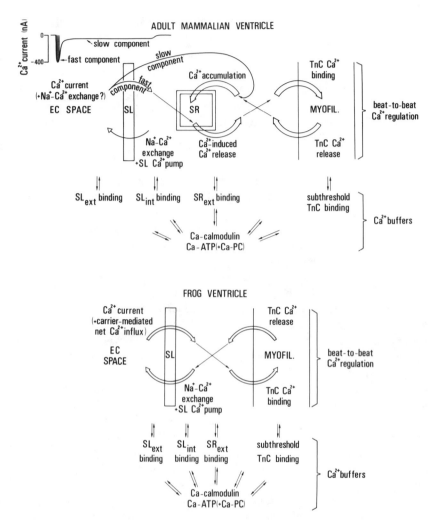

Fig. 1. Hypothesis of calcium-induced release of calcium from the sarcoplasmic reticulum during cardiac excitation–contraction coupling in adult mammalian ventricular cells, and absence of this process in the frog ventricular cell. SL, sarcolemma; SR, sarcoplasmic reticulum; myofil., myofilaments; PC, phosphocreatine; EC, extracellular; TnC, troponin C; subscripts ext and int, external and internal, respectively. [From Fabiato (1983), reprinted with permission of the American Physiological Society.]

coplasmic reticulum does play a physiological role in cardiac excitation–contraction coupling, the reaccumulation of calcium into the sarcoplasmic reticulum should be backed up by the outward transsarcolemmal movements of calcium by sodium–calcium exchange and the sarcolemmal calcium pump (Fig. 1). Only that calcium released from the sarcoplasmic reticulum would activate the myofilaments, and calcium released from the activated myofilaments would be reaccumulated into the sarcoplasmic reticulum, which is wrapped around individual myofibrils (Fig. 1). In addition to this beat-to-beat regulation of calcium, the resting level of free calcium would be regulated by a number of diffusible binding sites on calmodulin, ATP, and phosphocreatine and fixed binding sites on the sarcolemma, sarcoplasmic reticulum, and myofilaments.

The prominence of calcium-induced release of calcium among skinned cells from cardiac tissues varies with the species of animal as well as with the stage of embryonic and postnatal development or the aging process of a given cardiac tissue (Fabiato, 1982) in a manner consistent with the variations of excitation–contraction coupling in intact cardiac muscles (Chapman, 1983; Bers *et al.*, 1981; Sutko and Willerson, 1980). Calcium-induced release of calcium is completely absent in skinned cardiac cells from the frog ventricle (Fabiato, 1983), in which the activation of the myofilaments can be accomplished entirely by the transsarcolemmal influx of calcium, whereas the removal of calcium can be accomplished entirely by the transsarcolemmal processes of calcium extrusion: the sodium–calcium exchange and the sarcolemmal calcium pump (Fig. 1).

There is yet no steadfast argument against the hypothesis of a physiological role for calcium-induced release of calcium from the sarcoplasmic reticulum. This is not to say that such a hypothesis should be accepted, inasmuch as it relies almost entirely on experiments with skinned cardiac cells and can be criticized because of some unphysiological conditions that might be created by the preparation procedures. For this reason, the readers should not give excessive attention to this hypothesis and neglect alternative possibilities. This recommendation is especially important because, as is shown in the subsequent sections, new working hypotheses need to be sought inasmuch as all the other hypotheses appear to be unlikely, at least in their present form.

IV. HYPOTHESIS OF DEPOLARIZATION-INDUCED RELEASE OF CALCIUM FROM THE SARCOPLASMIC RETICULUM

The hypothesis of depolarization-induced release of calcium from the sarcoplasmic reticulum stipulates that the depolarization of the sarcolemma or the transverse tubules is transmitted to the sarcoplasmic reticular membrane causing a depolarization of the latter and opening channels through which calcium would flow down its concentration gradient from the lumen of the sarcoplasmic reticulum to the myoplasm. This hypothesis is not supported by experiments with skinned cardiac cells (Fabiato, 1985a). Electrical currents cause release of calcium from the sarcoplasmic reticulum only when the current density is sufficiently high to damage the sarcoplasmic reticulum (Fabiato, 1985a).

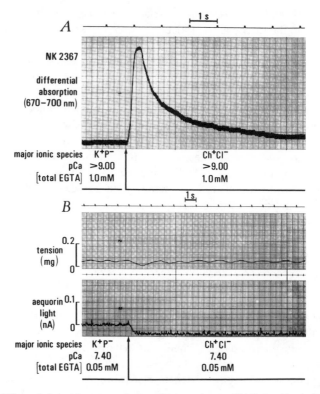

Fig. 2. Effect of the replacement of potassium propionate (K^+P^-) with choline chloride (Ch^+Cl^-) on the signal recorded with the potential-sensitive dye NK 2367 (A) and on the calcium release detected with aequorin (B) in two different skinned cardiac cells from the pigeon ventricle. Arrows indicate the time of solution change. Both skinned cardiac cells had been treated for 15 min with a solution of high ionic strength (0.510 *M*) to extract myosin and thereby eliminate the contraction artifact that would have been a major problem for the light absorption measurement with the potential-sensitive dye (Fabiato, 1985a). The solution used for the experiment itself had in both cases an ionic strength of 0.160 *M*. In panel (B) the pronounced downward deflection (direction opposite to that for a calcium release) of the aequorin light signal might correspond to a more depressive effect of 0.160 *M* ionic strength on the binding of calcium to aequorin when choline, instead of potassium, is the major cation. The slight downward movement of the tension trace caused by the solution change is related to the considerable increase of the compliance of the preparation resulting from myosin extraction. [From Fabiato (1985a), reprinted with permission of Academic Press.]

Figure 2 illustrates another method for attempting to depolarize the sarcoplasmic reticular membrane of skinned cardiac cells; this technique consists of a rapid substitution of ions in the bathing solution with anions and cations to which the membrane presents unequal permeabilities. Initially, the preparation is equilibrated in the presence of potassium propionate. The permeability of the sarcoplasmic reticular membrane is high for potassium but low for propionate.

After several minutes of equilibration, however, propionate penetrates inside the sarcoplasmic reticulum. The solution is then changed rapidly for one containing choline chloride. The permeability of the sarcoplasmic reticular membrane is low for choline but high for chloride. For a brief time after the ionic substitution, chloride ions enter the sarcoplasmic reticulum rapidly while propionate ions leave slowly, producing a transient increase of negative charge inside the sarcoplasmic reticulum. Simultaneously, potassium ions leave the sarcoplasmic reticulum rapidly while choline ions penetrate slowly; this results in a transient increase of positive charge outside the sarcoplasmic reticulum. Thus, both anionic and cationic substitutions should concur to render the outer surface of the sarcoplasmic reticulum more positive with respect to the inner surface than it was before the double ionic substitution. This would result in a depolarization of the sarcoplasmic reticular membrane if this membrane were polarized oppositely to the sarcolemma: negatively outside and positively inside.

Under conditions preventing any movement of calcium [i.e., the sarcoplasmic reticulum had been emptied by exposure to a very low free calcium concentration (pCa > 9.00) in the presence of a high total concentration of ethyleneglycol-bis(β-aminoethyl ether) $-N,N'$-tetraacetic acid (EGTA)], the double ionic substitution produced a transient signal that was detected with a potential-sensitive dye (Fig. 2A). Although these dyes detect changes of transmembrane potential in squid axon, it has not been possible to demonstrate that this transient signal does, indeed, correspond to a change of potential across the sarcoplasmic reticular membrane rather than to a mere change of surface potential.

The most definitive evidence against the hypothesis of depolarization-induced release of calcium from the sarcoplasmic reticulum is that the ionic substitution, which elicited a signal from potential-sensitive dyes, failed to induce any release of calcium from the sarcoplasmic reticulum that could be detected by recordings of tension or of aequorin bioluminescence, even when the sarcoplasmic reticulum was loaded optimally with calcium (by preequilibration in a solution at pCa 7.40) in the presence of a low total EGTA concentration (Fig. 2B).

V. HYPOTHESIS OF SODIUM-INDUCED RELEASE OF CALCIUM FROM THE SARCOPLASMIC RETICULUM

The hypothesis of sodium-induced release of calcium from the sarcoplasmic reticulum is that the transsarcolemmal influx of sodium occurring during the upstroke of the action potential triggers the calcium release. This hypothesis received initial support from experiments with fragmented sarcoplasmic reticulum (Palmer and Posey, 1967), but these early preparations were highly contaminated with fragmented sarcolemma and mitochondria, for which the competition between sodium and calcium is well established (Fabiato, 1986b). The hypothesis is still supported by indirect evidence obtained from intact frog atrial muscle (Vassort, 1973), even though the sarcoplasmic reticulum is poorly developed in this tissue (Fabiato, 1983). Extensive experiments in skinned cardiac cells have failed, however, to substantiate this hypothesis (Fabiato and Fabiato, 1976; Fabiato, 1986b). Partial substitution of sodium for potassium in a concentration range likely to occur during the action potential had no effect. The complete substitution of sodium for potassium depressed accumulation of calcium into the sarcoplasmic reticulum. Thus, subsequent releases of calcium by the calcium-triggered process were of smaller amplitude because they issued from a less-loaded sarcoplasmic reticulum. This total ionic substitution did not, however, induce a release of calcium from the sarcoplasmic reticulum, nor did it have any immediate direct effect on the release of calcium induced by the calcium-triggered process.

VI. HYPOTHESIS OF RELEASE OF CALCIUM FROM THE SARCOPLASMIC RETICULUM INDUCED BY A CHANGE IN pH

A change in pH has been proposed as a mechanism for release of calcium from the sarcoplasmic reticulum (Nakamaru and Schwartz, 1970; Shoshan *et al.*, 1981). The results in skinned cardiac cells have been totally negative (Fabiato, 1985b). As for the substitution of sodium for potassium, changes in pH appeared to affect the accumulation of calcium into the sarcoplasmic reticulum but not the release of calcium (Fabiato and Fabiato, 1978; Fabiato, 1985b).

VII. HYPOTHESIS OF RELEASE OF CALCIUM INDUCED BY MOVEMENT OF TRANSVERSE TUBULAR OR SARCOLEMMAL CHARGED PARTICLES LINKED MECHANICALLY TO SITES IN THE SARCOPLASMIC RETICULAR MEMBRANE

The contractile activation is controlled tightly by the potential imposed on the sarcolemma and, presumably, the transverse tubules of skeletal muscle (Costantin and Taylor, 1973). On the other hand, an electrical coupling between the transverse tubules and sarcoplasmic reticulum is not supported by available data

(Fabiato and Fabiato, 1979). Thus, it has been proposed that the coupling could be mechanical according to the following hypothesis.

Electrophysiological experiments in skeletal muscle have provided evidence for very low-level currents caused by the displacement of charged macromolecules embedded in the transverse tubular membrane (Chandler et al., 1976). It has been hypothesized that the charged particles in the transverse tubular membrane might be linked mechanically to sites in the sarcoplasmic reticular membrane that may correspond to foot processes made of electron-dense material (Franzini-Armstrong, 1975) or pillars made by a pair of electron-opaque lines bounding an electron-lucent interior (Somlyo, 1979), which have been seen in electron micrographs. A similarity was observed between the

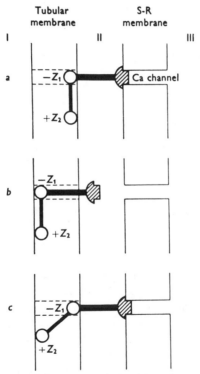

Fig. 3. A mechanical hypothesis for calcium release from the terminal cisternae of the sarcoplasmic reticulum of skeletal muscle. (I) denotes the lumen of the transverse tubules; the space labeled (II) is continuous with the sarcoplasm; and (III) indicates the inside of the terminal cisternae of the sarcoplasmic reticulum, where calcium is thought to be stored in skeletal muscle (Winegrad, 1979). Z_1 and Z_2 are charged molecules. Configuration a corresponds to the resting state, b to the activated state, and c to the refractory state. [Reproduced from Chandler et al. (1976), with permission of the authors and The Physiological Society.]

number of charged groups detected electrophysiologically and the number of foot processes determined by electron microscopy (Schneider and Chandler, 1973); however, recent data suggest that this relationship may be more complex than one charged macromolecule attached to each foot process (Schneider, 1981). Thus, the depolarization-induced movement of charged particles in the transverse tubular membrane would unplug a channel across the sarcoplasmic reticular membrane and allow calcium to flow down its concentration gradient (Fig. 3).

Tests of this hypothesis are very difficult in skeletal muscle and have not even been attempted in cardiac muscle. In the latter tissue, the charged particles might occur not only in the membrane of the transverse tubules, which are absent in some tissues, but also in that portion of sarcolemma forming diadic junctions with the sarcoplasmic reticulum.

VIII.   HYPOTHESIS OF RELEASE OF CALCIUM FROM THE SARCOPLASMIC RETICULUM INDUCED BY INOSITOL (1,4,5)-TRISPHOSPHATE

Inositol(1,4,5)-trisphosphate is an ubiquitous second messenger that induces release of calcium from the endoplasmic reticulum of nonmuscle cells (Streb *et al.*, 1983; Burgess *et al.*, 1984; Berridge, 1984) and from the sarcoplasmic reticulum of cardiac (Hirata *et al.*, 1984; Fabiato, 1986a), skeletal (Vergara *et al.*, 1985; Volpe *et al.*, 1985), and smooth muscle (Suematsu *et al.*, 1984; Somlyo *et al.*, 1985).

Experiments in skinned cardiac cells (Fabiato, 1986a) showed that inositol(1,4,5)-trisphosphate induces a slow release of calcium which causes a tension transient that increases from 3 to 10–15% of maximum tension, when the concentration of inositol(1,4,5)-trisphosphate is increased from 2 to 30 μM. If an optimum trigger for calcium-induced release of calcium is applied simultaneously with a near-optimum concentration of inositol(1,4,5)-trisphosphate, the tension transient resulting from the calcium release from the sarcoplasmic reticulum presents two distinct components: the inositol(1,4,5)-trisphosphate-induced release of calcium occurs much later than the calcium-induced release of calcium. This suggests that inositol(1,4,5)-trisphosphate-induced release of calcium is much less likely to be the primary mechanism of excitation–contraction coupling in cardiac muscle than calcium-induced release of calcium (Fabiato, 1986a). However, inositol(1,4,5)-trisphosphate-induced release of calcium may play a role in the modulation of calcium release by hormones or pharmacological agents. Note also that inositol(1,4,5)-trisphosphate enhances the spontaneous release of calcium that occurs when the sarcoplasmic reticulum is overloaded with calcium (Fabiato, 1986a).

These preliminary results with inositol(1,4,5)-trisphosphate are mentioned to examplify the continued consideration of alternative hypotheses for the mechanism of calcium release from the cardiac sarcoplasmic reticulum. The hypothesis of a calcium-induced release of calcium should not gain undue attention only because all other current hypotheses for the mechanism of calcium release from the sarcoplasmic reticulum appear to be unlikely.

ACKNOWLEDGMENTS

This review was supported by Grant HL 19138 from the National Heart, Lung, and Blood Institute and by Grant 83-667 from the American Heart Association.

REFERENCES

Affolter, H., Chiesi, M., Dabrowska, R., and Carafoli, E. (1976). Calcium regulation in heart cells. The interaction of mitochondrial and sarcoplasmic reticulum with troponin-bound calcium. *Eur. J. Biochem.* **67**, 389–396.

Antoni, H., Jacob, R., and Kaufmann, R. (1969). Mechanische reaktionen des frosch- und säugetier-myokards bei veränderung der aktionspotential-dauer durch konstante gleichstromimpulse. *Pflügers Arch.* **306**, 33–57.

Beeler, G. W., Jr., and Reuter, H. (1970). The relation between membrane potential, membrane currents and activation of contraction in ventricular myocardial fibres. *J. Physiol. (Lond)* **207**, 211–229.

Berridge, M. J. (1984). Inositol trisphosphate and diacylglycerol as second messengers. *Biochem. J.* **220**, 345–360.

Bers, D. M., Philipson, K. D., and Langer, G. A. (1981). Cardiac contractility and sarcolemmal calcium binding in several cardiac muscle preparations. *Am. J. Physiol.* **240**, H576–H583.

Burgess, G. M., Godfrey, P. P., McKinney, J. S., Berridge, M. J., Irvine, R. F., and Putney, J. W., Jr. (1984). The second messenger linking receptor activation to internal Ca release in liver. *Nature* **309**, 63–66.

Chandler, W. K., Rakowski, R. F., and Schneider, M. F. (1976). Effects of glycerol treatment and maintained depolarization on charge movement in skeletal muscle. *J. Physiol. (Lond.)* **254**, 285–316.

Chapman, R. A. (1983). Control of cardiac contractility at the cellular level. *Am. J. Physiol.* **245**, H535–H552.

Costantin, L. L., and Taylor, S. R. (1973). Graded activation in frog muscle fibers. *J. Gen. Physiol.* **61**, 424–443.

Fabiato, A. (1982). Calcium release in skinned cardiac cells: Variations with species, tissues, and development. *Fed. Proc.* **41**, 2238–2244.

Fabiato, A. (1983). Calcium-induced release of calcium from the cardiac sarcoplasmic reticulum. *Am. J. Physiol.* **245**, C1–C14.

Fabiato, A. (1985a). Appraisal of the hypothesis of the ''depolarization-induced'' release of calcium from the sarcoplasmic reticulum in skinned cardiac cells from the rat or pigeon ventricle. *In* ''Structure and Function of the Sarcoplasmic Reticulum'' (S. Fleischer and Y. Tonomura, eds.), pp. 479–519. Academic Press, New York.

Fabiato, A. (1985b). Appraisal of the hypothesis of a Ca^{2+} release from the sarcoplasmic reticulum induced by a change of pH in a skinned canine cardiac Purkinje cell. *Cell Calcium* **6**, 95–108.

Fabiato, A. (1986a). Inositol (1,4,5)-trisphosphate-induced release of Ca^{2+} from the sarcoplasmic reticulum of skinned cardiac cells. *Biophys. J.* **49**, 190a.

Fabiato, A. (1986b). Appraisal of the hypothesis of the sodium-induced release of calcium from the sarcoplasmic reticulum or the mitochondria in skinned cardiac cells from the rat ventricle and the canine Purkinje tissue. *In* ''Sarcoplasmic Reticulum in Muscle Physiology,'' Vol. 2 (M. L. Entman and W. B. Van Winkle, eds.), pp. 51–72. CRC Press, Boca Raton, Florida.

Fabiato, A., and Fabiato, F. (1976). Techniques of skinned cardiac cells and of isolated cardiac fibers with disrupted sarcolemmas with reference to the effects of catecholamines and of caffeine. *In* ''Recent Advances in Studies on Cardiac Structure and Metabolism,'' Vol. 9, ''The Sarcolemma'' (P.-E. Roy and N. S. Dhalla, eds.), pp. 71–94. University Park Press, Baltimore.

Fabiato, A., and Fabiato, F. (1978). Effects of pH on the myofilaments and the sarcoplasmic reticulum of skinned cells from cardiac and skeletal muscles. *J. Physiol. (Lond.)* **276**, 233–255.

Fabiato, A., and Fabiato, F. (1979). Calcium and cardiac excitation–contraction coupling. *Ann. Rev. Physiol.* **41**, 473–484.

Franzini-Armstrong, C. (1975). Membrane particles and transmission at the triad. *Fed. Proc.* **34**, 1382–1389.

Hirata, M., Suematsu, E., Hashimoto, T., Hamachi, T., and Koga, T. (1984). Release of Ca^{2+} from a non-mitochondrial store site in peritoneal macrophages treated with saponin by inositol 1,4,5-trisphosphate. *Biochem. J.* **223**, 229–236.

Koch-Weser, J., and Blinks, J. R. (1963). The influence of the interval between beats on myocardial contractility. *Pharmacol. Rev.* **15**, 601–652.

Kruta, V., and Bravený, P. (1968). Possible mechanisms involved in potentiation phenomena. *In* ''Paired Pulse Stimulation of the Heart'' (P. F. Cranefield and B. F. Hoffman, eds.), pp. 53–64. Rockefeller University Press, New York.

Langer, G. A. (1976). Events at the cardiac sarcolemma: Localization and movement of contractile-dependent calcium. *Fed. Proc.* **35**, 1274–1278.

Lewartowski, B., Pytkowski, B., Prokopszuk, A., Wasilewski-Dziubinska, W., and Otwinowski, W. (1982). Amount and turnover of calcium entering the cells of ventricular myocardium of guinea pig heart at single excitation. *In* ''Advances in Myocardiology,'' Vol. 3 (E. Chazov, W. Smirnow, and N. S. Dhalla, eds.), pp. 345–357. Plenum Press, New York.

Lüllmann, H., Peters, T., and Preuner, J. (1983). Role of the plasmalemma for calcium homeostasis and for excitation–contraction coupling in cardiac muscle. *In* ''Cardiac Metabolism'' (A. J. Drake-Holland and M. I. M. Noble, eds.), pp. 1–18. John Wiley & Sons, London.

McDonald, T. F. (1982). The slow inward calcium current in the heart. *Ann. Rev. Physiol.* **44**, 425–434.

Mensing, H. J., and Hilgemann, D. W. (1981). Inotropic effects of activation and pharmacological mechanisms in cardiac muscle. *Trends Pharmacol. Sci.* **2**, 303–307.

Morad, M., and Goldman, Y. (1973). Excitation–contraction coupling in heart muscle: Membrane control of development of tension. *Prog. Biophys. Mol. Biol.* **27**, 257–313.

Nakamura, Y., and Schwartz, A. (1970). Possible control of intracellular calcium metabolism by $[H^+]$: Sarcoplasmic reticulum of skeletal and cardiac muscle. *Biochem. Biophys. Res. Commun.* **41**, 830–836.

Palmer, R. F., and Posey, V. A. (1967). Ion effects on calcium accumulation by cardiac sarcoplasmic reticulum. *J. Gen. Physiol.* **50**, 2085–2095.

Schneider, M. F. (1981). Membrane charge movement and depolarization–contraction coupling. *Ann. Rev. Physiol.* **43**, 507–517.

Schneider, M. F., and Chandler, W. K. (1973). Voltage dependent charge movement in skeletal muscle: A possible step in excitation–contraction coupling. *Nature* **242**, 244–246.

Shoshan, V., MacLennan, D. H., and Wood, D. S. (1981). A proton gradient controls a calcium-release channel in sarcoplasmic reticulum. *Proc. Natl. Acad. Sci. U.S.A.* **78**, 4828–4832.

Somlyo, A. P., Somlyo, A. V., Shuman, H., Scarpa, A., Endo, M., and Inesi, G. (1981). Mitochondria do not accumulate significant Ca concentrations in normal cells. *In* "Calcium and Phosphate Transport across Biomembranes" (F. Bronner and M. Peterlik, eds.), pp. 87–93. Academic Press, New York.

Somlyo, A. V. (1979). Bridging structures spanning the junctional gap at the triad of skeletal muscle. *J. Cell Biol.* **80**, 743–750.

Somlyo, A. V., Bond, M., Somlyo, A. P., and Scarpa, A. (1985). Inositol trisphosphate-induced calcium release and contraction in vascular smooth muscle. *Proc. Natl. Acad. Sci. U.S.A.* **82**, 5231–5235.

Streb, H., Irvine, R. F., Berridge, M. J., and Schulz, I. (1983). Release of Ca^{2+} from a nonmitochondrial intracellular store in pancreatic acinar cells by inositol-1,4,5-trisphosphate. *Nature* **306**, 67–69.

Suematsu, E., Hirata, M., Hashimoto, T., and Kuriyama, H. (1984). Inositol 1,4,5-trisphosphate releases Ca^{2+} from intracellular store sites in skinned single cells in porcine coronary artery. *Biochem. Biophys. Res. Commun.* **120**, 481–485.

Sutko, J. L., and Willerson, J. T. (1980). Ryanodine alteration of the contractile state of rat ventricular myocardium. Comparison with dog, cat, and rabbit ventricular tissues. *Circ. Res.* **46**, 332–343.

Tsien, R. W. (1983). Calcium channels in excitable cell membranes. *Ann. Rev. Physiol.* **45**, 341–358.

Vassort, G. (1973). Influence of sodium ions on the regulation of frog myocardial contractility. *Pflügers Arch.* **339**, 225–240.

Vergara, J., Tsien, R. Y., and Delay, M. (1985). Inositol 1,4,5-trisphosphate: A possible chemical link in excitation-contraction coupling in muscle. *Proc. Natl. Acad. Sci. U.S.A.* **82**, 6352–6356.

Volpe, P., Salviati, G., Di Virgilio, F., and Pozzan, T. (1985). Inositol 1,4,5-trisphosphate induces calcium release from sarcoplasmic reticulum of skeletal muscle. *Nature* **316**, 347–349.

Wier, W. G. (1980). Calcium transients during excitation–contraction coupling in mammalian heart: Aequorin signals of canine Purkinje fibers. *Science* **207**, 1085–1087.

Wier, W. G., and Isenberg, G. (1982). Intracellular [Ca^{2+}] transients in voltage clamped cardiac Purkinje fibers. *Pflügers Arch.* **392**, 284–290.

Winegard, S. (1979). Electromechanical coupling in heart muscle. *In* "Handbook of Physiology," Section 2, "The Cardiovascular System," Vol. I, "The Heart" (R. M. Berne, N. Sperelakis, and S. R. Geiger, eds.), pp. 393–428. American Physiological Society, Bethesda, Maryland.

Wohlfart, B., and Noble, M. I. M. (1982). The cardiac excitation–contraction cycle. *Pharmac. Ther.* **16**, 1–43.

Wood, E. H., Heppner, R. L., and Weidmann, S. (1969). Inotropic effects of electric currents. I. Positive and negative effects of constant electric currents or current pulses applied during cardiac action potentials. II. Hypotheses: Calcium movements, excitation–contraction coupling and inotropic effects. *Circ. Res.* **24**, 409–445.

12

Calcium-Binding Proteins in the Regulation of Muscle Contraction

J. David Johnson, Elias J. Khabbaza, Brinda L. Bailey, and Theodore J. Grieshop

I. INTRODUCTION

One of the most vital functions of any excitable cell is to maintain its intracellular calcium ion concentration $[Ca]_i$ at certain discrete levels. Muscle is relaxed when $[Ca]_i$ falls below 10^{-7} M and contracts as Ca^{2+} rises above this level to several micromolar. The cell has the tremendous task of maintaining 10,000 extracellular calcium ions for each calcium ion that enters. This requires a very precise control and interplay of calcium influx and efflux mechanisms. Calcium homeostasis is regulated by membrane-bound calcium transporters, antiporters, channels, and ATPases. Some of these proteins occur in the sarcolemma or cell membrane of muscle, whereas others exist primarily in intracellular membranes that sequester calcium, e.g., the sarcoplasmic reticulum (SR) and mitochondria (MITO).

A schematic of the regulators of calcium homeostasis and contraction is shown in Fig. 1. Depolarization of the cell membrane occurs as Na^+ channels open allowing Na^+ to follow its concentration gradient ($[Na]_e = 140$ mM, $[Na]_i = 10$ mM) into the cell. With depolarization, the slow voltage-dependent calcium channels open, allowing extracellular calcium to enter. These calcium channels are the primary pathway by which extracellular calcium enters the cell; they can be inhibited selectively by calcium channel blocking drugs (calcium antagonists) such as nifedipine, diltiazem, and verapamil (see Janis and Triggle, 1983, for review). In many tissues, calcium channels have a $[Ca^{2+}]$ sensor or calcium-binding protein (CBP) that closes the channel as $[Ca^{2+}]_i$ rises (see Tsien, 1983,

CARDIAC MUSCLE:
THE REGULATION OF EXCITATION AND CONTRACTION

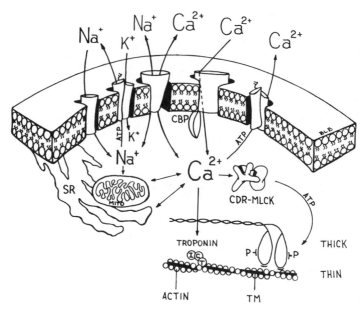

Fig. 1. A schematic representation of the transporters, antiporters, channels, ATPases, and contractile proteins that regulate calcium homeostasis and muscle contraction. Contractile mechanisms involved in both smooth muscle (calmodulin regulated) and skeletal cardiac muscle contraction (troponin regulated) are shown. Abbreviations include: SR, sarcoplasmic reticulum: MITO, mitochondria; CDR, calmodulin; MLCK, myosin light chain kinase; TM, tropomyosin; and CBP, calcium-binding proteins. See text for details of mechanisms.

review). We have suggested that these CBPs of the calcium channel are the receptors for some calcium antagonist drugs (Johnson, 1984; Johnson *et al.*, 1983) and have proposed a mechanism by which they block these channels (Johnson, 1984).

Two primary mechanisms for Ca^{2+} extrusion exist in the cell membrane. The first is a calcium ATPase, which actively extrudes intracellular calcium. The second is a $Na^+–Ca^{2+}$ antiporter. In the resting state (and to a lesser extent in the depolarized state), $[Na]_e$ is high, and the large Na^+ gradient favors entry of Na^+ and extrusion of calcium by the antiporter (see Fig. 1). A Na^+, K^+-ATPase is mainly responsible for actively transporting Na^+ out of the cell in exchange for K^+. Inhibition of this ATPase rapidly dissipates the Na^+ gradient. Under these circumstances, the $Na^+–Ca^{2+}$ exchanger can work in reverse: extracellular Ca^{2+} can enter (via its concentration gradient) and Na^+ can be extruded. Thus, when there is not a large extracellular $[Na^+]$ to pump against, the $Na^+–Ca^{2+}$ antiporter can be used as a mechanism for calcium influx.

Entry of calcium into the cell can presumably trigger the release of internal stores of calcium from the SR by a process known as calcium-induced calcium release (see A. Fabiato, Chapter 11 of this volume). The SR can actively reaccumulate calcium, a process that is mediated by a calcium-ATPase and is fundamental to relaxation of muscle. Although mitochondria accumulate calcium in a respiration-dependent manner and exhibit a Na^+-induced release of Ca^{2+} via a Na^+-Ca^{2+} antiporter (Vaghy et al., 1982), they probably play only a minimal role in regulating calcium homeostasis in normal muscle.

Calcium can be released from its internal stores by higher concentrations (μM) of contractile agonists such as histamine, serotonin, and catecholamines. These contractile agonists have effects that are tissue and species dependent, but, when they do elicit release from internal calcium stores, they can produce a contraction that is independent of extracellular calcium.

Once $[Ca^{2+}]_i$ reaches the range of $1-10$ μM, the contractile apparatus takes over to facilitate contraction. Skeletal and cardiac muscle contraction are regulated by the thin filaments. Troponin C (TnC) is the primary calcium receptor. Calcium binding produces structural changes in whole troponin (troponin I–troponin C–troponin T complex), which relieves a troponin I interaction with actin. This allows tropomyosin (TM) to roll back into the grooves of the F-actin superhelix, allowing the interaction of actin and myosin, actomyosin ATPase activity, and contraction (see Potter and Johnson, 1982). Removal of calcium from troponin C occurs with active sequestration of Ca^{2+} by SR and/or extrusion of cellular Ca^{2+} across the cell membrane, resulting in relaxation of cardiac and skeletal muscle.

Smooth muscle contractions are regulated by the thick filaments, and calmodulin, not troponin, is the primary calcium receptor. In smooth muscle, calcium binds to calmodulin (CDR of Fig. 1), causing structural changes that allow CDR to bind and activate myosin light chain kinase (MLCK). In the presence of calcium and calmodulin, this kinase phosphorylates a light chain of myosin. This results in structural changes in the thick filament, which then allow its interaction with actin, actomyosin ATPase activity, and smooth muscle contraction. Relaxation occurs when calcium is removed and calcium-insensitive phosphatases dephosphorylate the myosin light chains (see Adelstein, 1978).

Thus, while very similar mechanisms exist for regulating calcium homeostasis in cardiac, skeletal, and smooth muscle, rather dramatic differences exist in the mechanism of Ca^{2+} regulation of tension at the level of the contractile apparatus, the former two being thin filament (and troponin) regulated while the latter is thick filament (and calmodulin) regulated. Clearly, calcium-binding proteins at the level of the calcium channels, the Na^+-Ca^{2+} antiporters, the Ca^{2+}-ATPases, and the contractile apparatus (troponin and/or calmodulin) play a fundamental role in regulating muscle contraction. This family of proteins exhibits many structural similarities and is of primary importance not only in regulating calcium homeostasis within the cell but also in transducing the calcium signal into a contractile response. This chapter addresses the vital role of various calcium-binding proteins in the regulation of muscle contraction.

II. CALCIUM CHANNELS

A.   Structure

The slow, voltage-dependent calcium channel is the primary route for calcium entry in normal muscle cells. Until recently, very little was known about the structure of Ca^{2+} channels. With the advent of high-affinity radiolabeled calcium antagonists, structural information is becoming available. Recent data suggest that the calcium channel is a large multisubunit protein, MW = 210,000–278,000 that traverses the cell membrane.

Recently, Venter *et al.* (1983) used radiation inactivation to estimate the size of the Ca^{2+} channel (nitrendipine receptor) in smooth muscle as 278,000 Da. They used affinity labeling procedures to label covalently a 45,000-Da protein subunit of the channel with an analogue of nitrendipine. Campbell *et al.* (1984) used photoaffinity labeling with [³H]-nitrendipine to label covalently a protein subunit (MW = 32,000) of the calcium channel in cardiac sarcolemma and the ryanodine-sensitive fraction of cardiac sarcoplasmic reticulum.

More recently, Curtis and Catterall (1984) began solubilization and purification of the Ca^{2+} channels ([³H]-nitrendipine receptor) from transverse tubules of skeletal muscle. They have partially purified a glycoprotein with subunits of molecular weight 130,000, 50,000, and 33,000 as the nitrendipine receptor. Several lines of evidence from these laboratories indicate that the receptor for dihydropyridines (nitrendipine, nimodipine, nifedipine, or felodipine) is a protein of molecular weight in the range of 30,000–50,000.

B.   Calcium-Channel-Blocking Drugs

The effect of calcium antagonists or calcium channel blocking drugs on calcium currents and calcium channels has been discussed in detail by Kass (Chapter 2 in this volume). Much new and exciting information has come also from studies of binding of radiolabeled calcium antagonists to purified membranes from brain, heart, and smooth muscle. In vascular smooth muscle, these drugs bind with high specificity to calcium channels over a similar concentration range as they block calcium currents and relax tension (see Janis and Triggle, 1983; Gould *et al.*, 1982; Murphy *et al.*, 1983). Gould *et al.* (1982) have shown that in brain membranes, [³H]-nitrendipine binding is totally dependent on calcium. This strongly suggests that the protein component of the calcium channel that binds Ca^{2+}-channel blockers is a Ca^{2+}-binding protein. Several studies provide strong evidence that the Ca^{2+} antagonist receptor of the Ca^{2+} channel is an allosteric protein (see Murphy *et al.*, 1983, for review). Some drugs (e.g., diltiazem) can act through these allosteric mechanisms to enhance nitrendipine (dihydropyridine) binding, whereas other drugs (e.g., verapamil) noncompetitively inhibit nitrendipine binding. The Ca^{2+} channel has, therefore, several sites at which it binds various Ca^{2+}-channel blockers, and these different sites exhibit allosteric control over one another. Our best current picture of the Ca^{2+} channel is a multisubunit glycoprotein of MW = 280,000, of which one subunit (MW = 30,000–50,000) is a calcium-binding protein that exhibits allosterically related drug (Ca^{2+}-channel blocker) -binding sites.

C. Calcium-Induced Inactivation of Calcium Channels

In addition to their Ca^{2+}-dependent binding of dihydropyridines, many Ca^{2+} channels exhibit another Ca^{2+}-dependent process, that of Ca^{2+} inactivation. These Ca^{2+} channels close or inactivate as intracellular Ca^{2+} rises above the micromolar range. Through this process, the cell can presumably protect itself from the deleterious effects of very high intracellular calcium. As intracellular calcium rises, it binds to a calcium sensor or calcium-binding protein on the channel, producing structural changes in this CBP that result in channel blockade or inactivation. As intracellular calcium is reduced (e.g., during relaxation), calcium is removed from this CBP gate, relieving its inhibition of the channel and allowing the channel to open and facilitate influx of Ca^{2+} with the next depolarization.

There is evidence of calcium inactivation in skeletal muscle, paramecium, heart (see Tsien, 1983, for review), and smooth muscle (Godfraind, 1983). Teleologically, those muscle cells that are regulated by entry of extracellular Ca^{2+} (such as smooth and cardiac muscle) might be expected to use calcium inactivation to regulate entry of calcium and contraction.

Figure 2 shows a schematic representation of a Ca^{2+} channel under depolarized conditions. In Fig. 2A, the channel is open, allowing Ca^{2+} influx in support of contraction. As intracellular [Ca^{2+}] rises, it binds to a CBP region of the channel to close the channel via Ca^{2+} inactivation. Ca^{2+} binding (perhaps to this same CBP component of the channel) can promote the binding of dihydropyridines, such as nifedipine, to the calcium channel, resulting in channel blockade.

Thus, in this schematic, the CBP responsible for calcium inactivation of this channel is shown as the CBP that binds nitrendipine in a calcium-dependent manner and that is affected allosterically by other Ca^{2+} antagonists.

Because Ca^{2+} directs both calcium inactivation and dihydropyridine binding

A   B

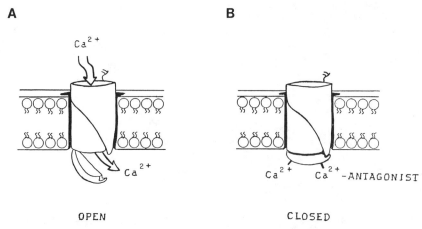

OPEN   CLOSED

Fig. 2. A schematic representation of a calcium channel under depolarized conditions (gates open). In (A), the channel is open, allowing calcium to enter the cell. As intracellular calcium rises (B), it binds to a calcium-binding protein subunit of the channel resulting in channel blockade. Calcium antagonists may bind to this same site, increasing its affinity for calcium and producing channel blockade. See text for details.

of Ca^{2+} channels, we believe that a single CBP (i.e., the CBP of Fig. 2) could be responsible for calcium inactivation and be the pharmacological receptor for some calcium antagonists. If this is the case, those tissues that are sensitive to calcium antagonist drugs should exhibit Ca^{2+} inactivation. We have tested this premise in coronary arteries, which are among the most sensitive to relaxation by Ca^{2+} antagonists. Coronary arteries were rinsed several times with a Ca^{2+}-free, physiological saline solution (PSS). These coronaries were depolarized by 35 mM KCl (to open the Ca^{2+} channels) and then titrated with Ca^{2+}. Tension as a function of added calcium is shown in Fig. 3. Tension increased to a maximum near 2.5 mM and declined in the presence of higher concentrations of Ca^{2+}. This decrease in tension was not caused by inhibition of the contractile apparatus, as a result of increased intracellular $[Ca^{2+}]$, but rather by a blockade of Ca^{2+} influx through Ca^{2+} channels, which thereby reduced cytosolic $[Ca^{2+}]$. That this is the case can be demonstrated by a histamine challenge of the coronaries under high-$[Ca^{2+}]$ (inactivation) conditions. Histamine was still fully effective in releasing Ca^{2+} from the internal Ca^{2+} stores and producing a full contraction in these Ca^{2+}-inactivated coronaries (data not shown). Thus, high $[Ca^{2+}]$ blocks entry of Ca^{2+} through Ca^{2+} channels, and, when Ca^{2+} is released into these cells from internal Ca^{2+} stores, contractions occur. This is consistent with our observation that the relaxation of tension in coronary arteries by Ca^{2+}-channel blockers can be circumvented by histamine's releasing Ca^{2+} from internal stores (Johnson and Fugman, 1983).

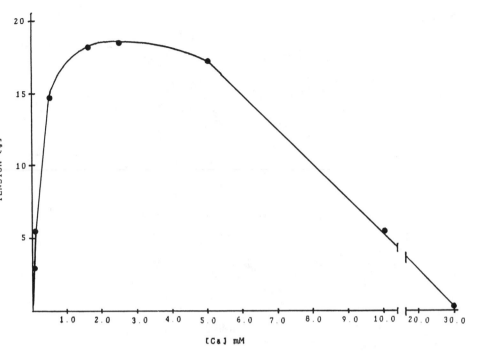

Fig. 3. Calcium-induced inactivation of calcium channels producing relaxation of tension in coronary arteries. Right, circumflex, porcine coronary artery segments (10 mm in length) were depolarized with 35 mM KCl in a calcium-free HEPES saline solution. Tension was recorded as a function of added calcium, as described by Johnson and Fugman (1983). This curve represents a typical titration and is the averaged data from two coronaries. After calcium-induced inactivation, subsequent challenge with 20 $\times$ 10^{-6} M histamine resulted in a full contraction.

Blockade of calcium channels by Ca^{2+} antagonists is *similar* to that by high extracellular [Ca^{2+}] in that both procedures relax tension by decreasing Ca^{2+} influx through the channel and thereby lower cytosolic [Ca^{2+}]. Furthermore, both types of blockade can be circumvented by release of Ca^{2+} from intracellular stores. These results suggest that coronary arteries have calcium channels that are inactivated or blocked by high concentrations of calcium. Godfrained (1983) and Van Breeman *et al.* (1981) have used measurements of ^{45}Ca influx to demonstrate calcium-induced inactivation of other types of vascular smooth muscle. Thus, those tissues (vascular smooth muscle) that are most sensitive to calcium-channel blockers appear to exhibit calcium-induced inactivation of their calcium channels. In contrast, the calcium channels of cells involved in excitation–secretion coupling do not show such inactivation nor calcium-antagonist blockade (see Hagiwara and Byerly, 1981).

III. CALMODULIN AND TROPONIN C

A. Calcium-Induced Structural Changes

Calmodulin and troponin C represent two additional CBPs that play fundamental roles in regulating muscle contraction. Calmodulin is a calcium receptor that is as essential to the contractile apparatus of smooth muscle as troponin C is to cardiac and skeletal muscle. Both calmodulin (Cheung, 1980; Cox *et al.* 1984, Klee and Newton, 1985) and cardiac and skeletal troponin (Potter and Johnson, 1982) are the subjects of recent reviews. Calmodulin appears to be a much more universal calcium-dependent regulatory protein than troponin C in that it is present in all eukaryotic cells; its structure is highly conserved, and it regulates more than twenty different proteins in a calcium-dependent manner (see reviews cited above).

In general, two types of calcium-binding sites exist in the troponin C super-family of CBPs. These are the higher-affinity $Ca^{2+}-Mg^{2+}$ sites ($K_a = 2 \times 10^7$ M^{-1}), which bind Ca^{2+} and Mg^{2+} competitively, and the lower-affinity calcium-specific sites ($K_a = 4 \times 10^5\,M^{-1}$). The binding of troponin I to troponin C and calmodulin increases the affinity of these CBPs for calcium by approximately 10-fold. The $Ca^{2+}-Mg^{2+}$ sites are always occupied by Ca^{2+} or Mg^{2+} and presumably serve only a structural role, whereas the Ca^{2+}-specific sites exchange Ca^{2+} rapidly and are presumably the sites at which Ca^{2+} initiates the process of muscle contraction (Johnson *et al.*, 1979). These sites have been called the Ca^{2+}-specific regulatory sites in troponin C (Johnson *et al.*, 1980). CBPs vary in the number of the Ca^{2+}-specific/$Ca^{2+}-Mg^{2+}$ sites that they possess; for example 2/2 for skeletal muscle TnC, 1/2 for cardiac muscle TnC, 4/0 for calmodulin, and 0/2 for parvalbumin. Because Ca^{2+} exchange with the $Ca^{2+}-Mg^{2+}$ sites is slow, only those CBPs with Ca^{2+}-specific sites can respond to rapid calcium transients and participate *directly* in the regulation of muscle contraction (Johnson *et al.*, 1979).

Calmodulin is unique among the CBPs discovered thus far in that all of its *four* calcium-binding sites are calcium specific (Dedman *et al.*, 1977), similar to the *two* calcium-specific sites on skeletal troponin C and the *single* calcium-specific site on cardiac troponin C (see Johnson *et al.*, 1980) that serve to regulate muscle contraction. These three proteins belong to a large superfamily of troponin C-like CBPs, and they share many similarities. In each case, calcium binding produces large structural changes that are reflected by increases in intrinsic tyrosine fluorescence, UV absorption, and α-helical content (Dedman *et al.*, 1977; Johnson *et al.*, 1978). Furthermore, calcium binding to the calcium-specific regulatory sites on these proteins results in the exposure or formation of hydrophobic sites on the surface of the protein (Johnson *et al.*, 1978; Johnson and Wittenauer, 1983; LaPorte *et al.*, 1980; Tanaka and Hidaka, 1980). Such hydrophobic sites are where these CBPs bind and interact with the proteins that they activate or regulate [see Johnson *et al.* (1981, 1982) and Potter and Johnson (1982) for calmodulin and troponin C, respectively]. The calcium-dependent exposure of active sites on these CBPs is, therefore, critical for transmission of the calcium signal.

These calcium-dependent hydrophobic sites also seem to be the sites where hydrophobic drugs can bind and inhibit the interaction of CBPs with other proteins. In this regard, calmodulin inhibitors, such as W-7 (Hidaka *et al.*, 1979), R24571 (Van Belle, 1981), and trifluoperazine (TFP; Levin and Weiss, 1978) can bind to specific sites on calmodulin and block or inhibit calmodulin's activation of proteins, such as myosin light chain kinase, adenylate cyclase, phosphodiesterase, and Ca^{2+}-ATPases.

We have examined calcium-dependent binding of the hydrophobic fluorescent probe ANS (anilinonaphthalene sulfonate) to a variety of CBPs. ANS binds in a calcium-dependent manner to calmodulin, cardiac and skeletal troponin C, and scallop CBP at concentrations of calcium at which the calcium-specific sites of these CBPs are occupied. No calcium-dependent binding was observed with parvalbumin, a protein with two calcium–magnesium sites and no calcium-specific sites. Furthermore, binding of magnesium to the calcium–magnesium sites of cardiac and skeletal troponin C and parvalbumin did not expose a calcium-dependent, hydrophobic ANS-binding site on these proteins. This suggests that binding of calcium to the calcium-specific regulatory sites on CBPs is perhaps required for the exposure or formation of these important hydrophobic interfacial sites.

B. Allosteric Interactions among Drug-Binding Sites on Calcium-Binding Proteins

Of the proteins that are bound by calmodulin and activated in a calcium-dependent manner, most bind half-maximally near pCa 6.0–6.1, with 1 : 1 stoichiometry. The question becomes then, how can calmodulin be directed with any degree of specificity toward any particular protein? Recently, we observed that the hydrophobic binding sites on calmodulin are allosterically related. That is, drug binding to some of these sites can potentiate drug binding to other sites (see Johnson, 1983; Mills *et al.*, 1985). We have found that the calmodulin inhibitor, R24571, and the calcium channel blocking drugs, prenylamine and diltiazem, can potentiate the binding of the fluorescent, dihydropyridine calcium channel blocker, felodipine, to calmodulin. This effect of prenylamine on felodipine binding (fluorescence) is shown in Fig. 4. At lower concentrations (10^{-7} to 10^{-5} M), prenylamine binds to calmodulin to promote felodipine binding (fluorescence); at higher concentrations, prenylamine can competitively displace felodipine from its binding site, resulting in the observed decrease in fluorescence. Our studies have shown that at 10 μM, prenylamine can increase

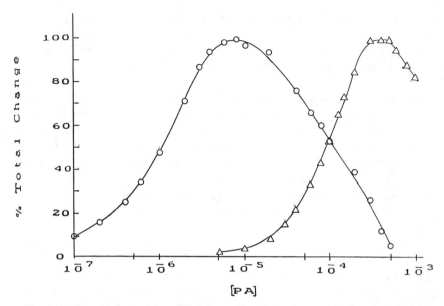

Fig. 4.   Effect of prenylamine on the fluorescence of felodipine binding to calmodulin (0) or cardiac troponin C (△). Solutions contained $1 \times 10^{-6} M$ felodipine in 10 m*M* MOPS, 90 m*M* KCl, 2 m*M EGTA, and 3mM* CaCl$_2$ at pH 7.0 with either $2 \times 10^{-7} M$ calmodulin or $2 \times 10^{-6} M$ cardiac troponin C. Prenylamine (PA) was added to give the concentrations indicated, and the change in fluorescence was monitored at 445 nm as described previously (Johnson, 1983).

the affinity of calmodulin for felodipine by approximately 20-fold through these allosteric mechanisms (Johnson, 1983). We examined several other CBPs and found that they too exhibit allosteric interactions among their hydrophobic drug-binding sites. The effect of prenylamine on cardiac TnC binding of felodipine is shown in Fig. 4. Here once again prenylamine and felodipine bound in a calcium-dependent fashion, and prenylamine potentiated felodipine's interactions through allosteric mechanisms similar to those observed on calmodulin. With both calmodulin and troponin C, calcium binding to the calcium-specific sites is required before these allosterically related drug-binding sites are exposed (i.e., magnesium will not produce the effect). It may be noted that although the affinities of prenylamine and felodipine are different for calmodulin and cardiac-TnC, a similar allosteric relationship still exists between the drug-binding sites in each CBP. These studies suggest that an allosteric relationship among the calcium-induced, hydrophobic, ligand (protein) -binding sites may be a general feature of the mechanism of action of many CBPs. Furthermore, calcium binding to the very important calcium-specific regulatory sites on these CBPs appears to activate these allosterically related sites.

Calcium binding to these regulatory sites is a prerequisite for these proteins to regulate muscle contraction and suggests a very important role for these allosterically related drug protein-binding sites in the regulatory action of CBPs. We believe, for example, that these allosteric mechanisms on calmodulin may serve to give it specificity for binding and activating certain proteins. Endogenous regulators might exist that could bind to calmodulin and potentiate its binding to phosphodiesterase rather than to other proteins, such as adenylate cyclase. Such control operating through allosteric mechanisms among the various protein-binding sites on calmodulin may allow selective activation of the many calmodulin-dependent processes in the cell.

C.   Alterations in Calcium Affinity

One additional feature of CBPs that need to be mentioned is that when drugs or proteins bind to their calcium-induced hydrophobic sites, the affinity of CBPs for calcium is often increased. This has been observed with cardiac and skeletal TnC, both of which exhibit 10-fold increases in their calcium affinities with TnI binding. Recently, large increases in calmodulin's affinity for calcium upon protein binding or TFP binding have been reported (Keller *et al.*, 1982; Forsen *et al.*, 1980). This phenomena is demonstrated by the calcium dependence of felodipine's binding to calmodulin. Felodipine binds half-maximally to calmodulin at approximately pCa 6.0 (Fig. 5). The addition of 2 μM R24571 altered the

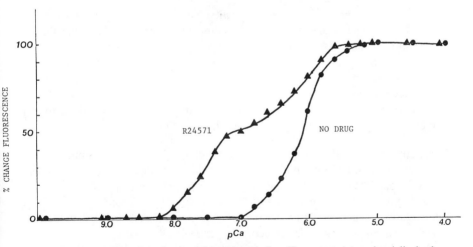

Fig. 5.   The calcium dependence of felodipine binding (fluorescence) to calmodulin in the absence and presence of calmodulin inhibitor R24571. Calcium titrations of felodipine ($1 \times 10^{-6} M$) and calmodulin ($1 \times 10^{-6} M$) in the absence of added drug and in the presence of $2 \times 10^{-6} M$ R24571 are shown. Calcium titrations were conducted in a 10 mM MOPS, 90 mM KCl, 2 mM EGTA buffer maintained at pH 7.0 as described previously (Johnson *et al.*, 1981).

calcium dependence of felodipine binding dramatically. In the presence of R24571, a class of calcium-binding sites that are occupied half-maximally at pCa 7.6 facilitated a portion of felodipine binding (Fig. 5). This suggests that binding of R24571 to calmodulin may increase the calcium affinity to some of its four calcium-binding sites by more than 40-fold. Thus, in calmodulin, troponin C, and probably many other CBPs, drug or protein binding to calcium-dependent sites can dramatically enhance the affinity of that CBP for calcium.

IV. SIMILARITIES BETWEEN THE CALCIUM-BINDING PROTEINS OF THE CONTRACTILE APPARATUS (TROPONIN C AND CALMODULIN) AND THE CALCIUM CHANNEL

From our examination of calmodulin as a model protein for the CBP of calcium channels, some rather interesting similarities appear:

1. Calcium in the micromolar range is required to regulate both the CBP of the channel and calmodulin.

2. Calcium is an absolute requirement for dihydropyridine drug binding to the CBP of the channel and to calmodulin.

3. Calcium protects the calcium channel and all CBPs from heat denaturation.

4. Some drugs that are selective for calcium channels bind and inhibit calmodulin and troponin C (see Johnson *et al.*, 1982, 1983).

5. Some drugs that are selective for calmodulin bind and inhibit calcium channels (see Johnson *et al.*, 1983).

6. Calcium channels, calmodulin, and troponin C all exhibit allosteric interactions among their calcium-dependent drug-binding sites. In fact, diltiazem can potentiate dihydropyridine binding to all three proteins.

All of these findings support our hypothesis that a CBP that is similar to but distinct from calmodulin and troponin C is the calcium-dependent gate of the calcium channel and a pharmacological receptor for some calcium channel blocking drugs. We believe that the 33,000- to 45,000-Da protein isolated from the solubilized and partially purified calcium channel is the CBP that binds calcium channel blockers in a calcium-dependent, allosteric manner.

Let us *assume* that this CBP, which gates the channel (calcium-induced inactivation) and binds calcium antagonists, is similar to calmodulin and troponin C in one additional way: with binding of calcium channel blockers, it also increases its affinity for calcium. If this is the case, as channel antagonists bind to this CBP (some in a calcium-dependent manner), they should increase this protein's affinity for calcium, causing it to bind more calcium and thereby close the channel through calcium-induced inactivation, perhaps even in the relaxed state. Thus, such antagonists might trick the calcium channel into premature inactivation by making it sense higher $[Ca^{2+}]$ than actually exists inside the cell. A schematic of this is shown in Fig. 2B. This hypothesis suggests that blockade of calcium channels by some calcium antagonists proceeds via a mechanism involving premature calcium-induced inactivation of calcium channels. In support of this, we note that those types of calcium channels that are most sensitive to calcium antagonists are indeed inactivated by calcium.

V. THE Na^+–Ca^{2+} ANTIPORTER AS A CALCIUM-BINDING PROTEIN THAT CONTROLS MUSCLE CONTRACTION

The role of Na^+–Ca^{2+} antiporters and Na^+–Ca^{2+} exchange mechanisms in regulating calcium homeostasis and tension is the subject of several chapters of this volume and will not be reviewed here. The Na^+–Ca^{2+} antiporter is, however, a CBP that is fundamental in regulating contraction. Its role in regulating tension in coronary arteries is shown in Fig. 6. In this figure, the Na^+, K^+-ATPase has been inhibited by two different mechanisms: by removal of extracellular K^+ and by addition of ouabain. In each case, inhibition of the Na^+, K^+-ATPase stops extrusion of Na^+ allowing dissipation of the large $[Na^+]$ gradient. Under these conditions, high extracellular Ca^{2+} can enter the cell by reversal of the Na^+–Ca^{2+} antiporter because there is no longer a large $[Na^+]$ gradient to pump against. As this calcium enters, tension rises (Fig. 6). Addition of 5 mM KCl to the constricted coronary artery produces rapid relaxation, presumably because extracellular K^+ reactivates the Na^+, K^+-ATPase, thereby reestablishing the $[Na^+]$ gradient. Thus, extracellular Na^+ enters once again through the Na^+–Ca^{2+} antiporter with the simultaneous extrusion of calcium, resulting in relaxation. Similar but irreversible effects are observed when the Na^+, K^+-ATPase is inhibited by ouabain (Fig. 6). Finally, these effects on tension, induced by inhibition of Na^+, K^+-ATPase (and mediated via Na^+–Ca^{2+} exchange) are observed even in the presence of calcium-channel blockade by verapamil, providing strong evidence that a large portion of the Ca^{2+} influx is via the Na^+–Ca^{2+} exchanger and not the Ca^{2+} channel. These data indicate that under conditions of Na^+, K^+-ATPase inhibition (such as digitalis treatment), coronary arteries may constrict from entry of calcium through a Na^+–Ca^{2+} exchanger. Such entry and the tension produced thereby (when extracellular $[Ca^{2+}]$ is high) cannot be blocked effectively by calcium antagonists. It is possible, therefore, that angina, which sometimes occurs in patients on digitalis, may not be relieved effectively by calcium channel blockers, because these

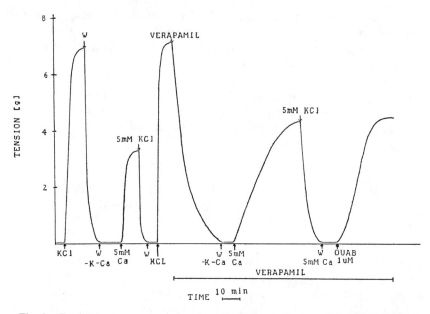

Fig. 6. Tension in coronary arteries produced by calcium influx through the calcium channels and the Na^+–Ca^{2+} antiporter. Average traces from two coronary arteries. Arteries were contracted with 35 mM KCl (KCl), washed with normal physiological saline solution (W), washed in KCl-free, $CaCl_2$-free saline solution (–K-Ca), contracted with 5 mM $CaCl_2$ (5 mM Ca), relaxed with 5 mM KCl (5 mM KCl), washed with normal physiological saline solution (W), contracted with 35 mM KCl, relaxed with 1×10^{-6} M verapamil, washed in KCl-free, $CaCl_2$-free saline solution, contracted with 5 mM $CaCl_2$, relaxed with 5 mM KCl, washed with normal PSS containing 5 mM $CaCl_2$, (W), and then subjected to 1×10^{-6} M ouabain to produce the observed contraction. Verapamil (1×10^{-6} M) remained in the bath at all times after its first addition.

antagonists are not effective in blocking entry of calcium via Na^+–Ca^{2+} exchange. Thus, although the Na^+–Ca^{2+} antiporter is a CBP that is generally involved in Ca^{2+} extrusion and relaxation, it may provide, under certain conditions (e.g., inhibition of Na^+, K^+-ATPase), a mechanism for the entry of calcium that is alternative to the voltage-dependent calcium channels.

VI. CONCLUSIONS

When we consider the role of calcium-binding proteins in the regulation of muscle contraction we can no longer focus our attention on troponin C and the contractile apparatus alone. It is clear that calcium receptors or CBPs must exist at many levels of the cellular architecture in order to conduct the calcium signal and regulate contraction. The voltage-dependent calcium channel, calcium AT-Pases, Na^+-Ca^{2+} antiporters, calcium uniporters, and the calcium-binding contractile proteins of skeletal and cardiac muscle (troponin C) and of smooth muscle (calmodulin) all share the common feature of having calcium-binding domains in their structures. Many studies suggest extensive homology among CBPs; therefore, understanding the mechanism of action of some of these proteins may increase our understanding of these calcium receptors in general. Our generalizations suggest that binding of calcium to the calcium-specific sites of some of these proteins expose hydrophobic drug and/or protein-binding sites. These are presumably the sites where calcium-binding proteins interface with other protein moieties to transduce the calcium signal. Furthermore, our evidence suggests that the various drug- or protein-binding sites on some of these CBPs are allosterically related. That is, drug or protein binding to one of these calcium-induced hydrophobic sites can affect binding to other drug- or protein-binding sites. Evidence of this type of calcium-dependent allosteric relationship is found in calmodulin, troponin C, and the calcium channel. In addition, we find evidence suggesting that drug or protein binding to these calcium-induced, hydrophobic binding sites can dramatically increase calcium affinity in many CBPs. This would effectively decrease the off-rate of calcium from these CBPs and increase the half-life of the activated $Ca^{2+}-CBP-protein$ complex during a calcium transient, because any change in calcium affinity must be reflected by changes in calcium exchange rates. Assuming that drug binding increases the calcium affinity of the calcium channel CBP, too, we have proposed a mechanism for inactivation of calcium channels by calcium and calcium channel blocking drugs.

When calcium binds to a CBP and exposes sites that are themselves related allosterically and when, in turn, occupancy of these sites (by endogenous regulators, proteins, or drugs) modulates calcium binding, the possibility of a very finely tuned control mechanism is obvious.

If the above generalizations hold true for each of the CBPs within the cell, then perhaps we are not being too optimistic in believing that some day we can control the important actions of calcium by specific pharmacological interventions at the level of each of these calcium receptors.

ACKNOWLEDGMENTS

This work was supported by grants from the American Heart Association, Central Ohio Affiliate, and the Muscular Dystrophy Association of America awarded to J. David Johnson. It was completed under the tenure of a Young Investigatorship awarded to J. David Johnson by the Central Ohio Affiliate of the American Heart Association. We gratefully acknowledge the Samuel J. Roessler Memorial Scholarship Fund for a summer scholarship to Theodore J. Grieshop.

REFERENCES

Adelstein, R. S. (1978). Myosin phosphorylation, cell motility and smooth muscle contraction. *Trends Biochem. Sci.* **3**, 27–30.

Campbell, K. P., Lipshutz, G. M., and Denney, G. H. (1984). Direct photoaffinity labeling of the high affinity nitrendipine-binding site in subcellular membrane fractions isolated from canine myocardium. *J. Biol. Chem.* **259**, 5384–5387.

Cheung, W. Y. (1980). Calmodulin plays a pivotal role in cellular regulation. *Science* **207**, 19–27.

Cox, J. A., Comte, M., Malnoe, A., Burger, D., and Stein, E. A. (1984). Mode of action of the regulatory protein calmodulin. *In* "Metal Ions in Biological Systems," Vol. 17 (H. Sigei, ed.), pp. 215–273. Marcel Dekker Inc., New York.

Curtis, B. M., and Catterall, W. A. (1984). Purification of the calcium antagonist receptor of the voltage-sensitive calcium channel from skeletal muscle transverse tubules. *Biochemistry* **23**, 2113–2117.

Dedman, J. R., Potter, J. S., Jackson, R. L., Johnson, J. D., and Means, A. R. (1977). Physicochemical properties of rat testis Ca^{2+}-dependent regulator protein of cyclic nucleotide phosphodiesterase. *J. Biol. Chem.* **252**, 8415–8422.

Forsen, S., Thulin, E., Drakenberg, T., Krebs, J., and Seamon, K. (1980). A ^{113}Cd NMR study of calmodulin and its interaction with calcium, magnesium and trifluoperazine. *FEBS Letters* **117**, 189–194.

Godfraind, T. (1983). Actions of nifedipine on calcium fluxes and contraction in isolated rat arteries. *J. Pharm. Exp. Ther.* **224**, 443–450.

Gould, R. J., Murphy, K. M. M., and Snyder, S. H. (1982). [^{3}H]Nitrendipine-labeled calcium channels discriminate inorganic calcium agonists and antagonists. *Proc. Natl. Acad. Sci. USA* **79**, 3656–3660.

Hagiwara, S., and Byerly, L. (1981). Calcium channel. *Ann. Rev. Neurosci.* **4**, 26–125.

Hidaka, H., Yamaki, T., Totsuka, T., and Asano, M. (1979). Selective inhibitors of Ca^{2+}-binding modulator of phosphodiesterase produce vascular relaxation and inhibit actin–myosin interaction. *Mol. Pharm.* **15**, 49–59.

Janis, R. A., and Triggle, D. J. (1983). New developments in Ca^{2+} channel antagonists. *J. Med. Chem.* **26**, 775–785.

Johnson, J. D. (1983). Allosteric interactions among drug binding sites on calmodulin. *Biochem. Biophys. Res. Comm.* **112**, 787–793.

Johnson, J. D. (1984). A calmodulin-like Ca^{2+} receptor in the Ca^{2+} channel. *Biophys. J.* **45**, 134–136.

Johnson, J. D., and Fugman, D. A. (1983). Calcium and calmodulin antagonists binding to calmodulin and relaxation of coronary segments. *J. Pharm. Exp. Ther.* **226**, 330–334.

Johnson, J. D., and Wittenauer, L. A. (1983). A fluorescent calmodulin that reports the binding of hydrophobic inhibitory ligands. *Biochem. J.* **211**, 473–479.

Johnson, J. D., Collins, J. H., and Potter, J. D. (1978). Dansylaziridine-labeled troponin C—A fluorescent probe of Ca^{2+} binding to the Ca^{2+}-specific regulatory sites. *J. Biol. Chem.* **253**, 6451–6458.

Johnson, J. D., Charlton, S. C., and Potter, J. D. (1979). A fluorescence stopped flow analysis of Ca^{2+} exchange with troponin C. *J. Biol. Chem.* **254**, 3497–3502.

Johnson, J. D., Collins, J. H., Robertson, S. P., and Potter, J. D. (1980). A fluorescent probe study of Ca^{2+} binding to the Ca^{2+}-specific sites of cardiac troponin and troponin C. *J. Biol. Chem.* **255**, 9635–9640.

Johnson, J. D., Holroyde, M. J., Crouch, T. H., Solaro, R. J., and Potter, J. D. (1981). Fluorescence studies of the interaction of calmodulin with myosin light chain kinase. *J. Biol. Chem.* **256,** 12194–12198.

Johnson, J. D., Vaghy, P. L., Crouch, T. H., Potter, J. D., and Schwartz, A. (1982). An hypothesis for the mechanism of action of some of the Ca^{2+} antagonist drugs: Calmodulin as a receptor. *In* "Advances in Pharmacology and Therapeutics II," Vol. 3 (H. Yoshida, Y. Hagihara, and S. Ebashi, eds.), pp. 121–138. Pergamon Press, New York.

Johnson, J. D., Wittenauer, L. A., and Nathan, R. D. (1983). Calmodulin, Ca^{2+}-antagonists and Ca^{2+}-transporters in nerve and muscle. *J. Neural. Trans. Suppl.* **18** 97–111.

Keller, C. H., Olwin, B. B., LaPorte, D. C., and Storm, D. R. (1982). Determination of the free-energy coupling for binding of calcium ions and troponin C to calmodulin. *Biochemistry* **21,** 156–162.

Klee, C. B. and Newton, D. L. (1985). Calmodulin: An Overview. *In* "Control and Manipulation of Calcium Movement" (J. R. Parratt, ed.), pp. 131–146. Raven Press, New York.

LaPorte, D. C., Wierman, B. M., and Storm, D. R. (1980). Calcium-induced exposure of a hydrophobic surface on calmodulin. *Biochemistry* **19,** 3814–3819.

Levin, R. M., and Weiss, B. (1978). Specificity of the binding of trifluoperazine to the calcium-dependent activator of phosphodiesterase and to a series of other calcium-binding proteins. *Biochim. Biophys. Acta* **540,** 197–204.

Mills, J. S., Bailey, B. L., and Johnson, J. D. 1985 Cooperativity among calmodulin drug binding sites. *Biochemistry* **24** 4897–4902.

Murphy, K. M., Gould, R. J., Largent, B. L., and Snyder, S. H. (1983). A unitary mechanism of calcium antagonist drug action. *Proc. Natl. Acad. Sci. USA* **80,** 860–864.

Potter, J. D., and Johnson, J. D. (1982). Troponin. *In* "Calcium and Cell Function," Vol. 2 (W. Y. Cheung, ed.), pp. 145–173. Academic Press, New York.

Tanaka, T., and Hidaka, H. (1980). Hydrophobic regions function in calmodulin–enzyme(s) interactions. *J. Biol. Chem.* **255,** 11078–11080.

Tsien, R. W. (1983). Calcium channels in excitable cell membranes. *Ann. Rev. Physiol.* **45,** 341–358.

Vaghy, P. L., Johnson, J. D., Wang, T., and Schwartz, A. (1982). Selective inhibition of Na^{+}-induced Ca^{2+} release from heart mitochondria by diltiazem and certain other Ca^{2+} antagonist drugs. *J. Biol. Chem.* **257,** 6000–6002.

Van Belle, H. (1981). R 24571: A potent inhibitor of calmodulin-activated enzymes. *Cell Calcium* **2,** 483–494.

Van Breeman, C., Hwang, O., and Meisheri, K. D. (1981). The mechanism of inhibitor action of diltiazem on vascular smooth muscle contractility. *J. Pharm. Exp. Ther.* **218,** 450–463.

Venter, J. C., Fraser, C. M., Schaber, J. S., Jung, C. Y., Bolger, G., and Triggle, D. J. (1983). Molecular properties of the slow inward calcium channel. *J. Biol. Chem.* **258,** 9344–9348.

Index